REACHING THE POOR

with Health, Nutrition, and Population Services

REACHING THE POOR

with Health, Nutrition, and Population Services

What Works, What Doesn't, and Why

Edited by
Davidson R. Gwatkin
Adam Wagstaff
Abdo S. Yazbeck

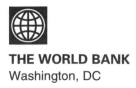

THE WORLD BANK
Washington, DC

ISBN-13: 978-0-8213-5961-7   eISBN 0-8213-5962-2
ISBN-10: 0-8213-5961-4   DOI: 10.1596/978-0-8213-5961-7

Library of Congress Catologing-in-Publication data
Reaching the poor with health, nutrition, and population services : what works, what doesn't, and why / [edited by] Davidson R. Gwatkin, Adam Wagstaff, Abdo Yazbeck.
        p.   cm.
    Includes bibliographical references and index.
    ISBN 0-8213-5961-4
    1. Poor – Medical care – Cross-cultural studies. 2. Poor – Medical care – Developing countries. 3. Health services accessibility – Cross-cultural studies. 4. Health services accessibility – Developing countries. 5. Poor – Nutrition – Cross-cultural studies. 5. Poor – Nutrition – Developing countries. 6. Human services – Cross-cultural studies. 7. Human services – Developing countries. I. Gwatkin, Davidson R. II. Wagstaff, Adam. III. Yazbeck, Abdo.

RA418.5.P6R43   2005
362.1'086'942 22

                                                          2005050781

Contents

FIGURES

ANNEX FIGURE

TABLES

ANNEX TABLES

Foreword

The poor suffer from far higher levels of ill health, mortality, and malnutrition than do the better-off; and their inadequate health is one of the factors keeping them poor or for their being poor in the first place. The health of the poor must thus be a matter of major concern for everyone committed to equitable development, from policy makers to service providers.

Health services can make an important contribution to improved health conditions among disadvantaged groups. Yet as the contents of this volume make clear, the health services supported by governments and by agencies like ours too often fail to reach these people who need them most.

This is not acceptable. Nor need it be accepted. The studies presented here point to numerous strategies that can help health programs reach the poor much more effectively than at present. In doing so, they strongly reinforce the messages of the 2004 *World Development Report* and other recent publications about the importance and possibility of making services work better for poor people.

Readers will no doubt form different views about which of these strategies are most promising for a particular setting—whether, for example, one would be best advised to follow Brazil's approach of seeking universal coverage for basic health services, Cambodia's strategy of contracting with non-governmental organizations, Nepal's use of participatory program development, or some other approach. This is to be expected and welcomed. We look forward to a vigorous and productive discussion on issues like these in order to build upon the important basic findings presented here that better performance is possible.

We also hope that readers will take to heart the equally important message that improved performance is needed. In light of the evidence presented here, it is clearly not safe to assume that the health projects important and intended for the poor are actually serving them. For example, poor women desperately need better delivery attendance than they are now receiving. But initiatives that reach primarily the better-off—like the institutional delivery program covered by the Bangladesh study in this volume—fall far short of filling this need. As this illustration shows, assumptions that programs reach the poor need to be replaced with vigilance in order to ensure that they do.

In brief, better performance in reaching the poor is both needed and feasible. These are the two messages from this volume that we shall be discussing with our colleagues. We are pleased to share these messages with other readers, as well, in the hope and anticipation that they too will find them valuable.

Jacques F. Baudouy, Director
Health, Nutrition, and Population
   Department
The World Bank

David Fleming, Director
Global Health Strategies
Bill and Melinda Gates Foundation

Anders Molin, Head
Health Division
Swedish International Development
   Cooperation Agency

Aagje Papineau Salm, Coordinator
Ministerial Taskforce, Aids and
   Reproductive Health
(Former Head, Social Policy Unit)
Netherlands Ministry of Foreign
Affairs

Preface

This volume presents eleven case studies that document how well or how poorly health, nutrition, and population programs have performed in reaching disadvantaged groups. The studies were commissioned by the Reaching the Poor Program, which was undertaken by the World Bank in cooperation with the Bill and Melinda Gates Foundation and the governments of the Netherlands and Sweden in an effort to find better ways of ensuring that health, nutrition, and population programs benefit the neediest.

The case studies, reinforced by other materials gathered by the Reaching the Poor Program, clearly demonstrate that *health programs can reach the poor far better than they presently do.* We hope that policy makers will take this message to heart and will find the experiences reported here helpful as they seek to develop the more effective strategies required to ensure that the poor share fully in health improvements.

Davidson R. Gwatkin, Adam Wagstaff, and Abdo S. Yazbeck

Acknowledgments

Many people and institutions have given invaluable assistance to the preparation of this volume. The Bill and Melinda Gates Foundation, the governments of the Netherlands and Sweden, and the World Bank's Research Support Budget provided generous financial support. Kathleen Lynch was an especially effective project editor, Jumana Qamruddin served with typical efficiency as the project's operations analyst, and Hugh Waters was generous with technical advice. Shanta Devarajan and Maureen Lewis contributed valuable inputs and support in their capacity as chief economists of the World Bank's Human Development Network; Jacques Baudouy and Christopher Lovelace were equally helpful and supportive as directors of the Bank's Health, Nutrition, and Population Department; and department sector managers Kei Kawabata and Helen Saxenian provided important assistance. Abbas Bhuiya, Hilary Brown, Norberto Dachs, and Tim Evans assisted in the selection of studies for inclusion in the Reaching the Poor Program. Reviewers of manuscripts produced under the program included Howard Barnum, David Bishai, Abbas Bhuiya, Christy Hanson, Kara Hanson, James Knowles, Michael Koenig, Saul Morris, David Sahn, William Savedoff, Cesar Victora, Eddy van Doorslaer, and Stephen Younger. Abbas Bhuiya, Frank Nyonator, Cesar Victora, and Hugh Waters were the members of an external review panel at the Reaching the Poor conference that undertook an early assessment of the study findings.

Acronyms, Abbreviations, and Data Notes

ADB	Asian Development Bank
ANC	Antenatal care
BCG	Bacille Calmette-Guérin (tuberculosis) vaccine
BIA	Benefit-incidence analysis
CHC	Community health center
CHRW	Community health research worker
CI	Concentration index
DH	District hospital
DHMO	District health and medical officer
DHMT	District health management team
DHS	Demographic and Health Survey
DOD	Difference of differences
DOTS	Directly observed treatment, short course (for tuberculosis)
DPT	Diphtheria, pertussis, and tetanus vaccine
ECHINP	Early childhood nutritional programs (Peru)
EmOC	Emergency obstetric care
EOC	Essential obstetric care
EPI	Expanded Programme of Immunization
EU	European Union
FCHV	Family and child health volunteer
FDH	Female district hospital
FP/RH	Family planning and reproductive health
FGD	Focus group discussion
FONCODES	Social Investment Fund (Peru)
FWV	Family welfare visitor
GBA	Greater Buenos Aires
HAART	Highly active antiretroviral therapy
H&FWC	Health and family welfare center
HDSS	Health and Demographic Surveillance System
IBGE	Instituto Brasileiro de Geografia e Estatística

ICDDR,B	International Centre for Diarrhoeal Diseases Research, Bangladesh
IFPRI	International Food Policy Research Institute
IFRC	International Federation of Red Cross and Red Crescent Societies
IIPS	International Institute for Population Sciences
IMCI	Integrated management of childhood illness
INDEC	Instituto Nacional de Estadística y Censos (Argentina)
ITN	Insecticide-treated net
KMET	Kisumu Medical and Educational Trust (Kenya)
LSMS	Living Standards Measurement Surveys
MCU	Maternity care unit
MCWC	Maternal and child welfare center
MDGs	Millennium Development Goals, United Nations
MICS	Multiple Indicator Cluster Survey (UNICEF)
MMR	Measles, mumps, and rubella vaccine
MMR	Maternal mortality ratio
NFHS	National Family Health Survey (India)
NGO	Nongovernmental organization
NMCC	National Malaria Control Centre (Zambia)
PACFO	Programa de Complementación Alimentaria para Grupos en Mayor Riesgo (Peru)
PAHO	Pan American Health Organization
PAI	Infant Feeding Program (Peru)
PAISM	Program of Integral Assistance to Women's Health (Brazil)
PANFAR	Nutritional Assistance Program for High-Risk Families (Peru)
PCA	Principal component analysis
PETS	Public Expenditure Tracking Survey
PHC	Primary health center
PNAD	National Household Sample Survey (Brazil)
PNC	Postnatal care
PROMUDEH	Ministerio de Promoción de la Mujer y Desarrollo Humano (Peru)
PRONAA	National Food Assistance Program (Peru)
PRONOEI	Programas no Escolarizados de Educación Inicial (Peru)
PRSP	Poverty reduction strategy paper (World Bank)
PSF	Family Health Program (Brazil)
RCV	Red Cross volunteer

RCH	Reproductive and child health
RH	Reproductive health
RPP	Reaching the Poor Program
SEA	Standard enumeration area
SES	Socioeconomic status
SEWA	Self-Employed Women's Association (India)
STPAN	Secretaría Técnica de Política Alimentaria Nutricional (Peru)
SUS	Sistema Único de Saúde (Unified Health System) (Brazil)
THC	Thana health complex
U5MR	Under-five mortality rate
UNFPA	United Nations Population Fund
UNICEF	United Nations Children's Fund
UPHSDP	Uttar Pradesh Health Systems Development Project
USAID	U.S. Agency for International Development
VCT	Voluntary counseling and testing
VDC	Village development committee (Nepal)
WHO	World Health Organization
WHS	World Health Survey (WHO)
ZRCS	Zambia Red Cross Society

All dollar amounts are current U.S. dollars unless otherwise indicated.

Part I

Introduction

1

Why Were the Reaching the Poor Studies Undertaken?

Abdo S. Yazbeck, Davidson R. Gwatkin, Adam Wagstaff, and Jumana Qamruddin

Few of the resources spent in the health sector reach the poor. This fact is gradually being recognized by health sector policy makers and by the international development community. A fast-growing body of empirical evidence has exposed as incorrect any assumption that spending on health necessarily means reaching and serving poor people.

The recognition that services are not reaching the poor, although a powerful motive for reform and change, does not by itself point toward a direction for change. To identify the type of change required, it is necessary to understand what works in reaching the poor, and why it works, in order to demonstrate to policy makers ways of making the health sector more equitable. The Reaching the Poor Program (RPP) is exploring these two issues—what works, and why—with the goal of identifying promising strategies.

The 11 case studies summarized in chapters 4 through 14 of this volume present the results of evaluation research commissioned by the RPP in an effort to fill gaps in knowledge about what types of program reach the poor most effectively. This chapter and the next two provide the context for the studies. Chapter 2 explains the empirical evaluation techniques used; chapter 3 surveys the types of program covered, gives an overview of the findings, and makes some suggestions about the policy implications.

The Spotlight of Empirical Evidence

Much of the earliest research on this topic dealt with the extent to which public spending on health care reaches the lowest income groups. Some of the first studies of this kind were done in East Asia, in Indonesia and Malaysia. The outcomes for the bottom 20 percent of the population—the poorest quintile—in these two countries were very different. Whereas in Indonesia in 1987 only 12 percent of all public expenditures on health went to the poorest quintile (van de Walle 1994), in neighboring Malaysia in 1984 the share was about 30 percent (Hammer, Nabi, and Cercone 1995).

Research in the Africa region undertaken during the early 1990s (analyzed in Castro-Leal and others 1999) confirmed that Indonesia's experience is much more typical for that region than is Malaysia's. Public spending on health was found to favor upper-income groups in Côte d'Ivoire (1995), Ghana (1992 and 1994), Guinea (1994), Kenya (1992), Madagascar (1993), South Africa (1994), and Tanzania (1992–93). The orientation of public health spending was not much different in South Asia, where studies in India (1994–95) and Bangladesh (2000) showed that spending patterns benefited primarily the better off (ADB–World Bank 2001; Mahal and others 2004).

A fuller but similar pattern emerged from *World Development Report 2004: Making Services Work for Poor People*. The report included a review and summary of all available studies on the extent to which publicly financed health and educational services reach different economic groups (Filmer 2003; World Bank 2003). The results for public spending on health are summarized in figure 1.1. In the 21 country studies, the best-off population quintile received, on average, around 25 percent of the subsidy from total government health care expenditures, while the poorest quintile received only around 15 percent. In 15 of the 21 cases, spending patterns favored the highest income groups. In only 4 countries (Argentina, Colombia, Costa Rica, and Honduras) did spending patterns show a larger subsidy going to the poor.

This reality that health services benefit primarily the better off emerges with equal clarity from recent examinations of the related assumption that programs which address the "diseases of the poor" are likely to benefit primarily the poor (Gwatkin 2001). The evidence on public spending for health summarized by Filmer (2003) shows that the services (loosely categorized as primary health care) which tend to focus on infectious diseases and on other maternal and child health issues that are particularly prevalent among disadvantaged groups favor the better off less than is the case for secondary and tertiary care. But although such services may generally be less pro-rich

Figure 1.1. *Proportion of Benefits from Government Health Service Expenc Going to the Lowest and Highest Income Quintiles, 21 Countries*

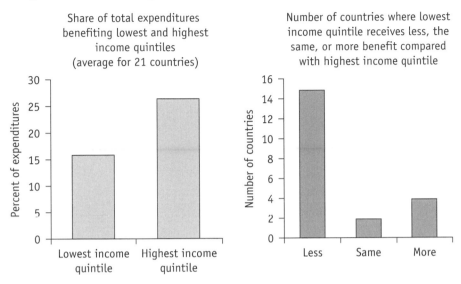

Share of total expenditures benefiting lowest and highest income quintiles (average for 21 countries)

Number of countries where lowest income quintile receives less, the same, or more benefit compared with highest income quintile

Source: Filmer 2003.
Note: The 21 countries covered are Argentina, Armenia, Bangladesh, Bulgaria, Colombia, Costa Rica, Côte d'Ivoire, Ecuador, Ghana, Guinea, Honduras, India (Uttar Pradesh), India (entire country), Indonesia, Kenya (rural), Madagascar, Nicaragua, South Africa, Sri Lanka, Tanzania, and Vietnam.

than others, only rarely are they pro-poor. Additional evidence comes from 45 Demographic and Health Surveys (DHSs) analyzed by the World Bank (Gwatkin and others 2000) which indicate that even services often given high priority in the name of equity (for example, oral rehydration for childhood diarrhea, attended delivery, and child immunization) are more likely to be captured by the well off than by the poor.

The World Bank recently completed a second-phase reanalysis of these and 33 additional DHS surveys, for a total of 78 surveys and 56 countries. An expanded list of more than a hundred indicators was used, covering a wide range of health, nutrition, and population outcomes; the use of health, nutrition, and population services; and the determinants of outcomes and service use. (Countries and indicators are listed in annexes 1.1 and 1.2.) For 22 of the 56 countries, more than one survey was analyzed, permitting a look at trends as well as levels.[1]

Figures 1.2 and 1.3, based on the most recent surveys available for the 56 countries, illustrate poor-rich gaps in health outcomes (child mortality) and use of a range of health services. It is clear that health outcomes and service

Figure 1.2. *Under-Five Mortality Rates among Lowest and Highest Economic Quintiles, 56 Countries*

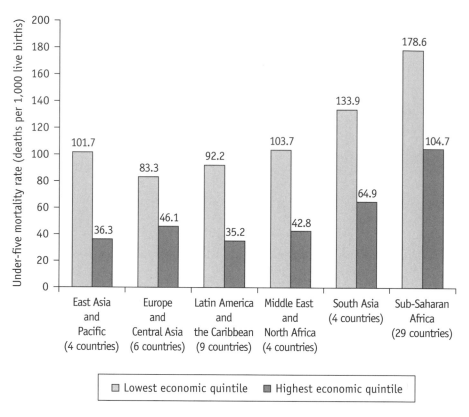

Source: Gwatkin and others 2005.
Note: Based on Demographic and Health Surveys conducted between 1990 and 2001; average date, 1997.

use are closely related to economic status. For outcomes (figure 1.2), the relationship is inverse: the lower a group's economic status, the higher is its under-five mortality rate (U5MR). In four of the six regions shown, under-five mortality (as measured by the unweighted average for countries in the region) was more than twice as high for the poorest 20 percent of the population as for the least poor quintile. The opposite pattern prevails for health service use, which is directly related to economic status: the lower a group's economic status, the less it uses health services. Although all of the eight services listed in figure 1.3 feature primary care interventions that are typically included in initiatives for reaching the poor, the coverage rate of each

Figure 1.3. *Use of Basic Maternal and Child Health Services by Lowest and Highest Economic Quintiles, 50+ Countries*

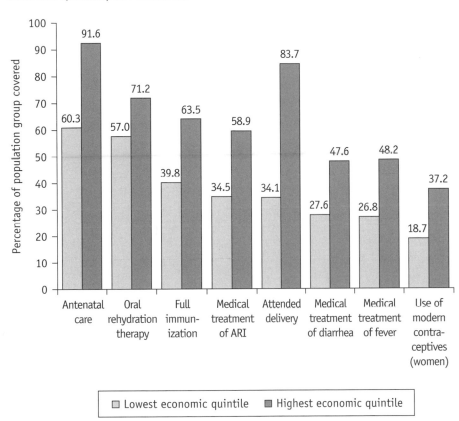

Source: Gwatkin and others 2005.
Note: Based on Demographic and Health Surveys conducted between 1990 and 2001; average date, 1997. Number of countries covered varies from 51 to 56, depending on the type of health service. ARI, acute respiratory infection.

is noticeably higher for the highest income group. On average, coverage of the eight services is about two-thirds higher for the least poor 20 percent of the population than for the poorest.

The studies on which figures 1.2 and 1.3 are based give little indication that such disparities are declining. Caution is called for in interpreting the information about trends in disparities, in light of the many different ways that disparities can be measured, the small size of the samples for some of the indicators of greatest interest, and the short time between survey dates (usually five years or less) in countries with two or more available surveys.

Yet such analysis as is possible gives only limited cause for optimism. For instance, a study using DHS data found that in the countries covered, the relative gap in U5MR between the least poor and poorest quintiles increased during the 1990s. "This uneven improvement in survival was due to the decrease of child mortality being much higher for the top quintile than for the bottom one. All too often the bottom quintile experienced no discernible improvement in U5MR" (Minujin and Delamonica 2004, 348). As disparities in health outcomes and in access to health services become evident, the question arises: what can be done about it?

From Evidence for Advocacy to Evidence for Action

Although not yet fully appreciated in health policy circles, the accumulating empirical evidence summarized in the preceding section has become well enough known to begin making itself felt. The result has been increased work on two issues: (a) the documentation and measurement of inequalities in health outcomes and in health service use, especially with regard to inequalities by economic status, and (b) the identification of strategies for reducing those inequalities.

Documentation of Inequalities

Work on documentation has been fueled by the discovery that information about household assets—for example, ownership of such common articles as bicycles and radios, and sources of water and fuel—can be used in place of income or consumption to assess families' economic status (Filmer and Pritchett 2001; for technical details, see chapter 2 in this volume). Because assets are far easier to measure through household surveys than income or consumption, this innovation made it feasible to examine economic inequalities in health status and service use. The previous focus on health inequalities attributable to gender, educational status, religion, and place of residence could therefore be broadened.

The application of the asset measurement method not only allowed the analysis of distribution of health outcomes and health system outputs in such surveys as the DHS-based studies of Gwatkin and others (2000); it also opened the door for other agencies to include asset questions in their surveys and thus undertake their own distributional analysis. Among the agencies sponsoring major household survey programs that have recently done so are the United Nations Children's Fund (UNICEF) and the World Health Organization (WHO). Over the past few years, asset questions have been added to UNICEF's Multiple Indicator Cluster Surveys (MICS) and to WHO's World Health Survey (WHS).[2] As of this writing, WHO plans soon to release WHS data on health status and service use information by economic quintile. This promises to be an important contribution, since the WHS contains a great deal of information about adult health and chronic diseases that is missing from the maternal and child health–oriented DHS. Distributional tabulations of data from the MICS, already available on the UNICEF website, provide much valuable information on countries and on topics such as child labor that the DHS and WHS do not include.[3]

Identification of Strategies for Reducing Inequalities

Concern among policy makers about improving health equity has grown faster than their knowledge of how to go about it. This dichotomy has intensified the need for and interest in policy and strategy options that can help policy makers realize their aspirations.

Illustrating both the promise and the limitations of the growing policy concern about health equity are two international initiatives: policy reduction strategy papers (PRSPs) and the Millennium Development Goals (MDGs).

PRSPs are prepared by the governments of poor countries to qualify for debt relief under the Heavily Indebted Poor Country (HIPC) program sponsored by the International Monetary Fund (IMF) and the World Bank.[4] These strategies are intended to focus on poverty alleviation to ensure that the additional resources made available are used for that purpose. Early assessments in the health sector, however, indicated that the health components of PRSPs were largely failing to focus on poverty. For example, an assessment of the interim versions of the first 23 PRSPs found that there was "limited emphasis on the poor, the supposed primary beneficiaries" (Laterveer, Niessen, and Yazbeck 2003, 138).

The eight Millennium Development Goals were adopted by the United Nations General Assembly in September 2000.[5] Poverty alleviation is the overall objective, but the three principal health goals are stated as national averages, and thus progress toward them could be achieved via progress by any income group, rich or poor (Gwatkin 2005).

The more receptive climate for pro-poor health strategies, symbolized and reinforced by initiatives such as the PRSPs and the MDGs, has given rise to a growing volume of research that seeks to go beyond diagnosis to the design of remedial policy and strategy options. The dynamic nature of such activities can be seen by noting some of the more prominent efforts of the past few years.

An early instance was the chapter on health, population, and nutrition in the World Bank's PRSP sourcebook. This chapter sought to draw together the abundance of knowledge about the development of pro-poor strategies in the health sector and related sectors and to present it in a form readily accessible to PRSP authors (Claeson and others 2002).

Another early activity, undertaken in a similar spirit, although from a somewhat different perspective, was the Global Health Equity Initiative organized by the Rockefeller Foundation and the Swedish International Development Cooperation Agency. The Initiative produced the well-known book *Challenging Inequalities in Health: From Ethics to Action* (Evans and others 2001). This 21-chapter volume is a collection of studies analyzing health gaps within and among countries and presenting the available tools and programmatic approaches for redressing persistent inequalities. The research disciplines represented include epidemiology, demography, and economics.

A more recent health research effort, also partially supported by the Rockefeller Foundation, is being conducted by the INDEPTH Network of demographic surveillance sites in developing countries.[6] The INDEPTH health equity project started as a purely diagnostic effort focused on inequalities in 13 member sites, with populations ranging from 8,000 to more than 200,000. The volume of studies produced by the initial phase covers inequalities in both health outcomes and health service use (INDEPTH Network 2005). Having found that inequality was much more prevalent than expected, INDEPTH added a remedial focus in the second round of the project by inviting proposals for assessing service delivery strategies aimed at reducing those inequalities. Thus far, it has funded five such assessments, all in Africa. Study topics include expanded outreach programs to encourage use by poor families of HIV/AIDS prevention and treatment services; targeted subsidies for insecticide-treated bednets; and child welfare grants to poor households.

A third Rockefeller-initiated activity, the Equity Lens Project, focused on strategy change from its beginnings in the early 1990s. The objective was to alert the leaders of prominent global health initiatives to the emerging documentation on coverage inequalities in the services they were supporting and to encourage them to develop more effective delivery strategies for reaching the poor. The project organized and supported a wide range of presentations, literature reviews, and similar activities in cooperation with global health initiative personnel working in six areas: child health, immunization, malaria, safe motherhood, trachoma, and tuberculosis. In September 2003 the Rockefeller Foundation, the World Bank, and the World Health

Organization concluded the project's initial phase with a consultation bringing together health equity specialists associated with the global initiatives. A second phase, featuring field experimentation with alternative strategies for reaching the poor, was being developed at this writing.

World Development Report 2004 (World Bank 2003) summarizes the growing evidence on how public spending on education, health, nutrition, water, sanitation, and electricity fails the poor in many low- and middle-income countries. It identified a number of public sector shortcomings: failure, often, to allocate resources to address the needs of the poor; inefficient spending of the resources that are allocated; and failure to ensure that the teachers and health providers who are paid to provide services actually are providing them and that the public knows about services and demands them. The evidence collected for the report goes a long way toward confirming suspicions that widespread assumptions about health spending reaching the poor are not supported by empirical evidence. The report offers alternative ways of improving the efficiency and equity of health and social sector expenditures by examining and strengthening the relationships between poor people, policy makers, and service providers and by strengthening accountability mechanisms.

The emphasis on health services in *World Development Report 2004* and other recent activities has recently been complemented by the focus on the social and economic determinants of health inequalities adopted by a commission established in March 2005 by the World Health Organization. Like some other activities described here, the WHO Commission on Social Determinants of Health will compile evidence and will propose agendas for action based on that evidence. In doing so, the commission, chaired by eminent epidemiologist Sir Michael Marmot, hopes to develop a "third major thrust" that can complement health system development and poverty relief by finding ways of reducing social disparities (WHO 2005).[7]

The Reaching the Poor Program

The Reaching the Poor Program (RPP), the source of the case studies in this volume, seeks to further the work described above. It is an effort to document coverage inequalities more fully and carefully than in the past. It seeks to do this for two reasons. The first is to increase awareness that many programs do not effectively reach the poor, in order to stimulate awareness of a need for improvement. The second, much more important, reason is to identify programs that *are* successful in serving disadvantaged groups, in order to provide guidance for policy makers wishing to reduce these inequalities and improve coverage among the poor. In providing such documentation, the RPP hopes to demonstrate the value of the benefit-incidence approach (described below and, more fully, in the next chapter) in assessing and monitoring the distribution of program benefits.

Background

The RPP was initiated in 2001 by the World Bank Health and Poverty Thematic Group, which brought together members of various Bank units who shared a concern for the health of the poor. The program grew out of interest on the part of group members and other Bank health personnel, stimulated by the emerging evidence about health coverage disparities and especially by the publication and dissemination of an analysis of 45 DHS-based studies (Gwatkin and others 2000) that had been undertaken on the group's behalf.

The DHS-based studies gave rise to a desire for improved diagnosis because they raised the possibility that health service projects, including programs supported by the Bank, were not succeeding in reaching the poor. But the study findings—that most countries' health outcomes and health system outputs are heavily skewed toward the better-off—were too general to apply to any specific project. Nor did the findings provide any basis for thinking that Bank-supported projects might perform any worse in this regard than those supported by other donors or by governments themselves. Even so, the suggestion that Bank-assisted health activities might not be pro-poor was unsettling, in light of the Bank's widely advertised antipoverty mission. It thus triggered an interest in refined diagnostic approaches that could go straight to the question of just who benefits most from specific projects.

More important, the DHS studies and the other evidence invalidating the conventional wisdom about the pro-poor nature of health activities began to raise hard-to-answer questions about what could be done to remedy the coverage inequalities being revealed. These concerns took the form of increasingly frequent requests for guidance from Bank staff members exasperated at being told that the projects on which they were working were unlikely to achieve their objectives. Bank personnel wanted to know not just that something needed to be done but what could be done. The reviews of the literature were of some use in responding to such queries, but because of the general nature of the recommendations then available and the limited empirical evidence underlying most of these recommendations, the practical guidance to be gleaned from them proved limited.

Thus, the RPP was established to take up specific issues of immediate concern to those responsible for ensuring that World Bank lending to health services—typically between $1 billion and $2 billion annually—was serving its intended beneficiaries. Because policy makers in national governments and in other external assistance agencies struggle with this same issue, it was hoped that the RPP findings would be useful to them as well.

Approach

In their search for a suitable approach for identifying the chief beneficiaries of health services, the RPP organizers drew on their familiarity with a particularly relevant analytical technique used by public finance specialists in the World Bank and elsewhere. This technique, *benefit-incidence analysis,* had been developed over the preceding 20 years to determine how overall government expenditures benefit different economic groups. It first caught the attention of the economic development community in the late 1970s, when landmark studies on Colombia (Selowsky 1979) and Malaysia (Meerman 1979) were published, and it became a standard technique for economic analysis.

More recently, health economists have become aware of the benefit-incidence approach, and findings from its use in assessing government health expenditures constitute the basis for the evidence presented above. Not many such studies have been done, however, and outside the health economics community, the technique is still poorly known. For example, almost all public health specialists are now aware of *cost-effectiveness analysis,* the economic technique used to measure the volume of health program outputs produced from a given volume of inputs. This method has been featured in *World Development Report 1993,* on health, and in other publications. Yet discussions with leading equity specialists in public health indicate that most of them have not heard of benefit-incidence analysis, the analogous technique that can determine how outputs are distributed among poor and better-off segments of the population.

Although the direct relevance of the benefit-incidence approach was the primary factor behind its adoption, its unfamiliarity in the health field was an important additional plus. It meant that by featuring the approach in a set of case studies, the RPP might be able not only to produce valuable findings but also to spread awareness about a technique that others might apply in subsequent investigations.

The basic approach featured in the RPP studies is very much in the benefit-incidence tradition, but it is a version that has been modified for use in the health, nutrition, and population fields. For example, as noted in the next chapter, the outputs whose distribution is assessed are usually not financial subsidies but rather service outputs such as clinic visits, children immunized, and people reached through home visits. Furthermore, the scope of activities covered is not limited to government-provided services, as was the original benefit-incidence work, but often deals, in addition or instead, with services obtained through private for-profit or not-for-profit providers. Another difference is that the studies do not often consider *net benefit*—the cost of service to the provider less the amount service recipients pay in taxes, out-of pocket payments, and insurance premiums; more frequently, the focus is on simple coverage differences across groups.

Limitations

The specific focus and approach adopted by the RPP has important advantages for dealing with the particular issue addressed: how well health services reach the poor. But they also mean that the RPP cannot claim to constitute or even approximate a complete approach to health equity. It has consciously chosen not to cover many important issues.

For instance, the RPP does not deal with the myriad social and economic factors that are arguably more important than health services in determining inequalities in health status. These issues have been and are being well addressed by many others, such as the WHO Commission on the Social Determinants of Health, whose efforts should be complemented, not duplicated. The RPP's complementary focus on health services is warranted in order to improve the distribution of benefits from the $380 billion spent annually on such services in low- and middle-income countries (World Bank 2004). Given the magnitude of this figure, an improvement in the distribution of health service benefits is sufficiently important to justify a significant effort, even should the maldistribution of those benefits constitute only a small part of the total health equity problem.

Neither does the RPP cover the political considerations that are important causes of inequalities in service coverage. Although this is a significant limitation, technical analyses like those produced through the RPP can nonetheless make an important contribution to policy development. For one thing, they are necessary if political commitment is to be translated into effective action. Without accurate empirical information about the distribution of program benefits, even ardently pro-poor policymakers with strong political support can too easily go astray. This seems to have been happening in the health field because of reliance on the incorrect assumption that programs are reaching disadvantaged groups. Technical information can also be useful tools in the hands of those wishing to increase political commitment.

Readers will also note the heavy emphasis on the economic dimension of health inequalities. Although obviously significant, this is but one of the many dimensions of health inequity and is not necessarily more important than, for example, gender, religion, or race. The justification for the special attention paid here to the economic aspect lies not in its greater importance but in the improved ability to analyze it and thus begin dealing with it. The measurement of differences in health status or service use along with the other dimensions mentioned has always been relatively straightforward, given the ease of determining an individual's gender, religion, or race. Until recently, however, determining a person's economic status has been a major challenge, as explained in the next chapter. As a result, assessment of health inequalities by economic status lagged behind assessments in terms of inequality's other dimensions, especially gender and education. But with the recent reduction in the difficulty of measuring economic status, that need no longer be the case.

Organization

To achieve its objectives, the RPP program was structured in three phases.

PHASE 1: KNOWLEDGE GENERATION. Case studies were commissioned through an international competitive bidding process. Researchers interested in documenting whether and why services reach the poor were asked for proposals. Although the grants were small (between $20,000 and $40,000), nearly 150 applications were received. Nineteen were selected for funding by a panel of technical specialists from the World Bank, the Rockefeller Foundation, the Pan American Health Organization, and the International Centre for Diarrhoeal Disease Research, Bangladesh.

After work had begun, a meeting of investigators was organized in October 2002 to give the researchers an opportunity to share their experiences and to review the ongoing research. The first phase ended with another peer review process in which technical experts reviewed the first drafts of each research activity financed. Peer reviewer comments were then made available to assist the researchers in completing the final drafts of their papers.

PHASE 2: KNOWLEDGE SYNTHESIS. A global conference held in February 2004 brought together researchers financed by the RPP program and investigators who had done similar work financed by other sources. (See annex 1.3 for a list of papers and authors.) In addition to the presentation of RPP and non-RPP papers, the conference activities included training on the data and methodological issues that arise in monitoring and evaluating the distribution of program health benefits, as well as group work by participants to begin drawing policy implications from the conference discussions and the research presentations.

PHASE 3: KNOWLEDGE DISSEMINATION. The final phase of the RPP program consists of several components. Among the most prominent are:

- This book, which presents 11 of the 19 case studies supported by the RPP.
- A special issue of the World Bank Institute journal *Development Outreach* designed for a policy audience and featuring briefer and less technical versions of some of the more interesting conference presentations, designed for a policy audience.
- Dissemination seminars for policy makers. The first, for English-speaking Africa, took place in Livingstone, Zambia, in January 2005.

Vigilance and Hard Work

As noted at the outset, simplistic assumptions about spending and health services for the poor have led to programs that served the better off. The Reaching the Poor Program seeks to replace these assumptions with empirical evidence on what really does reach the poor and why. In this way, it hopes to point the way toward more promising approaches.

The complex nature of the root problem and the concerted effort needed to solve it mean that careful research is needed for this purpose. "Poverty" is a complex and contextual problem that has proved immune to simple answers and policy fads. Inequalities in the health sector, stemming in large part from poverty, are also complex and contextual. Counteracting inequalities in the use of health services will take constant vigilance and hard work. We hope the RPP , in addition to identifying better strategies through its own work, will help others do the same by providing tools for policy makers to strengthen programs aimed at reaching the poor and for researchers to measure how well those programs do so.

Annex 1.1. Countries Covered by the Second Phase of the World Bank Health and Poverty Country Report Program

Note: Dates of the studies are given in parentheses.

East Africa and Pacific
Cambodia (2000)
Indonesia (1997)
Philippines (1998)
Vietnam (1997, 2000)

Europe and Central Asia
Armenia (2000)
Kazakhstan (1995, 1999)
Kyrgyz Republic (1997)
Turkey (1993, 1998)
Turkmenistan (2000)
Uzbekistan (1996)

Latin America and the Caribbean
Bolivia (1998)
Brazil (1996)
Colombia (1995, 2000)
Dominican Republic (1996)
Guatemala (1995, 1998–99)
Haiti (1994–95, 2000)
Nicaragua (1997–98, 2001)
Paraguay (1990)
Peru (1996, 2000)

Middle East and North Africa
Egypt, Arab Rep. of (1995, 2000)
Jordan (1997)
Morocco (1992)
Yemen, Republic of (1997)

South Asia
Bangladesh (1996–97, 2000)
India (1992–93, 1998–99)
Nepal (1996, 2001)
Pakistan (1990–91)

Sub-Saharan Africa
Benin (1996, 2001)
Burkina Faso (1998)
Cameroon (1991, 1998)
Central African Republic (1994–95)
Chad (1996–97)
Comoros (1996)
Côte d'Ivoire (1994)
Eritrea (1995)
Ethiopia (2000)
Gabon (2000)
Ghana (1993, 1998)
Guinea (1999)
Kenya (1998)
Madagascar (1997)
Malawi (1992, 2000)
Mali (1995, 2000)
Mauritania (2000)
Mozambique (1997)
Namibia (1992, 2000)
Niger (1998)
Nigeria (1990)
Rwanda (2000)
Senegal (1997)
South Africa (1998)
Tanzania (1996, 1999)
Togo (1998)
Uganda (1995, 2000–2001)
Zambia (1996, 2001)
Zimbabwe (1994, 1999)

Annex 1.2. Indicators Covered by the Second Phase of the World Bank Health and Poverty Country Report Program

Note: BCG, bacille Calmette-Guérin (tuberculosis) vaccine; DPT, diphtheria, pertussis, and tetanus vaccine.

Outcome Indicators

CHILD ILLNESS AND MORTALITY
Infant mortality rate
Under-five mortality rate
Prevalence of fever
Prevalence of diarrhea
Prevalence of acute respiratory
  infection

FERTILITY
Total fertility rate
Adolescent fertility rate

NUTRITIONAL STATUS
Children
Moderate stunting
Severe stunting
Moderate underweight
Severe underweight
Mild anemia
Moderate anemia
Severe anemia

Women
Malnutrition
Mild anemia
Moderate anemia
Severe anemia

FEMALE CIRCUMCISION
Prevalence of circumcision
Girls
Women

Prevalence of occlusion
Girls
Women

SEXUALLY TRANSMITTED DISEASE
Prevalence of genital discharge
Women
Men

Prevalence of genital ulcer
Women
Men

Service Indicators

CHILDHOOD IMMUNIZATION
BCG coverage
Measles coverage
DPT coverage
Full basic coverage
No basic coverage
Hepatitis B coverage
Yellow fever coverage

TREATMENT OF CHILDHOOD
ILLNESSES
Fever
Medical treatment of fever
Treatment in a public facility
Treatment in a private facility

Acute respiratory infection (ARI)
Medical treatment of ARI
Treatment in a public facility
Treatment in a private facility

Diarrhea
Use of oral rehydration therapy
Medical treatment of diarrhea
Treatment in a public facility
Treatment in a private facility

ANTENATAL AND DELIVERY CARE
Antenatal care visits
To a medically trained person
To a doctor
To a nurse or trained midwife
3+ visits to a medically trained
  person

Antenatal care content
Tetanus toxoid
Prophylactic antimalarial treatment
Iron supplementation

Delivery attendance
By a medically trained person
By a doctor
By a nurse or trained midwife
In a public facility
In a private facility
At home

CONTRACEPTIVE SERVICES
Contraceptive prevalence
Women
Men

Source of contraception: public sector
Women
Men

Source of contraception: private sector
Women
Men

TREATMENT OF ADULT ILLNESSES
Genital discharge, ulcer, sore
Women
Men

*Genital discharge, ulcer, sore treated in
public medical facilities*
Women
Men

*HIV/AIDS voluntary counseling and
testing*
Women
Men

Household Indicators

HYGIENIC PRACTICES
Disposal of children's stools
Sanitary disposal

Hand washing
Hand washing prior to food preparation
Hand washing facilities in household

BEDNET OWNERSHIP AND USE
Bednet ownership
Bednet ownership
Treated bednet ownership

Bednet use
By children
By pregnant women

BREASTFEEDING
Exclusive breastfeeding
Timely complementary feeding
Bottle-feeding

MICRONUTRIENT CONSUMPTION
Iodized salt
Availability of iodized salt in household

Vitamin A
Children
Women

TOBACCO AND ALCOHOL USE
Tobacco
Women
Men

Alcohol
Women
Men

SEXUAL PRACTICES
Nonregular sexual partnerships
Women
Men

Condom usage with nonregular partner
Women
Men

DOMESTIC VIOLENCE
Experience of violence, ever
Experience of violence in past year

EDUCATION
School completion
Women
Men

School participation
Girls
Boys

EXPOSURE TO MASS MEDIA
Newspapers
Women
Men

Radio
Women
Men

Television
Women
Men

KNOWLEDGE AND ATTITUDES ABOUT
HIV/AIDS
Knowledge about sexual transmission of HIV
Women
Men

Knowledge about mother-to-child transmission of HIV
Women
Men

Attitudes toward HIV
Women
Men

STATUS OF WOMEN
Household decision making
Can seek own health care
Can seek children's health care
Can make daily household purchases
Can make large household purchases
Can make meal-related decisions

Freedom of movement
Can travel to visit family and relatives

Other decision making/attitudes
Can decide how to spend own money
Can decide whether to have sex
Justifies domestic violence

ORPHANHOOD
Paternal orphan prevalence
Maternal orphan prevalence
Double orphan prevalence

Annex 1.3. Presentations at the Reaching the Poor Conference, February 2004

Child Health: National Programs

Maternal and Child Health Services of the Argentine Government
  *Mónica Panadeiros, Fundación de Investigaciones Económicas
  Latinoamericanas*
The Brazilian Government's Family Health Program
  Aluísio Barros, Federal University of Pelotas
Services Provided through Argentina's PROMIN Maternal and Child
Health Program
  Sebastián Galiani, Universidad de San Andrés

Child Health: Immunization

Measles Immunization in Zambia
  Joel Selanikio, American Red Cross
Immunization Coverage in the States of India
  G. N. V. Ramana, World Bank (India)
Immunization Coverage in Bangladesh
  Mushtaque Chowdhury, Bangladesh Rural Advancement Committee

AIDS, Tuberculosis, Malaria: AIDS and Malaria

Voluntary Counseling and Testing for AIDS in South Africa
  Michael Thiede, University of Cape Town
  Natasha Palmer, London School of Hygiene and Tropical Medicine
Distribution of Insecticide-Treated Bednets in Ghana and Zambia
  Joel Selanikio, American Red Cross
Social Marketing of Insecticide-Treated Bednets in Tanzania
  Rose Nathan, Ifakara Health Research and Development Centre

AIDS, Tuberculosis, Malaria

Tuberculosis Program of the Self-Employed Women's Association, India
  Mittal Shah, Self-Employed Women's Association
  Kent Ranson, Self-Employed Women's Association
Tuberculosis Control Services in Kenya
  Christy Hanson, World Health Organization
National Tuberculosis Programme in Lilongwe, Malawi
  Gillian Mann, Liverpool School of Tropical Medicine

Nutrition

Three Child Food Programs in Peru
  Martin Valdivia, Grupo de Análisis para el Desarrollo

Three Children's Feeding Programs in Argentina
Mónica Panadeiros, Fundación de Investigaciones Económicas Latinoamericanas
The Micronutrient and Health Project in Ethiopia and Malawi
Harry Cummings, University of Guelph

Reproductive Health
Emergency Obstetric Care in Rural Bangladesh
Iqbal Anwar, International Centre for Diarrhoeal Disease Research, Bangladesh
Reproductive Health Camps of the Self-Employed Women's Association, India
Mittal Shah, Self-Employed Women's Association
Kent Ranson, Self-Employed Women's Association
Participatory Reproductive Health Programs for Youth in Nepal
Anju Malhotra, International Center for Research on Women
Sanyukta Mathur, International Center for Research on Women

Health Systems: Overall Performance
Findings from 21 Country Studies of Who Benefits from Government Health Spending
Deon Filmer, World Bank
Beneficiaries from Public Health Care in Six Asian Countries
Aparnaa Somanathan, Equity in Asia-Pacific Health Systems Network
Bangladesh Health and Population Sector Programme
Anne Cockcroft, CIET International

Health Systems: Service Delivery Innovations
Contracting with Non-Governmental Organizations in Cambodia
J. Brad Schwartz, University of North Carolina
Indu Bhushan, Asian Development Bank
Upgrading the Government Health System in Uttar Pradesh, India
David Peters, Johns Hopkins School of Public Health
Krishna Rao, Johns Hopkins School of Public Health
Networking Private Providers of Reproductive Health Services in Kenya
Martha Campbell, University of California at Berkeley

Health Systems: Experiences from Other Sectors
Programs Providing Targeted Cash, Food, Services and Employment in 48 Countries
Margaret Grosh, World Bank
Microcredit Projects
Manohar Sharma, International Food Policy Research Institute

Social Funds in Six Countries
  Laura Rawlings, World Bank

Health Systems: Better Ways to Identify Poor Individuals
Conditional Cash Transfers through Mexico's PROGRESA Program
  Deon Filmer, World Bank
  David Coady, International Food Policy Research Institute
Targeted Subsidies for Health Insurance in Colombia
  Tarsicio Castañeda, Consultant in Health and Economics
Increasing Service Access by the Poor through Chile's Puente/Solidario Program
  Veronica Silva, Fondo de Solidaridad e Inversión Social

Health Financing: Insurance
Vietnam's Health Insurance Program
  Adam Wagstaff, World Bank
Thailand's Universal Insurance Coverage Initiative
  Chutima Suraratdecha, Health Systems Research Institute
Rwanda's Micro-Insurance Program
  Pia Schneider, Abt Associates

Health Financing: Vouchers and Fee Waivers
Indonesia's Healthcard Program
  Fadia Saadah, World Bank
  Menno Pradhan, World Bank
Hospital Equity Fund in Cambodia
  Bruno Meessen, Institute of Tropical Medicine, Antwerp
  Wim Van Damme, Médecins sans Frontières, Phnom Penh
Extension of the Eligibility for Free Health Services in Armenia
  Edmundo Murrugarra, World Bank
  Nazmul Chaudhury, World Bank

Notes

1. Further information about this reanalysis of DHS studies, including all the data produced, is available in the "Country Data" section of the World Bank Poverty and Health Website, www.worldbank.org/povertyandhealth.

2. For further information see, for the MICS, http://www.childinfo.org/ and for the WHS, http://www3.who.int/whs/.

3. For tabulations of MICS data on health status, service use, and related topics by economic quintile, see www.childinfo.org.

4. Further information about PRSPs can be found at http://www.imf.org/external/np/prsp/prsp.asp. Additional information about the HIPC program is available at http://web.worldbank.org/WBSITE/EXTERNAL/TOPICS/EXTDEBTDEPT/0,,contentMDK:20260411~menuPK:528655~pagePK:64166689~piPK:64166646~theSitePK:469043,00.html.

5. A fuller presentation of the Millennium Development Goals is available at http://www.developmentgoals.org.

6. Further information about the INDEPTH Network is available at http://www.indepth-network.org.

7. More on the commission can be found at its website, http://www.who.int/social_determinants/en.

References

ADB (Asian Development Bank)–World Bank. 2001. Bangladesh poverty assessment: Benefit incidence analysis—education and health sectors. Washington, DC.

Castro-Leal, Florencia, Julia Dayton, Lionel Demery, and Kalpana Mehra. 1999. Public social spending in Africa: Do the poor benefit? *World Bank Research Observer* 14(1): 49–72.

Claeson, M., C. Griffin, T. Johnston, M. McLachlan, A. Soucat, A. Wagstaff, and A. Yazbeck. 2002. Health, nutrition, and population. In *A sourcebook for poverty reduction strategies,* ed. Jeni Klugman, vol. 2, 201–29. Washington, DC: World Bank.

Evans T., M. Whitehead, F. Diderichsen, A. Bhuiya, and M. Wirth, eds. 2001. *Challenging inequities in health: From ethics to action.* New York: Oxford University Press.

Filmer Deon. 2003. The incidence of public expenditures in health and education. Background note to *World Development Report 2004,* World Bank, Washington, DC. http://www-wds.worldbank.org/servlet/WDS_IBank_Servlet?pcont=details&eid=000160016_20031020130801.

Filmer, Deon, and Lant H. Pritchett. 2001. Estimating wealth effects without expenditure data—or tears: An application to educational enrollments in states of India. *Demography* 38(1): 115–32.

Gwatkin, D. 2001. The need for equity-oriented health sector reforms. *International Journal of Epidemiology* 30: 720–23.

Gwatkin, D. 2005. How much would poor people gain from faster progress towards the millennium development goals for health? *Lancet* 365: 813–17.

Gwatkin, Davidson, Shea Rutstein, Kiersten Johnson, Rohini Pande, and Adam Wagstaff. 2000. Socio-economic differences in health, nutrition, and population—45 countries. Health, Nutrition, and Population Department, World Bank, Washington, DC. http://web.worldbank.org/WBSITE/EXTERNAL/TOPICS/

EXTHEALTHNUTRITIONANDPOPULATION/EXTPAH/0,,contentMDK: 20216957~menuPK:400482~pagePK:148956~piPK:216618~theSitePK:400476,00 .html.

Gwatkin, Davidson, Shea Rutstein, Kiersten Johnson, Eldaw Suliman, Adam Wagstaff, and Agbessi Amouzou. 2005. Socioeconomic differences in health, nutrition, and population. 2nd ed. World Bank, Washington, DC. http://web .worldbank.org/WBSITE/EXTERNAL/TOPICS/EXTHEALTHNUTRITIO- NANDPOPULATION/EXTPAH/0,,contentMDK:20216946~menuPK:400482~p agePK:148956~piPK:216618~theSitePK:400476,00.html.

Hammer, Jeffrey, Ijaz Nabi, and James Cercone. 1995. Distributional effects of social expenditures in Malaysia, 1974 to 1989. In *Public spending and the poor: Theory and evidence,* ed. Dominique van de Walle and Kimberly Nead, 521–54. Baltimore: Johns Hopkins University Press.

INDEPTH Network. 2005. *Measuring health equity in small areas: Findings from demographic surveillance sites.* Aldershot, UK: Ashgate Publishing.

Laterveer L., L. Niessen, and A. Yazbeck. 2003. Pro-poor health policies in poverty reduction strategies. *Health Policy and Planning* 18(2): 138–45.

Mahal, Ajay, Abdo S. Yazbeck, David Peters, and G. N. V. Ramana. 2003. The poor and health service use in India. In *Fiscal policies and sustainable growth in India,* ed. Edgardo M. Favaro and Ashok K. Lahiri, 217–39. New Delhi: Oxford University Press. http://www.oup.com/isbn/0-19-566600-3?view=in.

Meerman, Jacob. 1979. *Public expenditures in Malaysia: Who benefits and why.* New York: Oxford University Press.

Minujin, Alberto, and Enrico Delamonica. 2004. Socio-economic inequalities and health in the developing world. *Demographic Research,* special collection 2, article 13. http://www.demographic-research.org/?http://www.demographic-research .org/special/2/13/ (accessed May 15, 2005).

Selowsky, Marcelo. 1979. *Who benefits from government expenditures? A case study of Colombia.* New York: Oxford University Press.

van de Walle, Dominique. 1994. The distribution of subsidies through public health services in Indonesia, 1978–87. *World Bank Economic Review* 8(2): 279–309.

World Bank. 1993. *World development report 1993: Investing in health.* New York: Oxford University Press.

World Bank. 2003. *World development report 2004: Making services work for poor people.* New York: Oxford University Press.

World Bank. 2004. *World development indicators.* Washington, DC: World Bank.

WHO (World Health Organization). 2005. Commission on Social Determinants of Health: Imperatives and opportunities for change. Geneva. http:www .who.int/social_determinants/strategy/stratdoc18Feb05/en/.

2

How Were the Reaching the Poor Studies Done?

Adam Wagstaff and Hugh Waters

All of the studies in this volume are concerned with one broad question: how well do specific health programs reach the poor? Yet they vary in a number of respects—in the countries and types of program studied, of course, but also in the methods used. In part, this reflects variation in the exact question asked, but there are also methodological differences among studies that ask the same question. This chapter provides a tour of the methodologies used in the volume and explores the meaning of some of the terms used.

Snapshots, Movies, and Experiments

Although all the studies look at the broad issue of how well programs reach the poor, they take different approaches, which can be divided into three general categories. The first group uses the *snapshot approach* and asks, for example: How do rates of utilization of services delivered by the program differ between the poor and the less poor? Are the users of the program services drawn disproportionately from the poor? Such questions are clearly of interest, as many programs are designed explicitly in the hope that the poor will be the primary beneficiaries, and evidence that the use of program services is higher among the less poor should cause policy makers to worry. The snapshot approach is the least demanding in terms of data; data are needed for only one point in time, to capture the *current* distribution of utilization by the poor and the less poor.

The second group of studies asks: has inequality between the poor and the less poor in the use of services increased or decreased over time? This approach lets the film roll for two or more periods and then halts and reviews the trend over time. It may find that in each "frame," contrary to what the program's designers had hoped, the poor are not the heaviest users of program services. But as the frames roll forward, it may turn out that the inequality, or *gradient*, narrows over time, and knowing this would be some consolation, even though there is scope for improvement. This *movie approach* is more data demanding than the first. Now data are needed at two points in time, capturing the distribution of utilization by income (or some other measure of living standards) as it was and as it is.

There remains a third question: is the distribution of service use more equal (or less unequal) under the program than it would have been without the program? This begs the question of the *counterfactual*—what the world would have been like in the absence of the program. For example, the research may be examining a large program financed and delivered by the government, and one extreme counterfactual would be what the supply of and demand for health care would have been under a pure private market. Or the program under study may be run by a nongovernmental organization (NGO), and a plausible counterfactual would be what the government would have done in the absence of the NGO. In this approach, the researcher takes a snapshot of the actual situation and then disappears into the art studio to paint a picture of what he or she thinks the distribution would have looked like without the program. The two are then compared.

This third approach—the snapshot coupled with an artist's impression of an unknown world—is the most data demanding of the three. Data are now needed on the extant distribution and on the distribution in the counterfactual. Of course, this second distribution is never observed, so the researcher must not only be explicit about the scenario he or she has in mind but must also have some way of generating data that approximate the chosen scenario. There are various nonexperimental ways this can be done, but in this volume the tool used to generate the counterfactual data is the *experiment*. The data are collected before the experiment starts and again after it has been running for a while.

In the studies reported on here, the intervention groups and the control groups have been assigned on the basis of geography; some areas are under the program, and some are not. Ideally, this assignment would be random, and some chapters (for example, chapter 8, on the Cambodian health service reform) do report the results of a randomized experiment. More often than not, however, the assignment is not random. Evaluators are generally measuring the effects of the programs on participants only and do not know what effect the program would have had on nonparticipants. Because nonparticipants differ from participants in ways that might influence the outcome, it cannot be assumed that they would have been affected in the same manner or to the same extent.

Biases may result. Suppose the intervention and control groups differ in certain key factors that influence the outcomes being measured. Insofar as these are observable to the researcher, methods such as regression analysis and propensity score matching can be used to reduce selection on observables. This leaves the possibility that there may be selection on unobservables. Individuals who self-select into a program may have unobservable characteristics related to preferences or health status that make them more likely than others to join the program and also influence their use of health services or other positive outcomes (Waters 1999). But by focusing on differences in changes over time between the treatment and control groups, researchers can reduce this bias to the extent that the unobservables in question stay constant over time.

Table 2.1 shows how the three categories apply to the chapters in this volume. Most chapters are "snapshots" of a single time period in which equity is measured. The second-largest group consists of "experiments" that attempt to measure the results of various interventions, while two of the chapters are "movies" that examine changes in equity over time.

Targeting, Leakage, and Benefit Incidence

Before turning to the practicalities of undertaking studies in this field, some additional terms and concepts need to be introduced.

Let us suppose we are assessing a program designed to reach the poor. The administrators of such a program would be happy if the poor were indeed benefiting from the program and if, as intended, the nonpoor were *not* benefiting from it. The term *leakage* is used to describe instances where the nonpoor benefit from the program (a type II error); a "leaky" program is a poorly targeted program. The administrator would also want to know about people who are supposed to be beneficiaries but are not being reached. The term *undercoverage* describes instances where, contrary to the program's goal, the poor do not benefit from the program (a type I error).

Figure 2.1 illustrates the hypothetical case of a fee waiver program intended only for the poor. People in the top left-hand cell are poor and, correctly, receive the waiver. People in the top right-hand cell are also poor but do not receive the waiver (undercoverage). People in the bottom left-hand

Figure 2.1. *Leakage and Undercoverage in Targeting in a Fee Waiver Program*

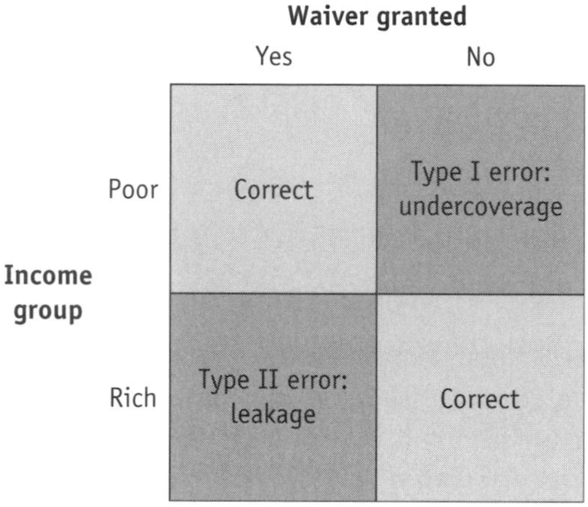

cell, although not poor, nonetheless are granted the waiver (leakage). People in the bottom right-hand cell are not poor and do not receive the waiver—the correct outcome.

These concepts can also be applied to an analysis of program beneficiaries. Leakage would then mean the fraction of program beneficiaries who are nonpoor, and undercoverage would mean the fraction of the poor who do not benefit from the program. Where all program beneficiaries benefit equally from a program, presenting the data along these lines makes sense.

Chapter 13, by Barros and colleagues, provides an example of this methodology. Among the four health and nutrition programs in Brazil that were evaluated is one targeted to very poor families (the Pastorate of the Child) and another that was initially implemented through a targeted approach but was designed to expand over time (the Family Health Program). The chapter begins by testing the hypothesis that considerable leakage and undercoverage exist in both programs. It then takes up the more interesting issue of what structural, programmatic, or social factors may be behind the inequitable distributions observed. Utilization and coverage data are presented across wealth quintiles. The implications of the analysis are particularly important for the wholly targeted program, since its coverage takes in a relatively wide wealth distribution even though its objective is to focus on children who are either undernourished or from extremely impoverished families.

The analysis by Valdivia in chapter 14 evaluates the targeting success of several nutritional programs in Peru. Using data from the Living Standards

Table 2.1. Questions Asked by the Studies Reported in This Volume

Study type	Question	Chapter and topic
1. Snapshot	How unequal is the distribution of service use between the poor and the less poor?	5. Reproductive health training program for private medical providers in Kenya
		6. HIV counseling and testing services in public clinics in South Africa
		9. Utilization of health services provided by the Self-Employed Women's Association (SEWA) in India
		13. Two universal and two targeted health programs in Brazil
		14. Targeted early childhood nutritional programs in Peru
2. Movie	Has inequality between the poor and the less poor in the use of services increased or decreased over time?	7. Utilization of maternal health services across socioeconomic status groups within a rural community in Bangladesh between 1997 and 2001
		12. Changes in the targeting of health and nutrition programs in Argentina between 1997 and 2001
3. Experiment	Is the distribution of service use more equal (or less unequal) under the program than it would have been without the program?	4. Integrated program of vaccination and bednet distribution in Ghana and Zambia
		8. Comparison of primary health services in Cambodia delivered through contractors with those delivered directly by the government
		10. Utilization and patient satisfaction related to a multifaceted health reform initiative in Uttar Pradesh State, India
		11. Participatory approach to reproductive health among rural and urban adolescents in Nepal

Measurement Surveys (LSMSs), Valdivia initially shows the proportions of beneficiaries who are within and outside eligibility thresholds. He then moves on to a valuable examination of marginal incidence to explore whether expansion of the programs would produce equity results on the margin similar to those produced on average. Two of the initiatives evaluated—a school breakfast program and the Vaso de Leche (Glass of Milk) program—showed favorable pro-poor results at the margin despite suboptimal targeting on average, suggesting that even where initiatives have significant leakage (with between 40 and 50 percent of beneficiaries outside the target group), their expansion may lead to disproportionately pro-poor results.

But what if "the program" consists of the government's entire spending on the health sector? Can we really analyze the extent to which the program reaches the poor by using the concept of a program beneficiary? Is someone who uses a government clinic just once a year as much a beneficiary as someone who makes extensive use of primary care, outpatient, and inpatient facilities? We could get a highly distorted picture if the poor, or the nonpoor, make much more extensive use of the program's services than does the other group.

The idea in *benefit-incidence analysis* (BIA) is to calculate the benefits associated with the program and see how they are distributed across the population, paying particular attention to the distribution between the poor and the better off.[1] Benefits, usually expressed in monetary terms, are based on records of service utilization. For example, if "the program" in question is the government's entire spending program for the health sector, the study would ask how many primary care visits, how many hospital outpatient visits, and how many hospital inpatient days each individual or household had in the period covered by the study. Each of these would then be converted to a monetary amount by multiplying the number of visits or days by the amount of government spending or subsidy involved. This may vary from one individual to the next—for example, poorer individuals may be exempt from fees at government facilities, so their subsidy per visit is larger than the subsidy to better-off people who have to pay toward the cost of the visit.

Armed with a measure of benefit accruing to each person, we can compute leakage in terms of program benefits, and this would indicate the share of program benefits accruing to nonpoor people. BIA studies often present the complement of this number—the share of program benefits going to the poor, sometimes known as the *benefit-incidence ratio*. This is a direct measure of targeting success. (Leakage is in a sense an *indirect* measure because a higher number indicates worse targeting performance.)

In chapter 12, Gasparini and Panadeiros employ BIA as part of their broader examination of individuals who use publicly financed health and nutrition programs, but rather than convert benefits into monetary terms, they integrate their findings into a gradient that expresses the degree of inequality. It is to this technique that we now turn.

Gradients and Inequalities

Sometimes the focus is not so much on juxtaposing the experiences of the poor and the nonpoor as on examining a gradient. It could be a gradient in health outcomes, or in service utilization, or in the benefits from government subsidies, and it could span the distribution of income or wealth or some other measure of living standards. But the common concern is with a gradient that captures *inequality*.

Let us suppose we have a living standards measure. (We take up the question of how to obtain such a measure in the next section.) We rank households according to the measure, starting with the poorest, and divide the sample into equal groups—say, five equal groups, or quintiles. Our interest is then in the gradient in the given health indicator across the five quintiles at a particular time, or in changes in the gradient over time, or in differences in the gradient between the actual situation and the situation under the hypothetical counterfactual.

Looking at gradients at a moment in time is fairly straightforward. Figure 2.2 shows rates of underweight across four income groups, using data

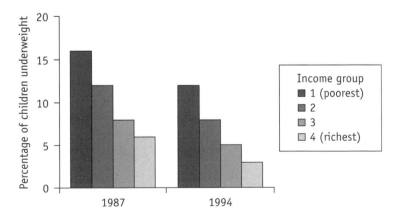

Figure 2.2. *Changes in the Distribution of Underweight Children, Ceará, Brazil*

Source: Based on Victora and others (2000).

from Ceará, Brazil, for 1987 and 1994. In both years there is an appreciable income gradient in the probability of child underweight, with poorer children suffering substantially higher rates of undernutrition. This much is easy to see. We could produce similar charts for health outcomes such as malnutrition, or for measures of utilization such as visits to hospital or full immunization of a child. When the variable is a measure of service utilization and the gradient is downward-sloping, the program is said to be pro-poor.

The analysis of South African voluntary counseling and testing (VCT) programs described in chapter 6 by Thiede, Palmer, and Mbatsha is an example of this approach. The authors present the distribution of VCT clinic utilization across wealth quintiles. Other studies in this volume that use these types of graphic representation include chapter 10, which analyzes health improvements in India, and chapter 4, which evaluates an integrated bednet and vaccination campaign.

Looking at figure 2.2, it is easy to say that in both years a gradient in malnutrition favored the better off. It is harder to say whether the gradient became steeper or shallower between 1987 and 1994. A similar problem might arise when comparing the distribution of utilization under a particular program with utilization in a counterfactual case. One device that makes it easier to answer such questions is the *concentration curve*.[2] In figure 2.3 the x-axis shows the cumulative percentage of the sample (children, in this case) ranked by per capita income, wealth, or whatever measure of living standards is being used, starting with the poorest. On the y-axis is plotted the cumulative percentage of whatever variable is being investigated (in this case, underweight), corresponding to the cumulative percentage of the sample. So, if the poorest 20 percent of children accounts for 30 percent of all underweight children, the ordinate for the y-axis is 30 percent. If the variable being investigated has higher values among the poor (as it does in this example), the resultant curve—the *concentration curve*—will lie above the 45 degree line. The latter is known as the *line of equality* because this is the shape the concentration curve would take if everyone had the same value of the indicator whose distribution we are investigating.

If the health indicator being considered is an undesirable outcome such as being malnourished, a concentration curve above the line of equality is a bad thing from the point of view of equity. If the health indicator is a good outcome, then, arguably, from the point of view of equity we would want the concentration curve to lie above the line of equality.[3] The farther from the line of equality the concentration curve is, the worse things are from an equity standpoint. So, figure 2.3 provides an answer to the question of

Figure 2.3. Concentration Curves Showing Changes in the Distribution of Underweight Children, Ceará, Brazil

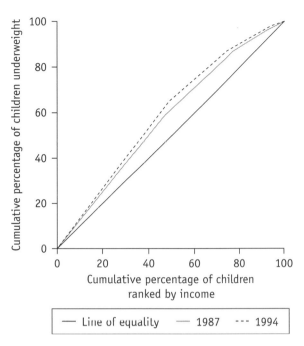

Source: Authors' calculations based on Victora and others (2000).

whether inequality in undernutrition in Ceará had decreased or increased; the answer is that it had increased.

Chapter 9 by Ranson and colleagues provides an example of this approach. The authors examine a health program of the Self-Employed Women's Association (SEWA) in India to assess whether services are in fact utilized by the poor. Frequency distributions of utilization by socioeconomic status are presented, and concentration curves are used to assess equity of utilization of the services offered by SEWA. Rather than display changes across time, the concentration curves in this study allow for comparisons of equity between SEWA's mobile reproductive health units, tuberculosis detection and treatment services, and women's education services in urban and rural communities.

Comparing two concentration curves is straightforward, but comparing multiple concentration curves is a little hard on the eyes. The curves may also cross, making comparison difficult. The *concentration index* is a useful way of reducing the strain on the eye, and it acts as a tiebreaker in the event of intersecting concentration curves. The index, quite simply, is twice the area between the curve and the line of equality.[4] The convention is to use a minus sign in front of the index when the curve is above the line of equality and a plus sign when it is below the line of equality. Of course, whether a negative concentration index is good or bad from an equity standpoint depends on whether the variable in question is something good, such as receiving health care when needed, or something bad, such as being malnourished.

The analysis in chapter 9, for example, presents concentration indexes for each of the SEWA program's health services, using the minus sign convention. All three services had concentration curves of utilization above the line of equality, yielding indexes in the range of –0.33 to –0.37. In chapter 8, Schwartz and Bhushan use concentration indexes to analyze the level of inequality for selected health service indicators in Cambodia. Here, the authors are primarily interested in whether contracting out health services affects ineqaluity.

Measuring Living Standards: Pitfalls for the Unwary

To obtain numbers for leakage and undercoverage and to graph a gradient and a concentration curve, we first need to know how to measure the variables underlying these concepts. For most readers, the measurement of living standards will be the big unknown (by contrast, measuring health service utilization, health outcomes, and so on will be fairly familiar), and so it is on this that we focus. Four approaches to measurement are possible, using income, expenditure, consumption, or a wealth proxy.[5]

The *income approach* is, on the face of it, straightforward and appealing. Many surveys ask respondents a simple question along the lines of how much was your household income in the past year? Respondents might be asked to place their income in a bracket rather than report the exact amount. Both practical and conceptual issues arise. Will people respond truthfully, especially if they think their answers may leak back to the authorities? Will respondents be able to recall accurately all household members' incomes, from all sources, for the past year? Should the question be asked in stages, focusing first on labor income and then on unearned income, including transfers? How should in-kind income such as gifts of food from neighbors be treated? Should income be measured before or after taxes? Should expenses associated with running the family business be deducted from income to derive net income, and if so, how are data on such expenses to be collected? How should the expenses associated with a piece of equipment such as a tractor be handled? The information collected to date on household income in developing countries is typically of poor quality, not least because of these problems.

Chapter 12, by Gasparini and Panadeiros, provides an example of a useful income approach to measurement when neither expenditure nor consumption data are available. The authors utilize two large living standards surveys to obtain data on utilization of targeted health and nutrition programs in Argentina. Although these surveys do not provide insight into expenditure, the authors estimated household welfare using household income, adjusting for household size through an "equivalence" scale. Utilization rates for the programs were then analyzed across the distribution of this income measure.

It is not clear, conceptually, whether income is the best measure of living standards. Income simply tells us how much money is coming into the household; it may not give an accurate picture of the household's living standard. Take the case of pensioners. In the developing world, any pension is probably small, and so even if people have pension income, they may be using up their savings in their old age.

An alternative that gets around this problem is to look at *expenditure.* Many surveys ask about household spending patterns and aggregate up to a total spending figure for the household. But here too there are technical and conceptual issues. Over what period should expenditure be measured? A week? A month? A year? Should the period vary according to type of purchase? How should "lumpy" purchases, such as a car or a television set, be handled?

A big problem with the expenditure approach is that many households in the developing world grow a great deal of the food they consume, and food can make up a large fraction of total consumption. A household may look poor from an expenditure standpoint because it gets its food from its own plot. Yet it may enjoy a reasonable standard of living. Another problem is that subsidies may give a distorted picture of living standards. For example, one household may be able to live rent free because the head of household is a doctor at the village clinic or a state-enterprise worker. Judged by expenditure, the household would appear poor because it pays no rent, but that would be the wrong inference.

For these and other reasons, the World Bank's Living Standards Measurement Study (LSMS) decided early on to measure living standards in terms of *consumption* instead of income or expenditure (Deaton and Grosh 2000; Deaton and Zaidi 2002).[6] A household's food consumption is defined as the sum of its own produce and any produce it buys from others or is given by others. A similar principle applies to other items of consumption; if, for example, the household has a small business producing handicrafts and keeps some for its own use, these products are counted as consumption, and the proceeds from sales of the remaining products show up in the household's consumption of other items (for example, school uniforms bought from the proceeds). The consumption approach does not measure expenditures on consumer durables; rather, it attributes to each durable a use value that depends on the purchase price and the expected life of the durable. It does not look at the amount of rent a family pays for its accommodations but at the imputed rent—the amount it would have had to pay had it rented its accommodations at the market rate. Everyone, whether living in a rent-free government house, a home the person built and owns, or a rented house, is assigned a positive imputed rent.

The consumption approach pioneered by the LSMS overcomes many of the objections that can be leveled at the income and expenditure approaches to measuring living standards. But it has a major drawback: it is complex and time consuming. LSMS consumption questions typically stretch over many pages of a household survey questionnaire. This is fine if assessing living standards is the main goal of the exercise, but it is a little cumbersome if that is only one of the aims. It is perhaps partly for this reason that other large-scale household survey exercises such as the Demographic and Health Survey (DHS) have eschewed the consumption approach. In fact, the DHS, somewhat surprisingly, has eschewed *all* approaches to measuring living standards, leaving researchers in the frustrating position of having excellent household data on maternal and child health variables but no income, expenditure, or consumption data that would, for example, allow them to compare immunization rates among the poor with those among the better off.

This situation led researchers to look at the nonhealth information collected in the DHS and ask whether it could be used to construct an ad hoc proxy measure of living standards. They concluded that it could (Filmer and Pritchett 1999, 2001). A long list of variables was assembled from the DHS, covering attributes of the household's dwelling (type of floor; materials used for the roof and floor), water and sanitation facilities enjoyed by the household (piped water in the house, piped water in the yard, or water from a pump), and ownership of various household durables (radio, television set, bicycle, or car). The information allows researchers to construct a weighted sum of these indicators. Clearly, an infinite number of weighting schemes could be applied. For example, should a car be given twice or three times the weight of a bicycle?

To select the weights, researchers typically employ principal component analysis (PCA). In extracting the first principal component, the weights are selected in such a way that no other weighted sum of the living standards indicators has a larger variance. The same is done for the second principal component, except that this second linear combination must be completely uncorrelated with the first component just extracted. The same procedure is followed for the third and fourth principal components, and so on.

When PCA is used to generate a proxy living standards measure, researchers retain just the first principal component, and this becomes the proxy measure of wealth or living standards. So, for example, when the method is applied to DHS data for Indonesia, possession of a bicycle gets a weight of 0.0285, and possession of a car receives a weight of 0.07262, or 2.5 times that of the bicycle (see Gwatkin and others 2000). The weights that emerge from the PCA exercise vary from one country to the next and one year to the next, reflecting circumstances and customs, as well as the number and type of indicators available in the DHS or in whatever survey is being used.

The PCA approach to the measurement of living standards is the one most often used in the chapters in this volume. Some of the studies utilized actual DHS data to which the PCA approach was applied, while others computed living standards measured by applying the PCA approach to data sets other than those produced by the DHS. The studies of voluntary HIV/AIDS counseling and testing in South Africa (chapter 6) and of private sector reproductive health services in Kenya (chapter 5) are examples of the use of DHS information.

Given the specificity of the programs evaluated in this volume, the second approach—use of non-DHS data sets—is far more common. In chapter 13 the authors measure inequality by applying PCA to both the Brazil DHS and data from regional surveys to construct an asset measure. In chapter 8 Schwartz and Bhushan construct a household wealth index, using PCA applied to baseline and follow-up surveys in Cambodia. The study of reproductive health among Nepalese adolescents in chapter 11 applies the PCA approach to baseline and endline surveys of urban and rural communities where a targeted, community-based, participatory health program had been initiated for disadvantaged youths. The resulting asset measures were used to assess inequalities in the effectiveness of the youth programs. Chapter 10 utilizes the same PCA asset approach to construct a socioeconomic status indicator from a family health survey in Uttar Pradesh State, India, and chapter 7 applies PCA to 1996 census data collected from a rural area of the Ganges-Meghna Delta in Bangladesh. Given the diversity of data and research questions addressed in these chapters, the PCA approach to living standards measurement can be a very robust tool when using non-health-related data.

This ad hoc approach to living standards measurement—in contrast to the income, expenditure, and consumption approaches—does not produce a cardinal measure of living standards, let alone a monetary one. That is, it simply yields a normalized score with zero mean and a variance of one, not a number with a dollar (or other monetary) sign in front of it. This approach cannot be used to determine whether people are poor in the sense that they live on less than a dollar a day. Nor can we make comparisons across countries; we cannot say that a household with a score of –0.75 living in Indonesia is poorer than one with a score of –0.25 living in India. What we *can* do is to rank households within a country. We can say that within a specific sample a household with a score of –0.75 is poorer, according to this measure, than one with a score of –0.25. From the point of view of capturing inequalities in health outcomes between poor and less-poor people, the approach seems to work reasonably well.[7]

Where Do the Data Come From?

One issue remains: where do we get the data to operationalize these ideas? It would be a shame, after all, to have come this far and not be able to put the ideas into effect. Two approaches are possible: we could rely on nationally representative household survey data, or we could collect new data and, if necessary, use nationally representative survey data to put this new information in context.

Many studies in this field make use of routine national surveys. Examples include chapters 10 and 13, which draw on India's National Family Health Survey and the Brazil DHS, respectively. Such surveys contain the necessary information on use of services and living standards, allowing the requisite tables and graphs to be made. Table 2.2 displays the data sources for the studies in this volume.

Researchers who are able to make use of routine surveys are in luck—no data-collection costs are incurred, and the focus can be entirely on data analysis. The study of reproductive health in chapter 7, for example, relies solely on census data, birth records, and routine maternal health care utilization data. When, however, the objective is to assess a specific program, especially one that operates only at the local level, a routine national survey may be of little use. It may not include enough—or even any—households in the program area, and it may not ask about use of the program's services. Then, a different strategy is called for.

Table 2.2. Data Sources Used by the Studies, by Chapter

Chapter	Data sources
4. Ghana and Zambia: Achieving Equity in the Distribution of Insecticide-Treated Bednets through Links with Measles Vaccination Campaigns	Exit interviews at vaccination/bednet sites; follow-up community-based household surveys in both countries
5. Kenya: Reaching the Poor through the Private Sector—A Network Model for Expanding Access to Reproductive Health Services	Survey of health providers; exit interviews of individuals at both case and control sites; household interviews of women of reproductive age; Demographic and Health Survey (DHS) data for socioeconomic status measurement
6. South Africa: Who Goes to the Public Sector for Voluntary HIV/AIDS Counseling and Testing?	Survey of individuals at voluntary counseling and testing (VCT) sites; in-depth interviews and focus groups; South Africa DHS
7. Bangladesh: Inequalities in Utilization of Maternal Health Care Services—Evidence from Matlab	Local census data; birth records; maternal health service utilization database
8. Cambodia: Using Contracting to Reduce Inequity in Primary Health Care Delivery	Baseline (1997) and follow-up (2001) household surveys within case and control health districts
9. India: Assessing the Reach of Three SEWA Health Services among the Poor	Exit surveys of individuals at Self-Employed Women's Association (SEWA) clinics; focus group of nonusers; in-depth interviews of health workers; DHS data for socioeconomic status measurement
10. India: Equity Effects of Quality Improvements on Health Service Utilization and Patient Satisfaction in Uttar Pradesh State	Baseline (1999) and follow-up (2003) exit interviews of outpatients (for assessment of patient satisfaction); Uttar Pradesh data from the National Family Health Survey for socioeconomic status measurement
11. Nepal: The Distributional Impact of Participatory Approaches on Reproductive Health for Disadvantaged Youths	Small-scale baseline (1999) and endline (2003) surveys of households and adolescents within two rural and two urban areas
12. Argentina: Assessment of Changes in the Distribution of Benefits from Health and Nutrition Policies	Two large living standards surveys (1997 and 2001)
13. Brazil: Are Health and Nutrition Programs Reaching the Neediest?	Brazil DHS; three surveys of specific populations residing in the states of Santa Catarina, Sergipe, and Rio Grande do Sul
14. Peru: Is Identifying the Poor the Main Problem in Reaching Them with Nutritional Programs?	Living Standards Measurement Survey (LSMS)

In such a case, the program administrators could organize an exit survey of users and ask them about their dwelling type, their ownership of household durables, the water supply they use, and so on. As table 2.2 shows, this proved a useful tactic in several studies, since the specific experiences and characteristics of program users were important. Armed with these data, the administrator could apply the PCA weights from a national survey (for example, the country's DHS) and generate for each user of the program's facilities a score on a proxy wealth index. From the national survey, the administrator will know the cutoff points on the wealth index that separate the poorest quintile from the second poorest, the second poorest from the middle quintile, and so on. She can then place each user in the national wealth distribution and see what fraction of the program's users comes from the country's poorest quintile, what fraction from the second-poorest quintile, and so on. If, say, 65 percent comes from the county's poorest quintile and the rest from the second poorest quintile, the administrator should probably feel fairly satisfied that her program is indeed reaching the poor.

Or should she? Perhaps the administrator would want to check how the population her program serves compares with the national population. If 75 percent of the local population is in the country's poorest 20 percent, the fact that just 65 percent of her users comes from the nation's poorest quintile would be something of a disappointment. To find out whether this is so, the administrator would have to obtain data on the local population—not just users of her program's facilities but nonusers as well. The more local is the focus of the program, the harder this is likely to be. Suppose the program operates across an entire state of a large country. The administrator might be lucky and find a national survey that was conducted in her state and, moreover, is representative at the state level. She could then sort the state's population into state wealth quintiles and locate her users in the state's wealth distribution rather than the nationwide wealth distribution. But if the program is more tightly focused or there is no representative survey at the state level, she has little option but to conduct a household survey of her own, in addition to or instead of the user exit survey. The household survey would allow her to collect data from all sampled households on wealth indicators, use the national PCA-based weights to generate a wealth score for each sampled household, and form wealth quintiles for the local population. Using the cutoff points for this local distribution, she will be able to answer more satisfactorily the question of whether she is indeed reaching the poor in her locality.

Chapters 4, 8, and 11 are interesting examples of studies that grapple with these methodological issues. The study of Cambodia in chapter 8 uses baseline and follow-up surveys that were specific to the areas served by the contracting program being evaluated. Chapter 11, which has a tightly focused analysis, uses community-based surveys. Although the limited size of these surveys poses some analytical limitations, their use allows for more comprehensive qualitative analysis. In chapter 4 the household surveys carried out to follow up on the integrated program of vaccination and bednet distribution allow the authors to search for discrepancies between ownership and use of the bednets.

Conclusions

In designing and conducting program evaluations, researchers need to weigh the benefits and disadvantages of these different approaches. As this chapter makes clear, measurement of success in reaching the poor involves a series of trade-offs.

One relates to program design. Estimates of program distribution made at a single point in time (the snapshot approach) require just one set of data but are subject to potential bias related to changes over time and to the selection of participants. Data collection at more than one point in time (the movie approach) and estimation of the potential effect of the program on nonparticipants (the experiment approach) require more complex data collection and analytical techniques.

Another trade-off is in the measurement of living standards or economic status. Consumption is a more accurate indicator than income or expenditure, but it is more time consuming to construct and entails more complex data collection. Principal component analysis requires only data on household assets. It provides a proxy for living standards, but one that is relative only, with no information on absolute levels of well-being. As more information from household surveys becomes available, researchers can take advantage of these data to conduct increasingly accurate and insightful research that can inform policy aimed at reaching the poor with important health benefits.

In evaluating the relative equity of programs making special efforts to reach the poor, it is important to not lose sight of the overall value of the benefit—and the extra cost of the special efforts themselves. Indicators such as the benefit-incidence ratio and the concentration index measure relative distribution only. They do not take into account the absolute value of the benefit being transferred, the administrative cost of the transfer, or the opportunity cost of the resources used to finance the benefit and its transfer.

The financing source of the benefit is also important. Public funds have an opportunity cost, and the success or failure of programs should be viewed in this light. An appropriate question would be whether the results are more or less pro-poor than the results from alternative programs that might have been funded.

In brief, there is no such thing as a single ideal approach. This is no cause for despair; it simply reflects the world's complexity, as attested by the studies in this volume. Many methods now exist that provide highly illuminating assessments of how well health programs serve the disadvantaged groups we most want to reach. They need to be used more often.

We promised a tour of the numerous methodological issues that chapter authors have had to grapple with in preparing their Reaching the Poor studies. The tour has probably seemed a little dry—like being given a lecture on the key decisions in wine making without getting close to any wine. It is hard in such a situation to gain a sense of how any of it matters. Perhaps the best thing to do is to bookmark this chapter and refer back to it while reading the rest of the volume. We hope that, as with drinking wine, knowing what you are looking for will lead to greater appreciation.

Notes

1. On benefit-incidence analysis, see http://siteresources.worldbank.org/INTPAH/Resources/Publications/Quantitative-Techniques/health_eq_tn12.pdf.

2. On the concentration curve, see Wagstaff, van Doorslaer, and Paci (1989, 1991); Kakwani, Wagstaff, and van Doorslaer (1997). For a practical guide to working with concentration curves, see http://www1.worldbank.org/prem/poverty/health/wbact/health_eq_tn06.pdf.

3. Just how far above the line of equality the concentration curve should be depends on the distribution of need. The more heavily concentrated is need among the poor, the farther above the line of equality we would want the concentration curve to be. Much of the literature in the field—although not in this volume—juxtaposes distributions of use and need in an attempt to assess health equity (Wagstaff, Paci, and van Doorslaer 1991; Wagstaff, van Doorslaer, and Paci 1991; van Doorslaer and others 1992, 2000; Wagstaff and van Doorslaer 2000).

4. For a practical guide to computing concentration indexes and the associated standard errors, see http://www1.worldbank.org/prem/poverty/health/wbact/health_eq_tn07.pdf. A spreadsheet that implements the formulas is downloadable from   http://www1.worldbank.org/prem/poverty/health/wbact/concentration_index.xls.

5. For a guide to living standards measurement in the context of health equity, including the use of principal components, see http://siteresources.worldbank.org/INTPAH/Resources/Publications/Quantitative-Techniques/health_eq_tn04.pdf.

6. Further details on the LSMS may be found at http://www.worldbank.org/lsms/.

7. For example, the concentration indexes for child malnutrition are quite similar across 20 countries, irrespective of whether the children are ranked by consumption or by a PCA-based wealth index.

References

Deaton, Angus, and Margaret E. Grosh. 2000. Consumption. In *Designing household survey questionnaires for developing countries: Lessons from 15 years of the Living Standards Measurement Study,* ed. Margaret E. Grosh and Paul Glewwe. New York: Oxford University Press.

Deaton, Angus, and Salman Zaidi. 2002. *Guidelines for constructing consumption aggregates for welfare analysis.* Living Standards Measurement Study 135. Washington, DC: World Bank.

Filmer, Deon, and Lant H. Pritchett. 1999. The effect of household wealth on educational attainment: Evidence from 35 countries. *Population and Development Review* 25(1): 85–120.

Filmer, Deon, and Lant H. Pritchett. 2001. Estimating wealth effects without expenditure data—or tears: An application to educational enrollments in states of India. *Demography* 38(1): 115–32.

Gwatkin, Davidson, Shea Rutstein, Kiersten Johnson, Rohini Pande, and Adam Wagstaff. 2000. Socioeconomic differences in health, nutrition, and population—45 countries. Health, Nutrition, and Population Department, World Bank, Washington, DC. http://web.worldbank.org/WBSITE/EXTERNAL/TOPICS/EXTHEALTHNUTRITIONANDPOPULATION/EXTPAH/0,,contentMDK:20216957~menuPK:400482~pagePK:148956~piPK:216618~theSitePK:400476,00.html.

Kakwani, Nanak C., Adam Wagstaff, and Eddy van Doorslaer. 1997. Socioeconomic inequalities in health: Measurement, computation, and statistical inference. *Journal of Econometrics* 77(1): 87–104.

van Doorslaer, Eddy, Adam Wagstaff, S. Calonge, T. Christiansen, M. Gerfin, P. Gottschalk, R. Janssen, C. Lachaud, R. E. Leu, B. Nolan, and others. 1992. Equity in the delivery of health care: some international comparisons. *Journal of Health Economics* 11(4): 389–411.

van Doorslaer, Eddy, Adam Wagstaff, Hattem van der Burg, Terkel Christiansen, Diana De Graeve, Inge Duchesne, Ulf-G. Gerdtham, Michael Gerfin, José Geurts, Lorna Gross, Unto Häkkinen, Jürgen John, Jan Klavus, Robert E. Leu, Brian Nolan, Owen O'Donnell, Carol Propper, Frank Puffer, Martin Schellhorn, Gun Sundberg, and Olaf Winkelhake. 2000. Equity in the delivery of health care in Europe and the US. *Journal of Health Economics* 19(5): 553–83.

Victora, C. G., F. C. Barros, J. P. Vaughan, A. C. Silva, and E. Tomasi. 2000. Explaining trends in inequities: Evidence from Brazilian child health studies. *Lancet* 356(9235): 1093–98.

Wagstaff, Adam, and Eddy van Doorslaer. 2000. Measuring and testing for inequity in the delivery of health care. *Journal of Human Resources* 35(4): 716–33.

Wagstaff, Adam, Eddy van Doorslaer, and Pierella Paci. 1989. Equity in the finance and delivery of health care: Some tentative cross-country comparisons. *Oxford Review of Economic Policy* 5: 89–112.

Wagstaff, Adam, Pierella Paci, and Eddy van Doorslaer. 1991. On the measurement of inequalities in health. *Social Science and Medicine* 33: 545–57.

Wagstaff, Adam, Eddy van Doorslaer, and Pierella Paci. 1991. On the measurement of horizontal inequity in the delivery of health care. *Journal of Health Economics* 10(2): 169–205.

Waters, Hugh. 1999. Measuring the impact of health insurance with a correction for selection bias: A case study of Ecuador. *Health Economics* 8(5): 473–83.

3

What Did the Reaching the Poor Studies Find?

Davidson R. Gwatkin, Adam Wagstaff, and Abdo S. Yazbeck

The features of the programs covered by the case studies in this volume vary widely. However, most programs or program innovations favored the poor by achieving higher coverage among them than among the better off, or by producing greater coverage increases among disadvantaged than among more privileged groups and thereby reducing disparities.

This, the principal overall finding of the studies presented in following chapters, is in line with the results of other studies identified by the Reaching the Poor Program. Together, the findings and results indicate that much better distributional performance on the part of health, nutrition, and population programs is possible.

The wide variation among programs favoring the poor points toward the availability of multiple potentially effective approaches. The challenge is to find the approach that works best in a particular setting in dealing with a particular issue.

Program Features

Although all the Reaching the Poor studies employed the same basic research method described in chapter 2, the programs covered differ widely (see table 3.1). This resulted from a decision to spread the programs assessed across a broad range of topics and settings. The purpose was to demonstrate the versatility of the research method and to reach a broad audience rather than provide guidance applicable to only a few countries and a limited number of topics.

Table 3.1. *Characteristics of the Programs Covered in This Volume*

Country	Characteristics
Africa	
Ghana and Zambia	Bednet distribution linked to government measles vaccination campaigns, with outreach provided by a nongovernmental organization (NGO)
Kenya	Reproductive health services delivered by private for-profit providers
South Africa	HIV/AIDS counseling and testing through government clinics with NGO counselors
Asia	
Bangladesh	Essential obstetric care services delivered through the health facilities of an NGO
Cambodia	Primary health services provided through government facilities by NGOs working under government contracts
India (Gujarat State)	Reproductive health services, tuberculosis detection and treatment, and women's education provided by an NGO employing a range of delivery strategies
India (Uttar Pradesh State)	Improvements in the quality of services delivered through government facilities
Nepal	Participatory development and delivery of reproductive health and HIV/AIDS education programs by an NGO
Latin America	
Argentina	Government maternal and child health and nutrition services
Brazil	Primary health services delivered through four government and NGO programs
Peru	Nutritional supplements delivered to poor areas through government and NGO programs

Location

Most of the world's low- and middle-income regions were represented in the studies. Five of the studies were from Asia—Bangladesh; Cambodia; Gujarat State, India; Uttar Pradesh State, India; and Nepal. Three were from Africa (Ghana and Zambia, Kenya, and South Africa), and three from Latin America (Argentina, Brazil, and Peru).

However, two areas were not covered. No proposals were received from the Middle East and North Africa region. Only a few dealt with programs in

Eastern Europe or Central Asia; two of the proposals that did were selected and funded, but neither study came to fruition.

Topics

Applications were invited for studies of programs dealing with four broad health, nutrition, and population topics related to the Millennium Development Goals (MDGs): nutrition; infant and child health; reproductive health; and HIV/AIDS, malaria, and tuberculosis. This focus and the application review procedure produced a fairly even distribution of case studies across the four topics. A fifth topic, health systems and financing, although not explicitly mentioned in the invitation, was also studied.

Size and Type

Seven of the 11 studies covered large-scale operational programs. The remaining 4 dealt with controlled experiments in smaller areas.

The seven operational programs encompassed both well-established ones generally considered effective enough to justify continuation without major change, and also programs that had recently been reformed to overcome perceived shortcomings. Some of the well-established, ongoing programs were nationwide (government health and nutrition programs in Argentina, government immunization and antenatal care in Brazil, and child feeding in Peru). Others, although not nationwide, still covered populations of many millions of people (the Pastorate of the Child program in Brazil; projects of the Self-Employed Women's Association in Gujarat, India; and voluntary counseling and testing for HIV/AIDS in urban South Africa). Reformed programs included Brazil's new national Family Health Program and the upgrading of government services in Uttar Pradesh, India's most populous state.

The four controlled experiments looked at innovative approaches in much smaller populations: the shift from home obstetric delivery to institution-based delivery in Bangladesh, contracting with nongovernmental agencies in Cambodia, distribution of insecticide-treated bednets in Ghana and Zambia, and participatory project development in Nepal.

Objectives

All the programs studied tried to reach the poor, but in none was that the sole objective, and the degree of emphasis varied. In some cases reaching the poor was a central concern, but in others it was secondary to such goals as increasing coverage of the population as a whole, reducing unit costs of service delivery, or improving the therapeutic effectiveness of the services provided.

The Bangladesh case study, for example, examined the distribution of benefits from a strategy that emphasized facility-based delivery. That strategy had replaced an earlier one focused on home delivery, not because the earlier strategy had been thought inequitable but because it had been considered therapeutically ineffective. The Kenya case study dealt with a project designed to increase overall access to maternal care by strengthening the modern private, commercial sector—a segment of the health system typically associated with the provision of services to upper income groups.

Strategy

In programs where reaching the poor was a central objective, a number of strategies were employed. Some sought to provide universal coverage that, once achieved, would include the poor as well as the better off. Others used more selective, targeted approaches.

Examples of classic universal coverage strategies are those employed by the Brazilian immunization and antenatal care programs. Brazil's reorganized Family Health Program aspired to universal coverage but sought to ensure that the poor came first by beginning in poor areas before expanding into better-off settings. Other programs, such as the Argentine government's health services, tried to ensure universal coverage not by providing services to the entire population but by serving as a safety net for people who, unlike upper income groups, could not buy care in the private sector. In so doing, it implicitly employed the "soft" targeting strategy of self-selection.

The more consciously targeted approaches adopted by other programs varied widely. For instance, the Cambodia experiment featured contracts with nongovernmental organizations (NGOs) that set specific performance targets for coverage in the poorest half of the population. The Ghana and Zambia experiments sought to test the hypothesis that distributing bednets through mass immunization campaigns would produce higher coverage rates among disadvantaged groups than would social marketing. In Peru the highest priority was given to poor areas in selecting locations for the government's school breakfast programs and in determining the amount of food provided through the government's Vaso de Leche ("Glass of Milk") initiative. The Self-Employed Women's Association in Gujarat State, India, set up mobile reproductive health camps in an effort to reach the many poor people living in remote areas not served by traditional static facilities. It charged only token fees, and even these were waived in cases of extreme poverty. The Nepal project organizers developed a participatory development strategy that, it was hoped, could increase the empowerment of poor and disadvantaged population groups.

Implementing Agency

The programs covered were designed and implemented by various types of organizations: governments, NGOs, the commercial private sector, and research institutions. Some were cooperative ventures between governments and NGOs.

Government programs included the maternal and child health services provided by the Argentine government, the Brazilian government's immunization and antenatal care programs, the Peruvian government's child-feeding programs, and the primary and secondary care services provided by the government of Uttar Pradesh State in India. NGOs operated the programs assessed in Gujarat, India; one of the four programs studied in Brazil; and several of the nutrition projects in Peru. The Kenya study, as noted, examined a commercial private sector project.

Cooperation between governments and NGOs figured prominently in three programs. The Cambodia study dealt with government financing of NGO-provided services in government facilities. The services delivered through the Ghanaian and Zambian immunization and bednet distribution campaigns were provided by the governments of those countries, assisted by Red Cross fieldworkers who visited homes to encourage people to use the services offered. In South Africa's voluntary counseling and testing program for HIV/AIDS, NGO representatives provided the counseling in government facilities, and government nurses did the testing.

Research institutions played central roles in two other programs. The program in Bangladesh was implemented, as well as assessed, by the International Centre for Diarrhoeal Diseases Research, Bangladesh (ICDDR, B). In Nepal the International Center for Research on Women was one of the collaborating agencies.

Program Accomplishments

None of the programs assessed in the studies in this volume was flawless. However, several achieved coverage rates that were higher among disadvantaged groups than among the better off. In many other cases, where coverage equality was not fully achieved, the programs produced much larger increases among the poor than among the more privileged and thus notable reductions in intergroup disparities. Defining a program with results in either category as one that favors the poor, the 11 studies presented in this volume can be grouped as follows:

- In six (those in Argentina, Cambodia, Ghana and Zambia, Nepal, Peru, and South Africa), all the programs covered favored the poor.
- In two (Brazil and Gujarat, India), some but not all of the programs studied were favorable to the poor.
- In two (Uttar Pradesh, India, and Kenya), the distributional outcome of the programs assessed was ambiguous.
- In one (Bangladesh) the program unambiguously failed to favor the poor.

Programs Favoring the Poor

ARGENTINA: NATIONWIDE GOVERNMENT MATERNAL AND CHILD HEALTH, IMMUNIZATION, AND CHILD-FEEDING PROGRAMS. By 2001, after a period of severe economic crisis, the programs covered were less clearly focused on the poor than in 1997. But even in 2001, between 35 and 50 percent of the benefits from the maternal and child health programs went to the poorest 20 percent of the population, and between 60 and 95 percent of that group was covered. The three child-feeding programs studied were delivering between 40 and 75 percent of their benefits to the poorest 20 percent, with coverage rates of 5 percent in one program and 30 percent in the other two. The immunization programs were less focused on the poor, presumably reflecting an orientation toward serving the entire population rather than focusing on those not receiving services from other sources. But even here, between 20 and 50 percent of all government-administered immunizations were given to children in the poorest 20 percent of the population (1997 data, the latest available), depending on the particular immunization. Coverage of this group by the government immunization program ranged from below 15 percent for measles, mumps, and rubella vaccine to over 90 percent for tuberculosis and polio. In contrast, the top 20 percent of the population received less than 5 percent of the government maternal and child health services and government child-feeding activities, and below 5 to just under 20 percent of the government-provided immunizations.

CAMBODIA: FIELD EXPERIMENT WITH GOVERNMENT CONTRACTS TO NGOs TO DELIVER PRIMARY HEALTH CARE SERVICES THAT THE GOVERNMENT TRADITIONALLY PROVIDES DIRECTLY. Gains for the poor were especially large in districts where the NGOs were given full responsibility for service provision under contracts specifying coverage of the population's poorest 50 percent as well as the population as a whole (and providing extra compensation to cover higher staff salaries and technical assistance). For seven of the eight services monitored, coverage among the poor improved—and inequalities in use declined—more rapidly in those districts than in districts where the NGOs had less control or where the government provided services directly. Where the NGOs had the most control, average coverage of the poorest 20 percent of the population by the eight services rose from less than 15 percent to more than 40 percent, nearly two-and-a-half-fold the increase in the districts receiving standard government services (personal communication from study authors). While full equality was not achieved even in these districts, the result was a much larger reduction in coverage inequality than elsewhere.

GHANA AND ZAMBIA: FIELD EXPERIMENTS TO DISTRIBUTE INSECTICIDE-TREATED BEDNETS THROUGH GOVERNMENT–RED CROSS MASS IMMUNIZATION CAMPAIGNS. Bednet ownership in the poorest 20 percent of the population rose from less than 5 percent to more than 90 percent in Ghana and from less than 10 percent to almost 80 percent in Zambia. Ownership differentials between the poor and the better off were eliminated in Ghana and were greatly reduced in Zambia. In each country postcampaign net use (as distinct from ownership) was 10 to 15 percentage points lower among the poorest than in the least-poor quintile; but even in the poorest quintile more than half of all children were reported to be sleeping under the nets.

NEPAL: FIELD EXPERIMENT ORGANIZED BY A MULTIAGENCY CONSORTIUM, WITH A PARTICIPATORY APPROACH THAT INVOLVED PROSPECTIVE BENEFICIARIES IN THE DEVELOPMENT OF ADOLESCENT HEALTH PROGRAMS. The outcome of the program was a larger improvement among the disadvantaged than among the better off for all three indicators covered: prenatal care, attended deliveries, and knowledge about HIV. The change was especially notable for the last two. The proportion of first births delivered at a medical facility rose from 25 percent to more than 40 percent in the poorest half of the population while remaining unchanged in the other half. Knowledge of HIV transmission more than doubled in the poorest quarter of the population; by the end of the experiment, more than 70 percent of adolescents in this group knew about at least two modes of transmission, while in the best-off quarter of the population the increase was only about half as large. For all three indicators, some degree of disparity persisted, but a distinct reduction in inequality among economic groups was achieved. Inequality also decreased in the control areas, but the declines there were typically smaller.

PERU: THREE GOVERNMENT AND NGO FEEDING PROGRAMS FOR POOR CHILDREN. In each of the three programs covered, children belonging to the poorest population quintile accounted for well over 20 percent of the beneficiaries. For the three sets of programs together, more than 33 percent of the food recipients belonged to the poorest 20 percent of the population, almost 60 percent to the poorest 40 percent, and only around 6 percent to the top 20 percent. Each of the two government programs covered about 19 percent of children in the poorest 20 percent of the population; the third, smaller program provided services to around 3 percent of the population in the poorest group.

SOUTH AFRICA: VOLUNTARY COUNSELING AND TESTING SERVICES FOR HIV THROUGH A COOPERATIVE GOVERNMENT-NGO PROGRAM IN URBAN GOVERNMENT CLINICS. Clinic patients seeking voluntary counseling and testing (VCT) were heavily concentrated among the poorer groups of residents. For instance, more than half of the patients seeking VCT services were among the poorest 20 percent of residents in the townships that the clinics served, and about 35 percent belonged to the poorest 20 percent of South Africa's urban population. Individuals seeking VCT were poorer than patients attending the clinics for other services—although even patients coming for other services were poorer, on average, than the township or national urban populations.

Programs with Mixed Records

BRAZIL: GOVERNMENT NATIONAL IMMUNIZATION AND ANTENATAL CARE PROGRAMS; HOUSEHOLD-LEVEL HEALTH EDUCATION BY COMMUNITY VOLUNTEERS OF AN NGO; AND A RECENTLY REORGANIZED, COMMUNITY-ORIENTED GOVERNMENT NATIONAL PRIMARY HEALTH CARE PROGRAM INTRODUCED FIRST IN POOR AREAS. The four programs produced very different results. The one with the strongest record of including poor groups was the government's reformed primary health care program, especially in its initial stages. In the city of Porto Alegre, where the program had recently been introduced, more than 40 percent of clients were among the very poorest—that is, the poorest quintile in the areas where the program was active. Only 2 percent came from the least-poor 20 percent of the areas' population. Where the program was better established and had begun to spread into less-poor districts, as in the city of Sergipe, coverage rates among the poor were higher: coverage was 55 percent among the poorest 20 percent of the population, for example, compared with 19 percent in Porto Alegre. Coverage rates in Sergipe were higher among the poor than among higher-income segments, although the differential was much less marked than in Porto Alegre.

The much smaller health education program operated by the NGO was also oriented toward the poor, although to a lesser degree. The poor received a disproportionately high share of program benefits, with 22 percent of the total going to the poorest 20 percent of the population and 53 percent received by the population's poorest 40 percent. But at the same time, a significant share of the benefits went to higher-income groups; the best-off 40 percent of the population received almost a third of the total.

The national immunization and antenatal care programs were found to provide significantly lower coverage among the poor than among better-off groups. Nationwide, incomplete immunization was more than twice as prevalent among the poorest 20 percent of children as among the best-off 20 percent (33 and 15 percent, respectively). Among pregnant women in the bottom population quintile, 70 percent received inadequate antenatal care, compared with 14 percent in the top quintile.

INDIA, GUJARAT STATE: REPRODUCTIVE HEALTH, TUBERCULOSIS DETECTION AND TREATMENT, AND WOMEN'S EDUCATION SERVICES PROVIDED BY AN NGO. In urban areas the poor were the main users of all three services, with a third or more of the clients coming from the poorest 20 percent of the population. The best-off 20 percent accounted for no more than 1 to 2 percent of beneficiaries. In rural areas the record was notably different. For each of the two programs operating in those areas (reproductive health camps and education sessions), program users were clustered in the middle economic groups, with smaller numbers among the poor and the better off.

Programs with Ambiguous Records

INDIA, UTTAR PRADESH STATE: AN INITIATIVE BY THE STATE GOVERNMENT TO STRENGTHEN THE HEALTH SERVICES OFFERED THROUGH ITS FACILITIES. Two years after the inception of the multifaceted program supported by a $110 million World Bank loan, the total average monthly patient load at the facilities receiving support had increased by nearly 6 percent, while the load at unsupported facilities had declined by over 15 percent. The distribution of this change across socioeconomic classes depends on how class is defined. If it is defined in economic terms, as in most of the other studies in this volume, the upper 40 percent of the population benefited considerably more than the lower 40 percent. When class is defined in social terms, the opposite is true: the gain among lower castes was higher than among members of upper castes.

KENYA: NETWORK OF PRIVATE, FOR-PROFIT MEDICAL PROVIDERS PROVIDING MATERNAL AND CHILD HEALTH CARE. The program's focus depended upon the group taken as the reference population. At the community level, the program was class neutral in that the socioeconomic profile of the network members' clients was roughly similar to that of the population in the communities where the members practiced. However, the network's distributional performance looks quite different if the reference population is that of Kenya as a whole rather than the communities served: far more patients came from the top 20 percent of the national population than from the bottom 20 percent (around 67 and 20 percent, respectively). In other words, the socioeconomic status of network patients was about the same as in the communities where the members practiced, but many more participating network practitioners were located in better-off than in poor communities.

A Program Not Favoring the Poor

BANGLADESH: FIELD EXPERIMENT WITH FACILITY-BASED EMERGENCY OBSTETRIC CARE BY A RESEARCH INSTITUTION. This program produced an increase in facility-based deliveries among the population as a whole—from about 18 percent in 1997 to around 29 percent in 2001—but there was little change in the inequality of service use across economic class. For example, in each year during this period, a woman in the least-poor 20 percent of the population was about 3 to 3.5 times as likely to have an attended delivery as a woman in the poorest 20 percent.

Conclusions

The findings of the eleven studies just summarized, similar to those of other project assessments assembled by the Reaching the Poor Program, point toward two conclusions—one concerning how well the programs studied have reached the poor, the second about which types of program have proven most successful in doing so. The two conclusions suggest a strategy for helping the poor receive a larger share of the benefits provided by other health, nutrition, and population services.

How Well Did the Programs Reach the Poor?

As has been seen, most of the programs reviewed in this volume favored the poor by achieving higher coverage among the poor than among the better off, or by reducing coverage disparities between the two groups. Other studies presented at the Reaching the Poor conference reported similar results. For example, of the 27 programs with readily comparable data described in conference presentations, 18 were pro-poor in the sense that the poorest 20 percent of the population received more than 20 percent of the program benefits. For 7 of the 27 programs, the poorest 20 percent of the population received more than 40 percent of total benefits. Fourteen of the 27 programs achieved coverage rates of 50 percent or more among the population's poorest quintile (Gwatkin, Bhuiya, and Victora 2004).

To be sure, such findings are not unambiguous since, as always, there were limitations in the study approaches used. Some of these limitations have been noted in the preceding two chapters. For example, differences in the snapshot, movie, and experimental approaches outlined in chapter 2 complicate cross-study comparisons. The preferred information about performance relative to some prior situation and/or some more typical program is available only from the studies that employed a movie or experimental approach. For the studies using the snapshot approach, it is necessary to rely instead on absolute coverage levels achieved by only the program of interest at one point in time, which can produce a different impression.

Another limitation, noted in chapter 1, is the heavy emphasis on only one of the many important dimensions of health inequality. Other caveats include the possibility of producing a desirable outcome for an undesirable reason, such as achieving a pro-poor distribution of benefits by providing services that the better off perceive as of inadequate quality, as appears to have happened in South Africa and Brazil. A further consideration is that Reaching the Poor studies show only whether the poor receive services, not whether the services are of adequate relevance or quality to improve their health. Also, the studies contain few references to costs.

The list could be expanded. In the end, however, any final assessment depends on the basis of comparison. If the studies and the programs they assess are compared with the ideal, they are wanting. But if the studies are judged by the same standards as are applied to the evidence on which program decisions are currently being made, they are noteworthy for their rigor.

Seen in this light, the accomplishments of the programs that the studies covered are noteworthy. Certainly, by no means all the programs fully eliminated coverage disparities. None came close to the theoretical targeting ideal suggested by figure 2.1 in chapter 2—reaching 100 percent of the poor while excluding all nonpoor. Yet it is by no means clear that such an outcome is ideal in anything but theory, considering the need to win political support among upper income groups and the possible cost of reaching the very poorest. Compared with the record of most current health, nutrition, and population programs, as described in the opening chapter, most of the initiatives identified through the Reaching the Poor Program produced marked improvements in reaching the poor that sometimes approached the dramatic. Whereas the typical current program delivers perhaps 10 to 20 percent of its benefits to the poorest 20 percent of the population it serves, the programs assessed by the Reaching the Poor Program routinely provided between 30 and 40 percent of benefits to the population's poorest 20 percent and achieved coverage of 50 percent of this group.

In bringing about such improvements, the programs sharply challenge the sense of inevitability implied by what is widely known as the "inverse care law," which maintains that "the availability of good medical care tends to vary inversely with the need for it in the population served" (Tudor Hart 1971, 405). The highly inequitable distribution of benefits from health, nutrition, and population programs may be the norm. But the studies presented here show that it does not have to be.

Which Types of Program Reached the Poor Best?

The most important implication of the basic finding just presented is obvious: it is possible for health, nutrition, and population programs to reach the poor much better than they are doing at present. The next question concerns how best to achieve this improvement.

At first glance, the evidence from the programs covered in this volume and described at the Reaching the Poor conference may seem to offer little guidance. This is because they fail to point toward what policy makers so often want: a single, optimal approach or set of approaches that can be easily introduced to deal with any problem anywhere in the world.

Indeed, the encouraging experiences are notable for the wide variation in the strategies employed. They feature numerous examples of approaches that worked well in dealing with one particular type of disease or service in one particular setting: contracting with NGOs to provide primary care in Cambodia; delivering food through neighborhood mothers' committees in Argentina; distributing treated bednets through immunization campaigns in Ghana and Zambia. But most of these are unique, with no assurance that the approach concerned would be effective in some other setting or in dealing with some other disease or service.

One reason for the paucity of documented examples of success using a particular approach may simply be the limited number of documented experiences available. Study of the distribution of benefits remains in its infancy. Examination of additional program experiences might well identify common features that can point toward strategies that, if not universally valid, at least can be effective under a variety of circumstances. To some degree, this appears to be happening with respect to some of the techniques featured in Reaching the Poor conference presentations. For example, use of proxy means testing to identify the poor, as in Colombia and Mexico, appears to work well in some East European countries (Posarac 2003; Tesliuc 2003), and the conditional cash transfers pioneered in Mexico are being used elsewhere in Latin America with initially promising results (Morris and others 2004).

Yet even for approaches like these, effectiveness varies widely across countries (Coady, Grosh, and Hoddinott 2004). And even if those particular approaches do prove widely applicable, the great variety of encouraging experiences presented in this volume shows that they are by no means the only ones that deserve consideration. Rather, the range of promising possibilities is broad.

This suggests that a determined search for a few universally optimal strategies could well turn out to be misguided. The evidence available thus far points more toward the existence of many very different but promising approaches, with the suitability of each depending heavily on the characteristics of the setting, the disease or condition being addressed, and the available service delivery mechanism.

What Are the Policy Implications?

In light of all this, what is a policy maker to do? Two suggestions emerge from the foregoing discussion:

- *Recognize that better approaches to service delivery are needed if the poor are to be reached effectively—and that such improved approaches are feasible.* Though hardly spectacular, this suggestion addresses a central constraint on improved performance: the failure of policy makers to recognize that their current activities are not pro-poor. Significant change can begin only when health policy leaders become aware, because of evidence like that presented in chapter 1, that their programs exacerbate rather than redress health inequity and when they recognize, from the evidence summarized in this chapter and from similar studies, that doing better lies within their power.

- *Be determined but flexible in identifying and implementing more suitable service delivery strategies.* As emphasized above, the available evidence is insufficient to guarantee that a strategy that has proved effective in dealing with an issue in one setting will work elsewhere.

The second suggestion implies that those responsible for programs should seek to learn from and draw on what has worked elsewhere rather than to copy it. This might be done through a process that can be summed up in five words: study, adapt, experiment, monitor, and adjust.

- *Study* the approaches used in those projects that appear to have reached poor groups. Even approaches not directly applicable to a particular setting can be highly instructive. Investigate, as well, the reasons the poor do not use available health, nutrition, and population services. Understanding the constraints faced by the poor or imposed on them by current strategies can be an important first step in finding solutions.
- *Adapt* to local conditions the approaches used in successful experiences elsewhere, applying the knowledge gained through field experience and through study of the constraints facing the poor. Adaptation may often involve combining more than one strategy. Nearly everywhere, it is also likely to call for a liberal dose of common sense. Developing effective pro-poor approaches is an art, not a science.
- *Experiment* with the adapted approaches by implementing them in a few, but not too few, places to see how well they work. The populations served have to be large enough to ensure that implementation takes place under typical rather than optimal administrative conditions, to get a good idea of what might happen were the approach more widely introduced.
- *Monitor* the experience, using one of the relatively simple techniques available, to ensure an accurate understanding of how well or how poorly the approach performs. Monitoring does not have to be nearly as complicated as some evaluation specialists might lead one to

believe, and it is necessary for a sufficiently correct assessment of program performance. Program administrators relying on their informal impressions almost always greatly overestimate the effectiveness of their activities in reaching disadvantaged groups.

- *Adjust* the approach according to the monitoring findings. It is unlikely that any approach will work perfectly the first time around. At least one and possibly many rounds of adjustment will be needed. Or, if the prospects of eventual success appear hopeless, drop that particular approach and try something else.

References

Coady, David, Margaret Grosh, and John Hoddinott. 2004. Targeting outcomes *redux*. Presented at the Reaching the Poor conference, World Bank, Washington, DC, February 19.

Gwatkin, Davidson R., Abbas Bhuiya, and Cesar G. Victora. 2004. Making health systems more equitable. *Lancet* 364(9441): 1273–80.

Morris, Saul S., Rafael Flores, Pedro Olinto, and Juan Manuel Medina. 2004. Monetary incentives in primary health care and effects on use and coverage of preventive health care interventions in rural Honduras: Cluster randomised trial. *Lancet* 364(9450): 2030–37.

Posarac, Aleksandra. 2003. Armenia's experience with proxy-means testing. Presented at the World Bank Human Development Learning Week seminar on Lessons in Targeting, Washington, DC, November.

Tesliuc, Emil D. 2003. Romania: The minimum guaranteed income (MGI) program. Presented at the World Bank's Human Development Learning Week seminar on Lessons in Targeting, Washington, DC, November.

Tudor Hart, Julian. 1971. The inverse care law. *Lancet* 1: 405–12.

Part II

Africa Studies

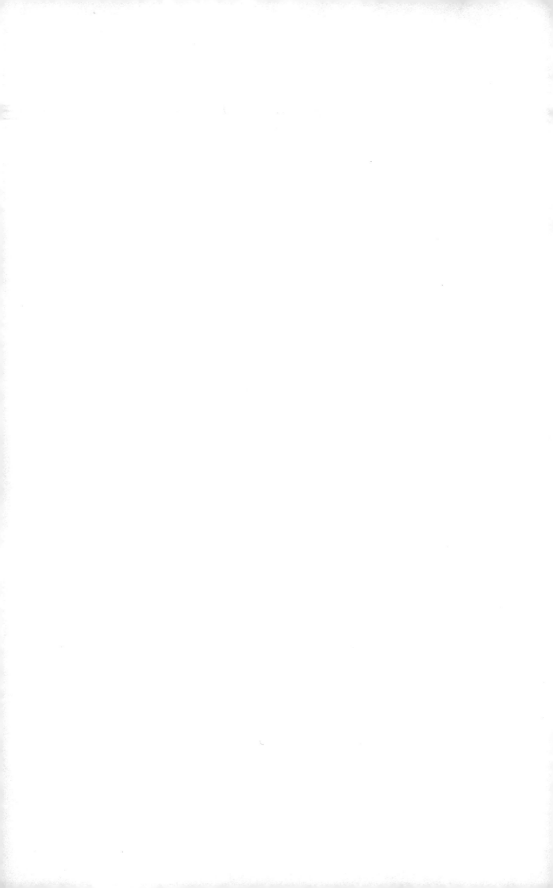

4

Ghana and Zambia: Achieving Equity in the Distribution of Insecticide-Treated Bednets through Links with Measles Vaccination Campaigns

Mark Grabowsky, Nick Farrell, John Chimumbwa,
Theresa Nobiya, Adam Wolkon, and Joel Selanikio

Providing insecticide-treated nets (ITNs) to 60 percent of children under five years of age is a key goal for malaria control in Africa (WHO 2000). Current delivery strategies, however, are falling well short of this mark. Among the 28 African countries for which comparable data are available between 1998 and 2002, ITN use by children under five was 5 percent or less in 23 countries, and the overall median rate was only 2 percent (Monasch and others 2004). Social marketing has shown some success in improving ITN coverage, and efforts are under way to introduce it on a larger scale. But the direct and indirect costs of marketing ITNs or using commercial distribution mechanisms may be barriers to equitable distribution. Although social marketing may not increase inequity for rural Africans (Nathan and others 2004), alternative methods of subsidy or distribution are needed to improve coverage and equity (Gallup and Sachs 2001).

In contrast to the low ITN coverage rates, childhood vaccination commonly achieves high coverage, particularly when vaccines are delivered through mass campaigns. Since 2001, the Measles Initiative has supported measles vaccination campaigns in 29 Sub-Saharan African countries. These campaigns typically take place over one week and target every child in the country regardless of prior vaccination status. Through 2004, more than 160 million children had received measles vaccination under this approach. Vaccination campaigns typically reach more than 90 percent of the target population, reduce virus transmission, and essentially eliminate measles deaths for up to three years (Biellik and others 2002; Grabowsky and others 2003). Measles campaigns are repeated every three to four years to reach subsequent birth cohorts and maintain low disease levels. The campaigns are highly effective in reaching all children regardless of their economic status. They have become particularly useful for serving children not reached through routine services that require contact with a health center.

In populations where measles vaccination campaigns are conducted, malaria is frequently the greatest health risk to children, particularly after the campaign reduces measles mortality. If each child vaccinated against measles during a campaign also received a treated bednet, ITN coverage would increase rapidly and equitably. The potential benefits of this approach have prompted recent global policy changes to encourage increased integration of ITN delivery and vaccination (WHO and UNICEF 2004). Linking ITN distribution with measles vaccination, however, presents many operational challenges.

To explore these challenges, we employed a three-phase approach aimed at developing and testing integrated campaigns for delivering both ITNs and measles vaccination to African children. Phase I was a small proof-of-concept experiment in one district in Ghana in December 2002. Phase II was a larger evaluation of operational and logistical requirements conducted in five districts in Zambia in June 2003. Phase III consists of an in-depth assessment of Togo's nationwide campaign undertaken in December 2004, looking at its impact on ITN coverage, malaria morbidity and mortality, and cost-effectiveness. In this chapter, we report on the phase I and II projects.

The Projects

The phase I project, in Ghana, was a small-scale proof-of-concept exercise to demonstrate the operational feasibility of combining measles vaccination and ITN distribution. The phase II (Zambia) study was a larger-scale evaluation of whether high and equitable coverage could be obtained in several districts simultaneously.

Ghana

During one week in December 2002, a mass measles campaign was conducted in Ghana, targeting 7.9 million children age 9 months to 15 years.

The area chosen for the study was Lawra District, located in the country's northwest corner, a rural area of extreme poverty with no ITN social marketing schemes. At the time, household ITN coverage in northern Ghana was estimated at 4.4 percent (Ghana Statistical Service 2000; NetMark Regional Africa Program 2000).

On the basis of population estimates and previous experience with polio campaigns, we estimated that approximately 29,000 children under five would be brought for vaccination. Experience with previous measles campaigns in Ghana suggested that each caretaker would bring an average of two children under five. To provide one ITN to each family that had one or more child under five, we estimated that 14,500 ITNs would be needed. In fact, 14,600 ITNs were obtained through Agrimat, Inc. (SiamDutch, Inc., Bangkok) and the Ghana country office of the United Nations Children's Fund (UNICEF). The total included 4,520 long-lasting nets (DAWA brand) and 10,080 nets pretreated with deltamethrin (2 milligrams per square meter). All nets were rectangular and extra large ($150 \times 180 \times 190$ centimeters).

Districtwide registration lists of children under five were available from a filariasis treatment campaign that had been conducted the previous year. The registration lists were updated and were made available at each vaccination and distribution post. Several days before the campaign, one Ghana Red Cross volunteer (RCV) attempted to visit every home in the post's catchment area to inform caretakers about the measles vaccination campaign, their eligibility for ITN distribution, and proper use of the ITNs. Local radio broadcasts, posters, and banners were used to advertise the measles campaign. Mass media (radio and posters) were not used to publicize ITN distribution because that might have attracted many people living outside the target district to the vaccination and distribution posts in the expectation of receiving ITNs. During the campaign, 28 vaccination and distribution posts operated in the district. Each served an average of 500 households (100 a day) and was staffed by a trained health worker or vaccinator, a recording clerk, and one or two RCVs. The fixed posts were typically at health centers, and the mobile sites targeted schools. Temporary posts were located at places convenient to the rural population (villages, markets, or churches). The Ghana Red Cross Society (GRCS) was responsible for transporting the ITNs to the district, and the district health management team (DHMT) handled logistics within the district in parallel to the vaccine cold chain. GRCS volunteers were present at all vaccination posts to provide additional help with campaign logistics.

All children 9 months to 15 years of age who came to a vaccination post received measles vaccinations, and each caretaker accompanying one or more children under five was given an ITN. The campaign integrated most aspects of ITN and vaccination operations, including program planning, social mobilization, health worker salaries, transportation for some personnel, and some supervision.

Zambia

During one week in June 2003, a mass measles campaign was conducted in Zambia, targeting 5,054,112 children age 9 months to 15 years.[1] The four rural districts chosen for the integrated measles-ITN campaign, Chilubi, Kaputa, Mambwe, and Nyimba, had a combined population of approximately 360,000, including about 65,000 children under five. Operational planning was intended to provide one ITN to each family with one or more children under five. The International Federation of Red Cross and Red Crescent Societies (IFRC) procured 75,000 long-lasting ITNs (LLITNs) for the four rural districts. The target was to provide 65,745 LLITNs. However, an additional 9,255 LLITNs were procured to ensure that stocks would be available throughout the campaign, since the number of children visiting health posts during immunization drives often exceeded the estimated national census figures used as the baseline because of influxes of refugees and underestimation of population sizes.

Planning meetings for incorporation of ITNs in the measles campaign were held weekly at the National Malaria Control Centre (NMCC) and at the Universal Child Immunization (UCI) offices from April to June 2003. The IFRC allocated funds to the NMCC for coordinating the ITN component of the measles campaign in all four districts. The support made available included microplanning meetings in each district, training of each district health management team by National Malaria Control trainers, and supervision during the campaign.

The logistics for the program consisted of transporting the ITNs from the central warehouse in the capital, Lusaka, to the districts and ensuring delivery to the vaccination and distribution posts. Each district held a planning exercise to determine the number of eligible children and families and to estimate the number of ITNs needed for full coverage. The districts also estimated the number of ITNs each vaccination post would need each day; on average, a post was expected to vaccinate approximately 300 children a day.

ITNs were delivered from the central level to the district health and medical officers (DHMOs) by the Zambia Red Cross Society (ZRCS). In three of the districts (Chilubi, Mambwe, and Nyimba), the DHMO was responsible for delivering the ITNs to each post. In Kaputa District, which presented a particularly difficult logistical challenge because of its isolation, poor roads, and widely dispersed population, ITNs were transported within the district by the ZRCS in coordination with the DHMO. Funds were provided to the DHMOs to pay allowances for district ITN managers, supervisors, and malaria agents (community health workers), hold orientation meetings, conduct the ITN component of the campaign, and transport personnel and supplies to the rural health centers and health posts.

Assessment Methods

In Ghana volunteers recruited by the Lawra District Red Cross conducted exit interviews with caretakers leaving vaccination and distribution sites. The volunteers were adults who could read and write English. They were instructed to choose field sites that met certain requirements: the sites had to be in a geographic area known to the volunteer, and they had to be community-based sites where ITNs were being distributed and at which caregivers would be present. (Schools were excluded because caregivers would not be there.) Some vaccination teams were mobile, and the assessors moved with them from site to site. Each volunteer visited about four sites in three days.

A single population-based survey was conducted in each country, five months after the campaign in Ghana and six months after the one in Zambia. The evaluation used a standard two-stage, cluster-sampling methodology (Henderson and Sundaresan 1982). In Lawra the clusters were drawn from population records maintained by the district health management team. For Zambia clusters were drawn from randomly selected standard enumeration areas (SEAs) within each of the five districts. The SEAs enabled the evaluation team to select clusters of 50 to 200 households from established divisions within each district.

In both surveys, wealth was measured by asking the head of household questions on household assets such as ownership of a bicycle, type of roofing material, and source of water. A scoring system was drawn from the Demographic and Health Surveys (DHSs) as developed and reported by the World Bank (Gwatkin and others 2000a, 2000b).[2] Each household was assigned a score for each asset; the score depended on whether the household owned that asset (or, in the case of sleeping arrangements, on the number of people per room). The scores were summed by household, and individuals were ranked according to the total score of the household in which they resided. The sample was then divided into population quintiles—five groups with approximately the same number of individuals in each.

In all the surveys, the volunteers used handheld computers—personal digital assistants (PDAs)—to read and record the survey questions. The PDAs were Visor Neos (Handspring, Inc.) that used the Palm Operating System, version 3.5 (Palm, Inc.) and were supplied by Satellife, Inc. Programming was done prior to shipment to the field, using Pendragon Forms 3.2. Data analysis specialists oversaw training and data collation and analysis. The assessment data were transferred from the PDAs to a laptop computer as an Access database using the synchronizing software and cradle supplied with the PDA. The Ghana data were analyzed in EpiInfo 6.0 and EpiInfo 2002. The Zambia data were analyzed using a combination of EpiInfo 6.0, SAS, Excel, and SUDAAN. Proportions were compared using chi-square tests.

To determine whether a child slept under the ITN, we assessed children who were 6 months to 59 months of age at the time of the campaign. A household was defined as the location where a single family group eats together. The index child was defined as the youngest child who usually slept in that household and who was 6 months of age at the time of the campaign. An ITN was defined as a pretreated, long-lasting ITN delivered during the campaign or a non-long-lasting net treated with insecticide within the previous six months. ITN retention was deemed to have occurred in those households where the surveyor saw a net that the caretaker reported having received. ITN hanging was defined as the surveyor's observation of the ITN over the bed where the caretaker said the child usually slept. A child was determined to have slept under an ITN if the caretaker reported that the child slept under an ITN the previous night. To assess whether an outcome measure was correlated with increasing wealth status, we considered each wealth quintile a separate stratum and applied the chi-square test for trend (EpiInfo 6.0). The equity ratio was defined as the ratio of ITN ownership in the lowest quintile to that in the highest quintile. Records with missing responses were excluded from the analyses.

Total ITN program component costs were defined as the cost of ITN procurement, including ITN purchase and delivery to the country, plus the operational cost of delivering the ITNs, including training, in-country transport, and community education. Costs that the measles campaign would have incurred in the absence of ITN distribution were excluded, as were the costs of external consultants and assessment. Cost information was taken directly from the funded budgets of the local Red Cross, the ministry of health, and the IFRC. All costs were expressed in 2003 U.S. dollars.

Results

Table 4.1 shows the distribution of households into wealth quintiles and the mean asset index score for each quintile for each of the three assessments. The number of households varied slightly across quintiles because more than one household score was at the breakpoint. The asset factor scores are not comparable between countries, as the factors derive from different national DHS surveys.

ITN Ownership

In both study areas the one-week campaign resulted in a large increase in ITN ownership. In Ghana overall household ITN ownership increased from 4.4 to 94.4 percent and in Zambia, from 16.7 to 81.1 percent (figure 4.1).

As table 4.2 shows, equity also improved in each area. Prior to the campaign, in both areas ITN ownership was low in all quintiles but was lowest in the poorest quintiles, with a statistically significant trend toward higher ownership in the wealthier quintiles. Precampaign ownership in Ghana, as assessed through exit interview surveys, showed a statistically significant positive association with household wealth status ($p < 0.01$). The ratio of the

Table 4.1. Distribution of Households within Districts by Wealth Quintile, Ghana (Phase I) and Zambia (Phase II)
(For wealth quintile columns, mean asset index score; number of households in parentheses)

	Wealth quintile					
Study and survey	1 (poorest)	2	3	4	5 (least poor)	All
Ghana						
Exit-interview survey	−0.398 (151)	−0.212 (157)	−0.089 (153)	0.384 (159)	1.026 (156)	0.147 (776)
Community-based survey	−0.317 (51)	−0.121 (50)	0.021 (49)	0.361 (50)	1.582 (48)	0.330 (248)
Zambia						
Community-based survey	−0.463 (342)	−0.352 (342)	−0.295 (340)	−0.223 (335)	0.117 (346)	−0.242 (1,705)

Source: Authors' calculations.

Figure 4.1. *Household Ownership of Insecticide-Treated Nets (ITNs) by Socioeconomic Status, Ghana and Zambia*

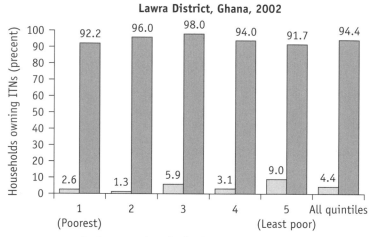

Source: Authors' calculations.

poorest to the least-poor households for ITN ownership was 0.29. The non-random sampling procedure used in the exit interview survey argues against attaching undue precision to these results, but they do support the consensus view among knowledgeable observers that precampaign possession in Ghana was negligible among all but the least poor. In Zambia the caretaker report of precampaign ITN ownership (measured by the survey carried out six months after the campaign), showed an association between ITN ownership and wealth ($p < 0.001$) and a poorest to least-poor ratio of 0.32 (table 4.2).

The postcampaign surveys showed an increase in ITN ownership among all wealth quintiles in both sites. In Ghana the community survey conducted five months after the campaign found no association between net ownership and wealth quintiles, and the ratio of poorest to least poor had risen to 1.01 (table 4.2). In Zambia too, the campaign led to a substantial increase in ITN coverage in all wealth groups (see figure 4.1). The ratio of poorest to least poor rose to 0.88, but the association between ITN ownership and wealth in Zambia remained statistically significant ($p < 0.001$).

ITN Use

As shown in table 4.3, in both study areas the rates of ITN use were lower than the rates of ownership. In Ghana 60.5 percent (150/248) of the index children slept under a net provided during the campaign. The equity ratio was high (0.85), and there was no statistically significant trend toward lower use by the poorest ($p = 0.69$). In Zambia 56.4 percent (962/1,705) of the index children slept under a net provided during the campaign. The equity ratio was high (0.79), but there was a statistically significant trend toward lower rates of use by those in the poorer groups ($p < 0.001$).

The most important factor contributing to the dropout from ownership to use was whether households hung up the ITNs they received. In Ghana 71.4 of households with an ITN did so. The equity ratio was high (0.84), and there was no statistically significant trend toward lower compliance by the poor. In Zambia 72.4 percent of households hung up their ITNs, with an equity ratio of 0.93 and a trend toward lower compliance among the poorest ($p = 0.03$). There was a smaller dropout from children not sleeping under a net hung over their bed. In Ghana 88.0 percent of children with an ITN hanging over their bed slept under it (equity ratio = 1.01; p-value for trend = 0.87); in Zambia the figure was 81.7 percent (equity ratio = 0.96; p-value for trend = 0.23).

Costs of ITN Delivery

In both studies the cost of procuring an ITN and delivering it to the country was $4.32. In Ghana the total cost of the ITN program component was $67,722: procurement costs for 14,600 ITNs of $63,072 and operational costs of $4,650.

Table 4.2. *Ownership of Insecticide-Treated Nets (ITNs), Reported Precampaign and Observed Postcampaign, by Wealth Quintile, Ghana (Phase I) and Zambia (Phase II)*

(For wealth quintile columns, number of owners divided by number in sample; percentages in parentheses)

| | Wealth quintile | | | | | | Equity measure | |
Study and timing	1 (poorest)	2	3	4	5 (least poor)	Total	p-value, chi-square test for trend	Equity ratio (poorest to least poor)
Ghana								
Precampaign	4/151 (2.6)	2/157 (1.3)	9/153 (5.9)	5/159 (3.1)	14/156 (9.0)	34/776 (4.4)	<0.01	0.29
Postcampaign	47/51 (92.2)	48/50 (96.0)	48/49 (98.0)	47/50 (94.0)	44/48 (91.7)	234/248 (94.4)	0.79	1.01
Zambia								
Precampaign	33/342 (9.6)	32/342 (9.4)	38/340 (11.2)	76/335 (22.7)	105/346 (30.3)	284/1,705 (16.7)	<0.001	0.32
Postcampaign	265/342 (77.5)	275/342 (80.4)	247/340 (72.6)	291/335 (86.9)	304/346 (87.9)	1,382/1,705 (81.1)	<0.001	0.88

Source: Authors' calculations.

Table 4.3. Distribution of Insecticide-Treated Net (ITN) Use by Wealth Quintile, Ghana (Phase I) and Zambia (Phase II)
(For wealth quintile columns, number of positive responses divided by number in sample; percentages in parentheses)

	Wealth quintile						Equity measure	
	1 (poorest)	2	3	4	5 (least poor)	Total	p-value, chi-square test for trend	Equity ratio (poorest to least poor)
Ghana								
ITN received	47/51 (92.2)	48/50 (96.0)	48/49 (98.0)	47/50 (94.0)	44/48 (91.7)	234/248 (94.4)	0.79	1.01
If ITN received, ITN hung over bed	34/47 (72.3)	36/48 (75.0)	31/48 (64.6)	28/47 (59.6)	38/44 (86.4)	167/234 (71.4)	0.61	0.84
If ITN hung, child slept under ITN	29/34 (85.3)	31/36 (86.1)	29/31 (93.5)	26/28 (92.9)	32/38 (84.2)	147/167 (88.0)	0.87	1.01
Child slept under ITN previous night[a]	30/51 (58.8)	31/50 (62.0)	29/49 (59.2)	27/50 (54.0)	33/48 (68.8)	150/248 (60.5)	0.69	0.85
Zambia								
ITN received	265/342 (77.5)	275/342 (80.4)	247/340 (72.6)	291/335 (86.9)	304/346 (87.9)	1,382/1,705 (81.1)	<0.001	0.88
If ITN received, ITN hung over bed	191/265 (72.1)	174/275 (63.3)	194/247 (78.5)	206/291 (70.8)	235/304 (77.3)	1,000/1,382 (72.4)	0.03	0.93
If ITN hung, child slept under net	158/191 (82.7)	141/174 (81.0)	144/194 (74.2)	172/206 (83.5)	202/235 (86.0)	817/1,000 (81.7)	0.23	0.96
Child slept under net previous night[a]	186/342 (54.4)	165/342 (48.2)	172/340 (50.6)	201/335 (60.0)	238/346 (68.8)	962/1,705 (56.4)	<0.001	0.79

Source: Authors' calculations.

a. Data refer to all children in the sample—both those who did not receive nets through the campaign and those who did—who were reported to have slept under a net, regardless of whether a net was observed over a bed.

The operational cost per ITN delivered was $0.32. In Zambia the total ITN program component cost was $315,788, with procurement costs of $292,697 for 67,754 ITNs and operational costs of $23,091. The operational cost per ITN delivered was $0.34. In both studies 93 percent of total ITN program component funds was spent on ITN procurement rather than operational costs.

Discussion

These findings suggest that integration of ITN delivery into measles vaccination campaigns achieves unprecedented levels of ITN ownership and equity at very low cost. In the study populations, the poorest families' ITN ownership rates were comparable to or exceeded those among the least poor. The increase in the equity ratio of ITN ownership in the poorest households compared with the least poor was substantial, rising from 0.29 to 1.01 in Ghana and from 0.32 to 0.88 in Zambia. Expressed as a difference rather than a rate, coverage among the poorest households in Ghana increased by 89.6 percentage points compared with 82.7 percentage points for the least poor. In Zambia the increase was 67.9 percentage points for the poorest and 57.6 percentage points for the least poor. This approach to ITN distribution resulted in a larger coverage increase among the poorest in both relative and absolute terms while ensuring high coverage levels for all wealth groups.

A major difference between vaccines and ITNs in achieving effectiveness is that whereas vaccines protect without any subsequent behavioral requirements on the part of the person vaccinated, ITN effectiveness requires ongoing proper use. We found that the two key factors contributing to lower use were whether the ITN was hung up and whether the child slept under it once it was hung. Our results indicate that these two use factors were not consistently related to wealth. The ratios of poorest to least poor for hanging the ITN and sleeping under it in Ghana were 0.84 and 1.01, respectively; in Zambia the ratios were 0.93 and 0.96. Seasonal factors were the most likely cause of lower use rates. In northern Ghana net use ranges from 99 percent in the rainy season, when mosquitoes are most prevalent, to 20 percent in the dry seasons (Binka and Adongo 1997). About half the homes in Zambia reported that they used nets during the rainy and hot season or when mosquitoes were numerous (Academy for Educational Development 2001). In our studies distribution and assessment were carried out over the dry season, and there was no intervening rainy season during the study period. Measuring ITN use during periods of high mosquito density following mass distribution will indicate what additional behavior change interventions may be required to increase use of the nets.

An important benefit of integration is that it promises to lower costs through cost sharing and operational efficiencies. The underlying cost of the nationwide measles campaign in Zambia was $0.89 per child, of which $0.57 was for operational costs (data from Ministry of Health, Zambia). The additional operational cost of adding ITNs in the study districts was $0.34 per child, and the cost per ITN was $4.32, making a total cost of $4.66 per ITN. So, commodities, rather than program costs, accounted for more than 93 percent of total project expenditures. Using this measure, the efficiency of mass distribution may be approaching the theoretical maximum because these costs were substantially below those reported for other approaches. In Zambia a community-based project was estimated to cost between $17 and $22 per net distributed (Hanson and others 2003), and a clinic-based revolving-fund approach in Mozambique cost $10 per net delivered (Dgedge and others 1999). A highly successful social marketing approach in Tanzania had a project financial cost of $8.30 per net delivered (Hanson and others 2003). As Hanson and others note, this figure excludes the contributions of users and does not reflect the true value of the resources consumed in delivering nets. Because the nets were distributed free of charge during the measles campaigns in Ghana and Zambia, there were no extra costs for caretakers, who were already coming to the service facilities to obtain measles vaccine. Furthermore, the campaigns reduced the travel time and thus the indirect costs of participants. Careful evaluation of a measles campaign in Kenya indicated that the campaign approach reduced direct costs to caretakers by 75 percent compared with travel to obtain routine vaccinations at a health center (KEPI and others 2002).

Although mass vaccination campaigns are relatively cost-effective as a means of achieving specific disease-control objectives (Uzicanin and others 2004), they can disrupt the routine delivery of other health services, mainly because of the high demands on health care workers for planning and conducting the campaigns. The campaign can also strain limited logistics capacity. Although possibly important, these adverse effects are difficult to measure and are rarely quantitatively studied. A complete assessment would include a comparison with the disruptions attributable to other distribution strategies such as social marketing. Mass campaigns integrating ITNs and other services are likely to be more disruptive than vaccination campaigns alone. Whether the additional gains in disease control justify these difficulties has not yet been evaluated. Although campaigns will always be somewhat disruptive, additional efforts are required to minimize the adverse impact of integrated campaigns, possibly through better coordination and planning.

There were no obvious constraints on using this approach in other campaigns. Measles campaigns are typically nationwide, and integrating ITN delivery into these larger efforts will present additional challenges as well as opportunities for additional efficiencies. The WHO–UNICEF strategy for measles control calls for "second opportunity" vaccination campaigns to be conducted in all countries where measles is endemic (WHO and UNICEF 2001). As practiced in the Americas and in Sub-Saharan Africa, campaigns are repeated every three to four years for children under five. Current plans call for vaccinating more than 150 million children a year in developing countries during these campaigns (Henao-Restrepo and others 2003). Each vaccination may represent a missed opportunity to deliver ITNs. The findings from these phase I and II studies suggest that integrating ITN distribution into vaccination campaigns can achieve higher and more equitable ITN coverage than other delivery strategies at a lower cost to both providers and consumers. Linking ITN distribution to measles campaigns presents an important opportunity for reaching malaria control goals and merits larger-scale implementation and evaluation.

Notes

The mass measles vaccination campaigns that provided the opportunity for this study were conducted by the ministries of health of Ghana and Zambia with support from the Measles Initiative (the American Red Cross, the UN Foundation, the U.S. Centers for Disease Control and Prevention, the United Nations Children's Fund, and the World Health Organization). In Ghana ITN distribution was conducted by the Ghana Red Cross with support from the Ghana Ministry of Health, the Lawra District Assembly, Rotarians against Malaria, Rotary/Ghana, the Rotary Foundation, the American Red Cross, the Ghana Red Cross, and the United Nations Children's Fund. The assessment was conducted by the American Red Cross with support from the Ghana Red Cross, the Ghana Ministry of Health, ExxonMobil, Satellife, Inc, and the World Bank. In Zambia distribution was supported by the Zambia National Malaria Control Program, the Zambia Ministry of Health, the Zambia Red Cross, NetMark, the Canadian International Development Agency, the International Federation of Red Cross and Red Crescent Societies, the U.S. Centers for Disease Control and Prevention, the World Bank, and Right to Play. The project was designed and managed by Mark Grabowsky, Nick Farrell, John Chimumbwa, and William Hawley. The assessment was designed and managed by William Hawley, Adam Wolken, and Joel Selanikio. Mark Grabowsky, Adam Wolkon, and William Hawley analyzed the data and wrote the first draft. All the investigators contributed to the interpretation of data, the review of the paper, and the writing of the final draft.

1. The target population included all children 9 months to 15 years of age (about 45 percent of the total population) plus an additional 10 percent for drop-ins such as

people outside the target age group or crossing the border from the Democratic Republic of the Congo. United Nations Development Programme (UNDP) population projections were refined using numerator data from previous polio campaigns. In all, approximately 4.7 million children were vaccinated.

2. Asset questionnaires and weighting of asset factor scoring for each country can be found at http://www1.worldbank.org/prem/poverty/health/data/ghana/ghana.pdf (accessed November 20, 2004).

References

Academy for Educational Development. 2001. NetMark formative qualitative research on insecticide treated materials (ITMs) in Zambia. Washington, DC.

Biellik R., S. Madema, A. Taole, A. Kutsulukuta, E. Allies, R. Eggers, N. Ngcobo, M. Nxumalo, A. Shearley, E. Mabuzane, E. Kufa, and J. M. Okwo-Bele. 2002. First 5 years of measles elimination in southern Africa: 1996–2000. *Lancet* 359:1564–68.

Binka. F. N., and P. Adongo. 1997. Acceptability and use of insecticide impregnated bednets in northern Ghana. *Tropical Medicine and International Health* 2(5): 499–507.

Dgedge, M., L. Kumaranayake, H. Cossa, B. Hogh, and J. Lines. 1999. Can the expansion of a subsidised ITN project become self-sufficient? The experience from an ITN project in Mozambique. Presented at the Second International Conference on Insecticide Treated Nets, Dar es Salaam.

Gallup, J. L., and J. D. Sachs. 2001. The economic burden of malaria. *American Journal of Tropical Medicine and Hygiene* 64(1–2 suppl.): 85–96.

Ghana Statistical Service. 2000. *Poverty trends in the 1990s.* Accra: Ghana Statistical Service.

Grabowsky, M., P. Strebel, A. Gay, E. Hoekstra, and R. Kezaala. 2003. Measles elimination in southern Africa (letter). *Lancet* 360(9334): 716.

Gwatkin, Davidson R., Shea Rutstein, Kiersten Johnson, Rohini P. Pande, and Adam Wagstaff. 2000a. Socio-economic differences in health, nutrition, and population in Ghana. HNP/Poverty Thematic Group, World Bank, Washington, DC.

Gwatkin, Davidson R., Shea Rutstein, Kiersten Johnson, Rohini Pande, and Adam Wagstaff. 2000b. Socio-economic differences in health, nutrition, and population in Togo. HNP/Poverty Thematic Group, World Bank, Washington, DC.

Hanson, Kara, Nassor Kikumbih, Joanna Armstrong Schellenberg, Haji Mponda, Rose Nathan, Sally Lake, Anne Mills, Marcel Tanner, and Christian Lengeler. 2003. Cost-effectiveness of social marketing of insecticide-treated nets for malaria control in the United Republic of Tanzania. *Bulletin of the World Health Organization* 81(4): 269–76.

Henao-Restrepo, A. M., P. Strebel, E. John Hoekstra, M. Birmingham, and J. Bilous. 2003. Experience in global measles control, 1990–2001. *Journal of Infectious Diseases* 187 (suppl. 1): S15–21.

Henderson, R. H., and T. Sundaresan. 1982. Cluster sampling to assess immunization coverage: A review of experience with a simplified sampling method. *Bulletin of the World Health Organization* 60(2): 253–60.

KEPI (Kenya Expanded Programme on Immunization); Division of Planning and Development, Central Bureau of Statistics; and Ministry of Finance and Planning. 2002. Vaccination coverage and economic evaluation of supplemental and routine measles immunization. Kenya Ministry of Health, Nairobi.

Monasch, R., A. Reinisch, R. Steketee, E. Korenromp, D. Alnwick, and Y. Bergevini. 2004. Child coverage with mosquito nets and malaria treatment from population-based surveys in African countries: A baseline for monitoring progress in Roll Back Malaria. *American Journal of Tropical Medicine and Hygiene* 71(2 suppl.): 232–38.

Nathan, R., H. Masanja, H. Mshinda, J. A. Schellenberg, D. de Savigny, C. Lengeler, M. Tanner, and C. G. Victora. 2004. Mosquito nets and the poor: Can social marketing redress inequities in access? *Tropical Medicine and International Health* 9(10): 1121–26.

NetMark Regional Africa Program. 2000. *Insecticide treated materials in Ghana: NetMark Regional Africa Program briefing book.* Washington, DC: Academy for Educational Development.

Uzicanin, A., F. Zhou, R. Eggers, E. Webb, and P. Strebel. 2004. Economic analysis of the 1996–1997 mass measles immunization campaigns in South Africa. *Vaccine* 22(25–26): 3419–26.

WHO (World Health Organization). 2000. Declaration, African Summit on Roll Back Malaria, Abuja, Nigeria, April 25. WHO/CDS/RBM/2000.17. Geneva.

WHO (World Health Organization) and UNICEF (United Nations Children's Fund). 2001. Joint statement on strategies to reduce measles mortality worldwide. WHO/V&B/01.40; UNICEF/ PD/Measles/01. Geneva: WHO.

———. 2004. Joint statement—malaria control and immunisation: A sound partnership with great potential. Geneva: WHO.

5

Kenya: Reaching the Poor through the Private Sector—A Network Model for Expanding Access to Reproductive Health Services

Dominic Montagu, Ndola Prata, Martha M. Campbell, Julia Walsh, and Solomon Orero

Our study, carried out in the summer of 2003, measured the effectiveness of a Kenyan program dedicated to increasing the availability of reproductive health services to the poor through training and networking of private medical providers. The Kisumu Medical and Educational Trust (KMET) program focuses on family planning services and encourages providers to add these services to the normal range of consultations, commodity sales, and clinical care they already provide. The study looked at the pool of potential clients of KMET members to evaluate which wealth group benefits from the subsidy given to private providers through the KMET. Analysis of actual KMET clients was used to better understand the program's success in providing quality reproductive health care.

Background

Kenya's population is estimated at 30.7 million, with 80 percent living in rural areas. Total fertility rates for women age 15–49 are 3.12 in urban areas and 5.16 in rural areas, and the contraceptive prevalence rate is 39 percent. The population growth rate is 1.9 percent a year, one of the lowest in Africa. The slow growth is attributable to family planning and to high mortality from HIV/AIDS (KDHS 1999; UNFPA 2002). Economic disparity is extreme: Nairobi's Kibera district is the largest urban slum in Africa.

According to the Kenyan Ministry of Health, the country has an estimated 27,000 midlevel providers (2,300 clinical officers and 24,600 nurses and nurse-midwives) and 3,300 physicians. The midlevel providers are found at all levels of the health system, in both rural and urban settings, while the doctors are concentrated in the larger towns and cities.

About 48 percent of health care outlets are outside the government structure and are run by for-profit private providers, by religious nonprofit organizations, or by humanitarian nongovernmental organizations (NGOs). Overall, 40 percent of all physicians in Kenya work in the private sector (Hanson and Berman 1998). The private sector is used increasingly for outpatient care, particularly by public sector employees, because of problems within the public sector and increases in National Hospital Insurance Fund (NHIF) rates. Private facilities, both for-profit and nonprofit, dominate certain types of medical institutions; 94 percent of clinics, maternity, and nursing homes and 86 percent of medical centers are private. The number of private health facilities has expanded greatly over the past 10 years, and such growth is expected to continue (World Market Research Centre 2003).

According to National Health Data, in 1997/98, 64 percent of total health care expenditure was private. Of that, 82 percent (53 percent of total expenditure) was out-of-pocket. Against this background, the study reported here looks at the effectiveness of an innovative NGO that supports the delivery of family planning and reproductive health services through private doctors and midlevel medical providers.

The Private Sector and Equity

The past decade has seen a movement toward examining the possible desirability of modifying the government's dual role in health care by separating the finance and delivery activities normal to national health systems. Much of this interest has been driven by a push to explore the potential for increased efficiency in service provision that might be realized by outsourcing some areas of health service delivery and support. Pressure on governments to do more with less in the context of sectorwide reform has led to greater integration of services provided by the public, private, and nonprofit sectors. Governments have begun to concentrate on areas within their core competencies and on the services that they are expected to provide: safety nets for disenfranchised groups, public health interventions, outbreak and disease monitoring, and the setting and enforcement of standards for provider training, facility quality, and medical inputs such as drugs and equipment.

Governments' growing recognition that the public sector cannot be the only, or even the principal, provider of direct health care for the poor is increasing the dependence on private nonprofit and for-profit health services. The continuing concern about private sector involvement in the provision of essential health care services is that natural market dynamics will lead to a focus on the better off and that services critical for public health will not reach the neediest.

Despite the risk of inequity, there are good reasons for trying to involve private providers in public health service delivery. The primary limitation on effective delivery of services for the poor is lack of infrastructure for close-to-client provision of care. The World Health Organization's Commission on Macroeconomics and Health estimated that globally, more than 23 percent of the cost of scaling up tuberculosis treatments and 25 percent of the cost of scaling up highly active antiretroviral therapy (HAART) treatment will be attributable to infrastructure (Mills and others 2002; Kumaranayake and others 2003). An important reason to consider the potential of private sector projects is their ability to leverage existing infrastructure, personnel, and provider-client relationships. Furthermore, the private sector's responsiveness to market forces and its employment flexibility have the potential to increase service efficiency through more rapid adaptation to changing demand than could be done within a government health system.

The study reported here examines the record of a Kenyan network of private practitioners with respect to reaching the neediest. The network is the Kisumu Medical and Education Trust (KMET), a nonprofit organization started in 1995 to increase access to maternal and child health services in and around the city of Kisumu in western Kenya. High rates of maternal mortality were being experienced in local hospitals, with mothers arriving after poor, nonexistent, or drastically delayed local care. The goal of the KMET network is to increase the accessibility of reproductive health and family planning services for the poor, using private providers to establish new, easily accessible service delivery points.

Providers joining the KMET are trained, supplied, and supported so that they can provide services they would not have offered prior to membership. By grouping private, for-profit health providers into a network with NGOs and the public sector, the KMET furnishes responsive training and support to many service delivery points that are theoretically accessible to the poor. Enrolled medical providers, limited to one per site, become part of the KMET network. Participating providers are required to meet specified facility standards. In exchange they receive free training, a free initial manual vacuum aspiration kit for early abortions and postabortion care, regular delivery of contraceptive commodities to their clinic, and a limited number of low-interest one-year loans. Network members also have access to yearly medical updates and networking events.

The KMET began by training both government and private sector doctors and consultants in safe abortion practices and postabortion care. The training program quickly grew to include midwives, clinical officers, and nurse practitioners. Since 2001, all new providers have come from these midlevel provider cadres. The total number of providers is 204, in five provinces. Of these, 65 are exclusively private, and 139 work at least part-time in missions or the public sector. Nurses and clinical officers make up about-two thirds of the KMET members, and physicians account for a third.

Research Questions and Study Design

Our research question, based on the goals set by the KMET network, is whether KMET provider programs for family planning access are benefiting the poor in Kenya. If they are, can the KMET model be replicated or expanded to promote equity and increase access to basic reproductive health services at affordable prices for the poorest segments of the Kenyan population? We attempt to answer these questions by examining the socioeconomic status of KMET providers' current and potential clients.

To provide the data needed for this purpose, we conducted a survey of KMET clients that was implemented by Steadman Research Incorporated, a private survey research group based in Nairobi, in May 2003. The survey had three major components: a provider survey, client exit interviews, and a household survey. The provider survey included both KMET members and matched nonmembers. Client exit interviews were conducted with clients of both members and nonmembers.

The Sample

From the KMET member roster of 204 providers, a systematic sample was drawn by selecting every second medical practitioner on the list. For each selected provider, exit interviews were conducted with three female clients: the first female client of the day; the first arriving after noon; and the first arriving after 5 PM. If no patients arrived after 5 PM, no replacement exit interviews were conducted.

To allow comparison of KMET member and nonmember services and types of client, all nonmember medical service providers located within 2 kilometers (in urban areas) or 5 kilometers (in rural areas) of every second network member in the sample were counted and numbered, starting from a randomly selected network provider.[1] From the nonmember providers at each locale, one was randomly selected for interview, yielding a total of 50—roughly, a 2:1 ratio of members to nonmembers. When possible, selected nonmember providers were matched with member providers according to their level of training. Where equivalence was not possible, nonmembers were selected from the next lower level of training. As with network members, three exit interviews with female clients were conducted, with the same limitation on third interviews as at the member sites. Table 5.1 shows types of provider by network membership status.

To explore the characteristics of potential clients, 500 household interviews with women of reproductive age were conducted. Households were randomly selected within 2 kilometers of each network provider. Given the challenges of counting every household within that radius for the subsequent random selection, we used the Expanded Programme on Immunization (EPI) quasi-probability sampling methodology. This approach enabled us to reduce costs by avoiding the creation of a sampling frame. Under the EPI method the geographic central point of the primary sampling unit (PSU) is first located on a map; this is the starting point for the selection of households. A random direction from the starting point is then chosen, using a spinning object such as a bottle.

For our study, we introduced a slight variation. From the selected provider location (the starting point), the interviewer walked about 5 min-

Table 5.1. Types of Health Care Provider Covered in Study
(Percentage of respondents in each category)

Type of provider	KMET member (N = 102)	Nonmember (N = 50)
Specialist (obstetrics/gynecology or other)	13	12
Doctor	17	14
Nurse	36	40
Nurse-midwife	17	4
Clinical officer	14	28
Pharmacist	0	2
Other	4	0
Total	100	100

Source: Provider survey.

utes in the direction of a specific cardinal point (for example, north). Having done this, the interviewer spun the bottle to point out the direction of the household to be interviewed. From the household thus identified, one woman of reproductive age was randomly selected for interview from the household roster, which listed all eligible women. For each sampling point, five household interviews were conducted, one or two in each cardinal direction. Supervisors made random checks biweekly during the survey process to verify the implementation of household and interviewee selection.

In all, 101 member providers and 50 nonmember providers were interviewed.[2] At four member sites, only two interviews were held, and at two member sites, only one interview. In all, 295 exit interviews were conducted with clients of members. Among the nonmember sites selected, at one site only two interviews were conducted, at one site only one interview was conducted, and at three sites no interviews were conducted, at the request of the provider. The total number of interviews with nonmember clients was 138. The household interviews numbered 500.[3]

Determination of Socioeconomic Status

Socioeconomic status was determined for all respondents by using the asset and factor score methodology that had earlier been applied to the 1998 Kenya Democratic and Health Survey, or DHS (Gwatkin and others 2000). Asset ownership was determined through client and household reporting. Table 5.2 gives summary statistics on ownership of assets among clients in the survey, community households in the survey, and the overall population of Kenya.[4] For each respondent, asset factor scores from the 1998 Kenya DHS were applied to the reported assets owned and were summed to yield a total asset score. Individuals were assigned to wealth quintiles using cutoff points based on the 1998 DHS (Gwatkin and others 2000). Wealth data were supplemented by client and household survey data on educational attainment.

Data Analysis

Socioeconomic status among respondents was compared using the *t*-test for comparison of two proportions. Statistical significance is reported for *p*-values less than 5 percent.

Logistic regression analysis was used to test for association between socioeconomic status and the choice of a KMET member provider. For the model, we constructed dummy variables for socioeconomic status. The model also controls for urban or rural residence, age, parity, and education.

Table 5.2. *Household Assets of Population Groups Covered in Study (Percentage of respondents in each category)*

Asset category	Clients of members (N = 295)	Clients of nonmembers (N = 138)	Households (N = 500)	Kenya average (DHS 1998)
Has electricity	31.6	23.1	45.8	11.7
Has radio	36.2	36.6	93.8	66.4
Has bicycle	11.6	10.1	36.2	28.3
Has car	10.9	8.8	7.2	5.0
Has telephone	42.8	48.4	21.6	2.7
Has piped water in residence	24.6	16.6	31.8	19.5
Uses piped water from public tap	25.4	29.5	40.4	9.4
Uses drinking water from inside well	18.1	17.6	8.2	8.0
Uses water from public well	9.4	6.4	4.2	12.7
Uses river or surface water	22.4	30.2	14.2	42.5
Uses own flush toilet	20.3	19.0	18.8	6.6
Uses shared flush toilet	2.2	6.4	3.2	3.2
Uses pit latrine	77.5	72.9	77.2	67.6
Uses bush or field as latrine	0.7	2.0	0.4	15.9
Has roof of natural material	11.8	8.2	2.8	29.6
Has roof of corrugated iron	79.7	80.0	89.6	66.4
Has roof of ceramic tile	5.4	9.4	5.6	2.9

Source: Household and exit interview surveys; Kenya Demographic and Health Survey (DHS), 1998.

Findings

We have studied use of two types of service. The first is the overall set of services available from the different types of provider covered. The second is that set of services dealing with reproductive health, which constitutes the focus of the KMET network.

Overall Service Use

Table 5.3 presents selected characteristics of household respondents and clients according to provider. The clients of member-providers are similar in many demographic and health characteristics to the clients of nonmember providers and to the populations of the communities. This is not surprising, since the clients of both member and nonmember providers are drawn from the same nearby community.[5]

Regarding educational attainment, member providers and nonmember providers in rural areas both cater to populations slightly less educated than in the surrounding communities. In urban areas both cater to slightly more educated populations than in the surrounding communities (table 5.4).

Figure 5.1 shows all household respondents by national wealth quintile. Two features are noteworthy:

- The pattern of wealth in the areas where the KMET providers are located appears considerably more polarized than in Kenya as a whole. Sixty-one percent of the total sample is in the highest quintile

Table 5.3. *Characteristics of Clients and Household Respondents Covered in Study (Percentage of respondents in each category unless otherwise specified)*

Characteristic	Clients of members (N = 295)	Clients of nonmembers (N = 138)	Households (N = 500)
Age (years)	28.5	28.7	29.0
Visited site before today for family planning	41	28	23[a]
Ever visited other site for family planning	34	49	64[b]
Currently using family planning	52	45	57
Currently using family planning (married respondents only)	53	56	57
Believe abortion services are easily available	21	18	18
Aware that current provider offers abortion services	11	7	n.a.

Source: Household and exit interview surveys.
a. Ever visited reference KMET site for family planning.
b. Ever visited any non-KMET site for family planning.

Table 5.4. Educational Attainment among Clients and Households Covered in Study (percent)

Educational level	Rural				Urban			
	Clients of members (N = 179)	Clients of nonmembers (N = 66)	Households (N = 212)	National average	Clients of members (N = 116)	Clients of nonmembers (N = 72)	Households (N = 288)	National average
No formal education	3	5	1	2	1	0	3	1
Some primary	27	18	26	26	3	7	13	10
Primary completed	41	51	37	41	32	30	32	31
Secondary completed	22	17	23	22	25	44	38	35
Technical/vocational	6	9	12	9	33	14	13	18
University and beyond	0	0	0	0	5	6	2	4
Total	100	100	100	100	100	100	100	100

Sources: Household and exit interview surveys for clients and households; Kenya Demographic and Health Survey (DHS), 1998 for national averages.

Figure 5.1. *Distribution of Residents of Areas Where KMET Members Are Located, by Wealth Quintile*

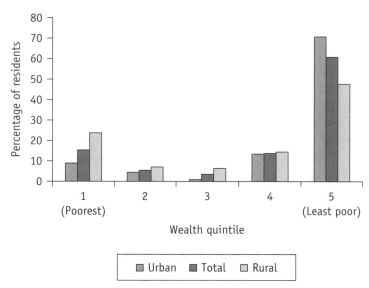

Source: Authors' calculations.

of the national population and 16 percent is in the lowest quintile. Very few respondents are in the middle three quintiles.

- Unsurprisingly, the respondents in the poorest quintile are predominantly rural and the least poor quintile is mainly urban.

Clients of both KMET members and nonmembers have similar wealth profiles. In both groups clients are skewed toward the low- and high-income quintiles, reflecting the household populations from which the clients come (figure 5.2). We found no statistically significant difference between the proportions of poorest-quintile clients going to members and nonmembers ($p < 0.5$). In brief, nonmember and member providers in both urban and rural areas serve clients who are broadly reflective of the communities where the providers practice.

Use of Reproductive Health Services

Overall, the percentage of clients who reported visiting KMET for reproductive health reasons (39 percent) does not differ significantly from the share for the nonmember providers (32 percent).[6] Although KMET members see a higher proportion of family planning and reproductive health (FP/RH)

Figure 5.2. *Distribution of KMET Member and Nonmember Clients, by Wealth Quintile*

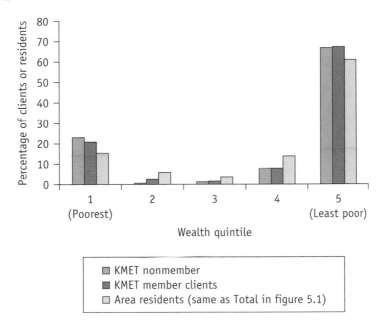

Wealth quintile

> ▨ KMET nonmember
> ▨ KMET member clients
> ☐ Area residents (same as Total in figure 5.1)

Source: Authors' calculations.

clients than do nonmember providers, the difference is not statistically significant after adjusting for wealth (p < 0.25).

Table 5.5 presents results from the multiple logistic regression analysis of household respondents who have ever visited a provider for FP/RH services. It indicates that household respondents who have used KMET providers for these services were more likely to be rural (odds ratio = 1.7; *p* < 0.03) and less educated (odds ratio for completing secondary school = 0.4; *p* < 0.00) than FP/RH users who had sought services from non-KMET providers. On other aspects—wealth, age, and parity—there is very little difference between household respondents who visit member providers and those who visit nonmember providers.

Limitations

This study suffers from a number of significant limitations. Most important, it uses cross-sectional data to examine correlation of socioeconomic status with the activities of an NGO. That being so, only correlations can be calcu-

Table 5.5. *Odds Ratios: Household Respondents Ever Having Visited KMET and Other Providers for Family Planning and Reproductive Health (FP/RH) Services (Dependent variable: report ever having visited KMET provider for FP/RH services)*

Independent variables	Odds ratio	Robust se	p > |z|
Economic group (quintile)			
1 (poorest)	Reference category		
2	1.228	0.741	0.734
3	0.734	0.555	0.683
4	2.055	0.972	0.128
5 (least poor)	1.988	0.770	0.076
Residence			
Urban	Reference category		
Rural	1.714	0.427	0.030
Age group (years)			
≤24	Reference category		
25–29	1.128	0.361	0.706
30–34	1.369	0.507	0.396
35+	1.197	0.538	0.688
Parity			
<2	Reference category		
3–4	0.760	0.244	0.392
5+	0.508	0.250	0.168
Education			
None/some primary	Reference category		
Primary complete	0.543	0.213	0.120
Some secondary	0.684	0.263	0.323
Secondary complete	0.415	0.149	0.014
Vocational	0.186	0.090	0.000
University	0.406	0.367	0.318
−2 log likelihood	216.300		
Number of observations	361		

Source: Household and exit interviews.

lated, and causality cannot be established. The measure of wealth—assets weighted according to eigen values calculated from national DHS data—is a measure of convenience, chosen to allow the broadest comparison of clients with national data. We use it while recognizing its limitations: asset ownership is not a true value of actual wealth or poverty, both of which are highly dependent on income flows and consumption.

The definitions of rural and urban followed local political usage, as was the case for the DHS, but the variation among rural areas in particular is much broader in national surveys than in the sample of sites. This difference stems naturally from the locations in which private medical practices are likely to exist—locales with sufficient population density and income level to provide a clientele. The result is to bias the sample sites toward a subset of rural populations wealthier sthan the national cross-section.

Clients and households were interviewed according to a set schedule, in our attempt to select a wide range of clients. It is possible, however, that a different group of clients visits the clinics only in the evenings, when many of the targeted clinics are open, and these clients would have been excluded from our sample.

As with respondent reporting of income, some asset ownership variables were likely to have been altered as a result of response bias. Selection bias may have been a factor as well. Twenty percent of our sampled providers had to be replaced, and 14 providers could not be found. Clients of the missing providers may have had different characteristics from those of the other selected providers.

Implications

In rural areas the average clients of both KMET providers and nonmember providers are somewhat poorer than the households in the nearby community. Both groups of providers serve a similar proportion of clients in the lowest socioeconomic stratum.

Because the KMET clients reflect an undifferentiated cross-section of socioeconomic status from the catchment area in which the clinics are located, defined here by the households surveyed, the success or failure of the KMET network to continue reaching the poor is likely to be determined primarily by the network's ability to identify and enroll more providers in rural settings. Our findings indicate that the KMET has succeeded so far in reaching rural clients, but we cannot draw a conclusion about whether this is attributable to provider differentiation or to program emphasis on rural placement.

The client and household surveys indicate that there are large differences between the better-off and the poor in the areas studied. The goal of KMET, then, must be to focus on the poor end of this dichotomous client population. The recent shift in enrollment priorities to midlevel providers is an important first step toward this goal because few doctors practice outside urban areas. Our research suggests that this shift in focus should be accelerated and that the KMET organization should place increasing emphasis on rural towns.

Concern about a potential decrease in equity associated with a shift in focus from public to private sector health services may be mitigated by the design of the KMET network. If the KMET continues to expand in rural areas using midlevel providers as planned, equity in access to care may be enhanced by increased availability of services equivalent to those already available in cities and larger towns. Our research does not provide strong evidence that this is now occurring, but it does support the contention that such a shift is likely.

Our central research question—does the KMET benefit the poor?—was answered positively but weakly. From our analysis, we can say that the KMET private provider program is "nondiscriminatory" with respect to the wealth of clients benefiting from improved access to FP/RH services in the communities where the clients live. Thus, the poor benefit as part of overall gains equally shared across all wealth quintiles. There is no evidence of a pro-nonpoor bias stemming from use of private providers in this program, but there is evidence that further efforts are necessary to target programmatic investments to the more needy and marginalized.

We take these results as an indication that empowering the private, for-profit health sector in rural settings may provide an opportunity for government to expand health care without the high infrastructure costs implied by direct government provision of care. This potential should continue to be evaluated, and programs that work through private for-profit providers should be considered for integration into national health planning when their missions are aligned with public health goals.

Notes

1. We limited ourselves to matching every second member provider because of budget constraints, and we accepted the limitation because nonmenber providers constitute a comparison group rather than the primary focus of the study.

2. Twenty of the providers were replacements for providers not located, dead, or no longer associated with the KMET. One provider refused to participate.

3. Survey instruments were based on private provider instruments used in other settings by the authors, with an additional asset survey section designed to match the questions on the 1998 Kenya Demographic and Health Survey (DHS). Anonymity was guaranteed to all respondents; provider names were coded, and the codes were held by the researchers. Client and household respondent names were not requested. Participation by respondents was voluntary. A small number of providers refused to participate, but the refusal rate for clients and household women was close to zero. This low rate was partially attributable to the careful selection of interviewers; in each region of Kenya, interviewers were selected on the basis of their match with the locally predominant tribal groups. No incentives were offered to any group for participation.

Data entry was carried out electronically using a scanning system and software in the Steadman Research offices in Nairobi, with 15 percent human entry verification. Because the instrument formats were standardized, language confusion was irrelevant for scanning entry. Data coding and cleaning were initially done in Nairobi using FoxPro software. All data were electronically transferred to the University of California at Berkeley for further cleaning and analysis using statistical software Stata Release 7.

4. Questions about livestock ownership were asked as well, for matching to an earlier World Bank study, but these are not used here because they are not among the asset measures used by the DHS.

5. Household respondents were exclusively married women. No marriage entry screen was used in client exit interviews. When limited to married respondents only, there is no statistical difference ($p = 0.277$) in the percentage of respondents at different locations who report current use of family planning. The married-women-only rates for use of family planning in member exit interviews, nonmember exit interviews, and households are 56, 53, and 57 percent, respectively.

6. Reproductive health includes family planning, abortion, antenatal care, and treatment of sexually transmitted infections.

References

Gwatkin, Davidson, Shea Rutstein, Kiersten Johnson, Rohini Pande, and Adam Wagstaff. 2000. Socio-economic differences in health, nutrition, and population in Kenya. HNP/Poverty Thematic Group, World Bank, Washington, DC.

Hanson, K., and P. Berman. 1998. Private health care provision in developing countries: A preliminary analysis of levels and composition. *Health Policy and Planning* 13(3): 195–211.

KDHS (Kenya Demographic and Health Survey). 1999. *Kenya facility survey, Demographic and Health Survey.* Calverton, MD: Macro International Inc.

Kumaranayake, L., C. Kurowski, L. Conteh, and C. Watts. 2003. Thinking long-term: The costs of expanding and sustaining priority health interventions in low and middle-income countries. Presented at the International Health Economics Association biannual meeting, San Francisco.

Mills, A., R. Brugha, K. Hanson, and B. McPake. 2002. What can be done about the private health sector in low-income countries? *Bulletin of the World Health Organization* 80(4): 325–30.

UNFPA (United Nations Population Fund). 2002. *Annual report*: New York: UNFPA.

World Market Resource Centre. 2003. Kenya health sector. www.wmrc.com (accessed May 28, 2003).

6

South Africa: Who Goes to the Public Sector for Voluntary HIV/AIDS Counseling and Testing?

Michael Thiede, Natasha Palmer, and Sandi Mbatsha

HIV/AIDS poses a fundamental threat to global health. South Africa is one of the worst-affected countries in the world, with an estimated HIV prevalence of 11.4 percent (Shisana and Simbayi 2002). Studies show that socioeconomic status is the principal determinant of exposure to HIV/AIDS, with poverty and social inequalities leading cofactors in HIV transmission (Farmer 2001; Gilbert and Walker 2002). Reaching disadvantaged groups is therefore crucial for both prevention and awareness campaigns. This chapter examines patterns observed in the socioeconomic status of individuals attending public sector clinics and receiving voluntary counseling and testing (VCT) in three township areas of Cape Town, South Africa.[1]

VCT for HIV/AIDS, combined with pretest and posttest counseling, has been promoted as a key motivating force for safer sexual behavior (Magongo and others 2002; UNAIDS 2002). VCT is a critical component of any national strategy to limit transmission of HIV (Forsythe and others 2002) and is a prerequisite for effective treatment, care, and support services, including programs to reduce mother-to-child transmission, preventive therapy for tuberculosis, and administration of antiretrovirals. The evidence is growing that VCT can bring about behavioral change and can improve the coping strategies of people with HIV, leading to reductions in reported risk behavior (Pronyk and others 2002).

Studies in Uganda (Matovu and others 2002; Nuwaha and others 2002) have explored reasons for obtaining VCT. Factors influencing VCT uptake included attitudes about the consequences of an HIV-positive result, the influence of a sexual partner, cost, accessibility, awareness, and the perceived risk of HIV infection. The features and quality of a counseling service also influence uptake by different groups. Matovu and others (2002) suggest that clients value confidentiality, regular availability of counseling (rather than "one-off" sessions), the possibility of receiving counseling without testing, presence of nonresident counselors (for greater confidentiality), and counseling outside the health center (at a "neutral site" such as a community center).

Research Questions

This study seeks to ascertain the socioeconomic status of individuals accessing VCT at public sector clinics in South Africa and the reasons for any unusual distribution of uptake. These aspects of VCT use are important to understand because VCT will increasingly be the entry point for a range of support and treatment services for people living with HIV. Any skewing of access to VCT in favor of certain socioeconomic groups will have implications for the equitable delivery of all these other services.

In addition to its public sector health clinics, South Africa has a thriving private sector. There is evidence that people from all socioeconomic groups use the private sector, believing that both the technical quality and the interpersonal quality of care are superior (Schneider and others 1999). In periurban settings such as those where this research was conducted, a network of public sector clinics offers primary care free of charge to the uninsured, who make up more than 80 percent of the South African population. In urban South Africa there is also a competitive market of private general practitioners (Chabikuli and others 2002) and a growing number of commercial clinic chains (Palmer and others 2003). VCT is free of charge in the public sector, and capacity to offer the service is slowly being established throughout Western Cape Province, although it is still rudimentary outside the Greater Cape Town area.

Methods

Three clinics with relatively well established VCT programs in the Greater Cape Town area were selected, in consultation with local health department personnel. :

- *Masiphumelele Clinic* is located in a settlement with a population of about 20,000 that has developed over the past 10 years on the outskirts of Cape Town.

- *Khayelitsha Site B General Clinic* is a big community clinic in Cape Town's largest township, which has an estimated population of 500,000.
- *Langa Clinic* serves the oldest township community within the Cape Town vicinity (population about 60,000). The clinic has implemented an integrated program to address the dual tuberculosis-HIV epidemic in cooperation with the ProTEST initiative. ProTEST is coordinated by the World Health Organization and the Joint United Nations Programme on HIV/AIDS (UNAIDS) in collaboration with four Sub-Saharan African countries. The underlying principle of the approach is that early detection prevents ongoing transmission of tuberculosis and slows the progression of the HIV infection. A key feature of the ProTEST initiative is that every patient who comes to a pilot site for tuberculosis services receives counseling about tuberculosis and HIV and is encouraged to take an HIV test (Godfrey-Faussett and others 2002).

The model for VCT delivery is similar in all three clinics. Counseling is provided by lay counselors from local nongovernmental organizations (NGOs). A nurse is responsible for testing and refers patients back to the counselor after informing them of the results.

An interview administered in the waiting room of each clinic was used to assess access to VCT services by various socioeconomic groups. In-depth interviews and focus group discussions with staff, clinic users, and local community groups were conducted to explore barriers to access and attitudes toward VCT.

To establish the socioeconomic status of the respondent, the waiting room questionnaire asked a series of brief, closed-ended questions about gender, race, education, employment status, sanitary and living conditions, and household assets. Many of these latter questions were taken from the South African Demographic and Health Survey (DHS) to allow comparison with that data set during the analysis phase of the study. Some questions about knowledge concerning VCT were also asked.

The waiting room interview was developed in English, translated into Xhosa, and then back-translated to check the quality of the translation. It was administered by a single fieldworker at all three sites. Systematic sampling was used, with every fifth adult (defined as above age 14) approached in the waiting room, as well as in any specific VCT waiting area, and asked to give informed consent to participate in the interviews. Interviews were split into two parts. The first was carried out in this initial phase, and the second was conducted once it had been established whether the person being interviewed would have VCT at that visit. For those who did attend VCT, reasons for electing to use the service were explored. For those who did not, more general questions were asked concerning sources of information about VCT and HIV.

Qualitative methods were used for in-depth interviews and for community and staff focus group discussions to explore attitudes toward VCT uptake and provision. Sets of detailed interview guidelines were developed for in-depth interviews as well as for focus group discussions with clinic staff and community groups. These interviews and discussions were conducted in both English and Xhosa by different members of the research team.

Participants in 15 extensive in-depth interviews were chosen in part from a subset of patients and in part randomly from the communities. Community focus group discussions were held with groups that were suggested by community members as representative (a community development group in Masiphumelele, a housing project group in Khayelitsha, and a church group in Langa). A further criterion for inclusion was knowledge about services at the local clinic, but group members did not have to be patients at the facility.

Nature and Sources of Data

The findings reported here are based on four sets of data:

- *Data from the waiting room surveys, described above, on the socioeconomic status of individuals (a) attending clinics and (b) receiving VCT.* In all, 540 waiting room interviews were conducted (50 in Masiphumelele, 270 in Khayelitsha, and 220 in Langa). After data cleaning, the final sample included 525 patients, 208 of whom had attended the clinics for VCT.

- *Data from the South African Demographic and Health Survey (DHS) on socioeconomic status of urban households.* To enable us to comment on any differences in socioeconomic status between those attending the clinic and receiving VCT and those within the catchment area of the clinic, a picture of the broader socioeconomic environment of the area was required. This was obtained by generating an asset index from South Africa's 1998 DHS. All urban households from the DHS were used to generate an asset index by means of principal component analysis ($N = 7,752$). Household characteristics and assets included in the generation of the index were the particular household's main source of drinking water, the type of toilet facility, flooring and wall material of the dwelling, access to electricity, and a range of household valuables such as a radio, television, or car. An asset score was thus assigned to all urban South African households included in the DHS.

- *Data on the socioeconomic status of 507 DHS households in townships around Cape Town and Johannesburg.* So that the socioeconomic status of individuals attending township clinics could be compared with those living in similar areas rather than with the urban population of South Africa as a whole, a subset of the South African DHS was selected. As the universal sample of households included in the DHS from townships in Greater Cape Town and Johannesburg, 507 households were chosen.[2] These households formed the group with which we compared the socioeconomic status of individuals attending the clinics and receiving VCT. This comparison group was ranked in quintiles on the basis of the asset scores generated from the whole DHS urban sample. The socioeconomic status of the 525 individuals included in the study who were receiving services (including VCT) was then compared with the reference population of 507 township households.
- *Qualitative information from in-depth interviews and focus group discussions.* The discussions and in-depth interviews were taped, transcribed, and analyzed by two authors independently for key themes, drawing on fieldwork diaries as an additional source of information.

Findings about the Distribution

Of the 525 people interviewed, 208 were attending the clinics for VCT. The socioeconomic characteristics of three groups were compared:

- a universal sample of the 507 Cape Town and Johannesburg township households in the DHS (the reference population)
- a systematic sample of 525 people attending three clinics for any service
- the 208 individuals (out of the 525) who were attending for VCT

Figure 6.1 illustrates how the 507 sample township households in the metropolitan areas of Johannesburg and Cape Town fit within the socioeconomic quintiles of the sample of all urban households in the South African DHS. Although the number of township households in the top quintile of all South African urban households is low, at 8.1 percent, it is still higher than would be expected for this type of periurban setting. One explanation lies in the broad range of socioeconomic backgrounds and income levels that make up the top quintile in South Africa, which has a highly unequal income distribution, as reflected by a Gini index of 59.3 (World Bank 2001). Under apartheid, black South Africans were restricted as to where they could live. Townships today therefore include areas of widely varying wealth.

The percentage of people falling into the lowest wealth quintile is also lower than might be expected. Whereas the township areas in the two metropolitan areas under investigation are of key importance for the study of social and economic transformation and relative deprivation in South Africa, they do not represent the economically worst off metropolitan neighborhoods in the country. A number of urban localities in other parts of South Africa are significantly more deprived. As can be expected, most of the township population falls into the middle three wealth quintiles, with a peak at 28.8 percent in the central quintile.

A first finding, therefore, is that the area in which the study was conducted is not worse off overall than the South African urban population in terms of relative distribution of household assets. A comparison that took

Figure 6.1. *Township Asset Scores Compared with Urban Demographic and Health Survey (DHS) Wealth Quintiles, South Africa*

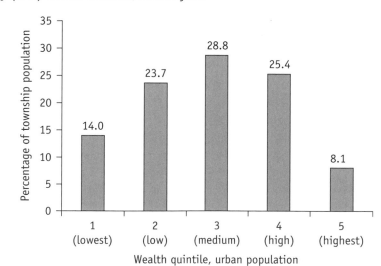

Source: Demographic and Health Survey (DHS), South Africa, 1998.

into account both urban and rural households would reflect the fact that township households are, on average, considerably better off than households in rural areas (Booysen 2002).

The systematic sample of patients from three township clinics around Cape Town reveals a clear pattern when analyzed in terms of asset scores. Figure 6.2 assigns the patient sample to South African urban wealth quintiles. The upper two wealth quintiles were underrepresented among both the patients visiting the clinics for general health services and those coming to the clinics for VCT. Only 1.9 percent of patients who came for general services and 1.0 percent of those who received VCT fell into the top quintile; 8.8 and 7.2 percent, respectively, belonged to the second-highest quintile. Within both subsamples the second-lowest quintile was best represented, with 38.5 percent of general patients and 38.9 percent of VCT users.

The most obvious differences between those attending these clinics for general services and those receiving VCT emerge in the lowest and central

Figure 6.2. *Patient Asset Scores Compared with Urban Wealth Quintiles, South Africa*

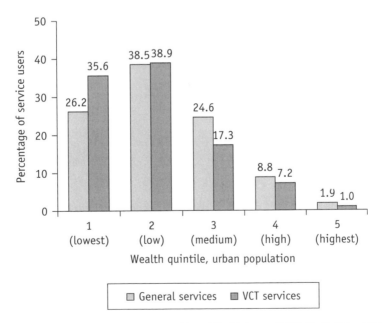

Sources: Waiting room interviews; Demographic and Health Survey (DHS), South Africa (1998).
Note: VCT, voluntary counseling and testing.

quintiles. Nearly a quarter of general patients fell into the medium wealth quintile (24.6 percent), while the percentage of VCT users from this category was substantially lower (17.3 percent). There is a corresponding discrepancy at the lower end of the wealth scale: 26.2 percent of general patients came from the lowest wealth quintile, whereas more than a third of VCT users (35.6 percent) belonged to this socioeconomic group. There is a significant relationship between township households' socioeconomic status and public sector VCT uptake (chi-square for trend, 6.713; $p = 0.00957$). This result requires further investigation, given such pronounced differences among socioeconomic groups in utilization patterns of general and VCT services.

The service utilization pattern becomes more intriguing when viewed within the socioeconomic spectrum of the township environment. For the purpose of this analysis, the factor scores generated for each asset on the basis of the urban DHS sample were used to define the wealth quintiles for this subsample of township households from the DHS.

Figure 6.3. *Patient Asset Scores Compared with Township Wealth Quintiles, South Africa*

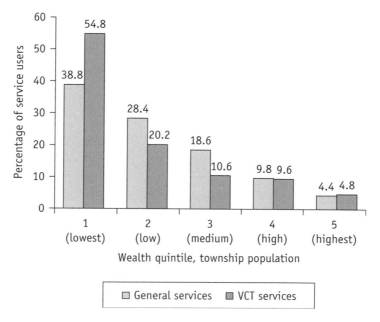

Sources: Waiting room interviews; Demographic and Health Survey (DHS), South Africa, 1998.
Note: VCT, voluntary counseling and testing.

Health service utilization across the wealth quintiles generated at the township level reveals a pattern in which public service utilization decreases with increasing wealth (figure 6.3). This is true for both general health services and VCT services offered at the township clinics, but the pattern is more pronounced for VCT services (chi-square for trend, 4.802; $p = 0.02843$). For general clinic utilization and uptake of VCT, representation of service users from both top quintiles is low: 4.4 percent of general patients and 4.8 percent of VCT patients fall into the top quintile, while 9.8 percent and 9.6 percent, respectively, can be assigned to the second-highest quintile. Between service categories, notable differences emerge in the socioeconomic structure of patients from the lower three wealth categories. The most remarkable result is that more than half of the VCT patients, 54.8 percent, falls into the lowest township wealth quintile. These results are unexpected because the services offered are targeted at the whole socioeconomic spectrum of public sector users.

Overall, the findings show that socioeconomic groups are not evenly represented in clinic attendance, and this pattern is even more exaggerated when it comes to VCT use. The least well off quintiles among the township population take up the services more than the others.

The waiting room survey gathered a wide range of data about people's knowledge concerning VCT and the motives for VCT uptake. Of the multiple reasons people gave for having a test, the leading ones were tuberculosis (explicitly mentioned by 30.0 percent of patients) and sexually transmitted diseases (explicitly mentioned by 28.0 percent). In both cases, nearly all the patients had been referred by a health worker. People also mentioned a range of general symptoms of illness—"because I am very sick," coughing, chest problems, loss of appetite, and similar complaints. Most of the younger age groups came for testing as a consequence of sexually transmitted diseases or because they simply wanted to know their status. In the older groups, tuberculosis was the key reason for testing.

Clinic health workers clearly play an important role in conveying information about HIV prevention services available at the clinic. Of the clients interviewed, 95 percent had received information from clinic health workers. The role of information transmitted via radio and television is also apparent; the impact of televised information had even reached beyond those living in households with television sets. Posters at clinics in the study setting reached more patients (63.7 percent of the sample) than did campaigns that used brochures and leaflets (14.8 percent of the sample). Community health workers had reached 42.8 percent of the people interviewed at the clinics.

Findings about Reasons for the Distribution

The quantitative analysis presented above suggests that certain groups within the community are more likely to access public sector clinics and VCT. To complement these findings and to explore reasons that may explain them, focus group discussions and in-depth interviews were analyzed.

Any discussion about voluntary counseling and testing is dominated by fears surrounding HIV/AIDS. The fear of an incurable disease is paired with the perceived risk of expulsion from the family or rejection by a partner. Lack of access to treatment was also given as a reason not to test:

> [If I tested positive,] . . . I would just feel like I am already dead because there is no cure for this. (*woman, Khayelitsha*)

> What makes people not come [to VCT services] is their background. Sometimes you get that their family do not accept a positive person. They see her as if she is someone who was misbehaving outside and then got positive. One is afraid to tell her husband because she is worried that the husband will divorce her. A mother who is not working is afraid of being left with the children to feed . . . Some people think when you touch them you going to make them positive. (*woman, Langa*)

> Positive people are not welcome in the family. (*woman, Langa*)

> People have a fear of knowing. They also say "Why must we test if the government does not treat us?" (*woman, Langa*)

In staff focus groups, counselors observed that these general fears lead many people to delay attending VCT unless they experience symptoms that might be AIDS related.

A big impediment people face in their communities is the stigma that leads people to shun anything related to HIV/AIDS. Resistance to outreach programs by counselors was voiced:

> If [the clinic counselors] would go outside to the community, it would be worse. People do not want that counselors be seen who come to their door. It is better if the counselors stay there, so they can counsel those who go to the clinic. (*woman, Khayelitsha*)

> We also don't want [the counselors] really to come to our places. (*man, Khayelitsha*)

> HIV/AIDS workshop is not very good because that name is scary. (*man, Khayelitsha*)

For the same reasons, people criticize the lack of anonymity in the clinics:

We are a small community. If you are seen [in the waiting area for VCT], there is some question mark above you. So people don't want to be seen there. They don't want to go local. HIV is often portrayed as misbehavior. (*woman, Langa*)

There's a problem with the clinic: the room where counseling takes place. Everyone in the waiting room can see it and from the public entrance. If you go in there everybody knows what you are there for. There's the stigma. (*woman, Langa*)

Closely linked to the issue of stigma is people's fear that their interaction with nurses and counselors is not confidential. Community members may travel to a clinic in a different part of town to have an HIV test. Some interviewees in the communities stated that they preferred to go to a private general practitioner for testing for reasons of confidentiality:

If my counselor is my neighbor, I think that maybe she can tell people about me and my status. Therefore I decide to go and do the test in Salt River and not here in Langa, you understand? (*woman, Langa*)

Sometimes people they go to another clinic. We fear each other. (woman, *Langa*)

We don't have any confidentiality here . . . for confidentiality we go to Wynberg. (*woman, Khayelitsha*)

False Bay is not safe anymore because the health workers do go there and come back and tell, so the only place I see is Fishhoek clinic, and Wynberg. People prefer going to places far away from here. (*woman, Masiphumelele*)

Breaches of confidentiality reported in the communities may not actually reflect reality. Rumors about what happens at the clinics echo people's fears:

There is a particular chair in the clinic that people know if you are seen sitting in it, you know that is for people who tested positive. (*woman, Masiphumelele*)

Overall problems having to do with waiting times and with rudeness and favoritism on the part of health workers were similar to those raised about primary care services generally in South Africa (Edgington, Sekatane, and Goldstein 2002). In a number of cases, lack of trust toward health workers is clearly expressed, although this often appears to be based on expectations of what would happen or on the experience of others rather than on individuals' own experience:

> I don't trust anyone. Because I just hear from the TV that they treat some people with needles that have been used by an HIV person. (*woman, Khayelitsha*)

> The people at the clinic do not have a nice way of dealing with the issues in a sensitive way . . . [tells a story about someone else] . . . the health worker visited the house and shouted at her. (*woman, Masiphumelele*)

> I don't know if this test is voluntary. (*woman, Khayelitsha*)

> These health workers do not make people confident because they turn around the folders and check the status of the people. (*woman, Masiphumelele*)

The level of distrust seems to be more an expression of uneasiness and anxiety associated with HIV/AIDS than a reflection of actual negative experiences with clinic staff and VCT services. People interviewed who revealed their HIV-positive status generally described a different experience than was expected by other respondents, and they reported kindness, support, and confidentiality on the part of the clinic staff:

> They treat them [those with HIV] good and advise us how to behave. (*woman, Langa*)

> The staff here care very much. (*HIV-positive woman, Langa*)

Issues surrounding information and the type of promotion of public VCT services were also discussed in the focus groups. Several participants mentioned radio, leaflets at the clinic, and LoveLife, a media campaign promoting reproductive health:

> The billboards are good but they must not be put on the freeway where you cannot see them. (*woman, Langa*)

> What about those who cannot read? They are people like us. How are they going to get this information? (*woman, Khayelitsha*)

The most marginalized parts of the townships—that is, informal settlements or squatter camps—were spoken of as those least likely to access services. Their residents were seen as high-risk groups for HIV but as more inclined to call on traditional healers. Reasons mentioned for the lack of interaction between squatters and public primary health services were economic (people spend their time looking for money and food), cultural, and related to language and education.

> They in the informal there, they suffer. (*woman, Khayelitsha*)

> [HIV awareness should] include people from the rural areas, who cannot read and also include our culture, the culture of the African people. According to our culture the elders are not allowed to talk with their children about sex. (*man, Khayelitsha*)

Limitations

As highlighted in the previous section, carrying out research on issues associated with HIV/AIDS is a highly sensitive task. Both the reluctance of people to be interviewed in depth and limitations on what they were willing to talk about in interviews hindered data collection. Because of the difficulties of recruiting people for interviews or focus groups, qualitative data are not drawn from a wide, community-based sample but from specific groups, and these groups' views may differ systematically from those of other members of the community.

The second set of limitations concerns the use of the South African DHS for the comparison data. The approach had two drawbacks. Because the DHS was conducted in 1998, the data are relatively old, and asset ownership patterns within townships in South Africa may have changed. The only clear development in asset ownership affecting households across the board, however, seems to relate to the possession of telephones as a result of the spread of mobile phones. The second weakness of the DHS data is the extent to which the asset ownership questions used in the DHS are appropriate for South African urban and periurban settings. Given the relatively high prevalence of many "basic" assets, a refined set of questions would probably have yielded superior results. Future work could benefit from a focus on more appropriate wealth indexes for specific settings.

The study design was highly focused and reveals a number of areas requiring further exploration. The study examined only relatively well resourced township clinics in the public sector. It thus highlights the need to know more about what is happening in more rural areas and about where else people might be going for VCT. Furthermore, our facility-based study design did not allow us to comment on the rate of uptake or of exclusion from the service in the community as a whole. Larger, more comprehensive (and hence more expensive) research designs would be required to shed light on these important questions.

Implications

The population of townships in Western Cape Province is relatively affluent compared with the rest of the South African population covered by the DHS. Public sector users in those townships are from the poorest quintiles, and public sector users of VCT are even more concentrated in those quintiles. Reasons for this are suggested by the qualitative findings, which consistently reflect a perception that public sector VCT is deficient in confidentiality—a key quality dimension for this service.

Health policy makers face a number of dilemmas related to access to services. The first is whether services reach the right population and in sufficient quantity. Related to this is the question of whether services are perceived to be of adequate quality and accessibility. Findings from this study suggest that VCT in public sector clinics reaches poor groups but that this may be happening as a result of negative attitudes toward the service rather than positive ones.

It is unlikely that the relatively wealthier groups choose not to obtain VCT at all; studies from other countries show that uptake of VCT is positively associated with socioeconomic status and education (Kowalczyk and others 2002). But we do not know where individuals who do not use the public sector for VCT are going. Evidence abounds that many urban South Africans go to the private sector for general primary health care services and that where conditions of greater sensitivity are involved, this is likely to be a very high percentage. For instance, more than 50 percent of patients with sexually transmitted infections use the services of private general practitioners (Rispel and others 1995; Wilkinson and others 1998). We can therefore hypothesize that some groups, especially wealthier ones, go to the private sector and that others may travel out of the area to obtain VCT in more anonymous settings in the public sector.

In light of high private sector utilization throughout the world, the perception of public sector health services as being of poor quality is a problem of increasing concern for those who can afford no alternative. It undermines many areas of health service delivery in the public sector and causes impoverishment of vulnerable households that pay for private services instead of using the public sector. Although the findings of this study suggest a progressive incidence of uptake of VCT, a more positive finding would have been an even distribution of VCT use across all socioeconomic quintiles, including the poorer groups.

VCT recipients who choose not to use the public sector incur costs of travel and time or private sector fees to access a service of tremendous public health importance that is available free of charge. Measures to address this situation could include improving the perceived confidentiality of services at public clinics through physical modifications such as changes in waiting areas and room allocations and by training health workers and helping to cultivate trust in health workers at the clinics. The physical environment at the clinics must be designed in a way that ensures confidentiality, and health workers and counselors must place higher value on patients' privacy. To be sure, the reputation of services, rather than their actual shortcomings, may keep many people away. The problem may be one of suspicion and perception as much as of real breaches of confidentiality. This points toward a need to address people's perceptions, as well as features of the service. If many people are using the private sector and are likely to continue doing so in the near future, the possibility of a voucher system for VCT could be explored if the private sector could offer good-quality counseling and testing that is more acceptable to clients and can be monitored for quality.

Finally, the study findings suggest a clear agenda for future research in this area. It is important to begin to understand the extent of exclusion from VCT in various service settings and areas. Research at the community level into uptake of VCT and choice of provider (and the associated costs) would be one next step toward advancing knowledge in this area. It should be coupled with more in-depth qualitative work aimed at understanding the key barriers to access to VCT by different vulnerable groups.

Notes

1. VCT as part of antenatal care was explicitly excluded because it is part of a broader service. Moreover, the uptake of services within a package focusing on the prevention of mother-to-child transmission is based on a different set of motivations.

2. Johannesburg townships in the DHS, similar to those in Greater Cape Town periurban areas, were included to increase the sample size of reference households.

References

Booysen, F. le R. 2002. Measuring poverty with data from the Demographic and Health Survey (DHS): An application to South Africa. *Studies in Economics and Econometrics* 26(3): 53–70.

Chabikuli, N., H. Schneider, D. Blaauw, A. Zwi, and R. Brugha. 2002. Quality and equity of private sector care for sexually transmitted diseases in South Africa. *Health Policy and Planning* 17: 40–46.

Edgington, M., C. Sekatane, and S. Goldstein. 2002. Patients' beliefs: Do they affect tuberculosis control? A study in a rural district of South Africa. *International Journal of Tuberculosis and Lung Disease* 6(12): 1075–82.

Farmer, P. 2001. Community based approaches to HIV treatment in resource-poor settings. *Lancet* 358: 404–9.

Forsythe, S., G. Arthur, G. Ngatia, R. Mutemi, J. Odhiambo, and C. Gilks. 2002. Assessing the cost and willingness to pay for voluntary HIV counseling and testing in Kenya. *Health Policy and Planning* 17: 187–95.

Gilbert, L., and L. Walker. 2002. Treading the path of least resistance: HIV/AIDS and social inequalities—a South African case study. *Social Science and Medicine* 54: 1093–110.

Godfrey-Faussett, P., D. Maher, Y. Mukadi, P. Nunn, J. Perriens, and M. Raviglione. 2002. How human immunodeficiency virus voluntary testing can contribute to TB control. *Bulletin of the World Health Organization* 80: 939–45.

Kowalczyk, J., P. Jolly, E. Karita, J. Nibarere, J. Vyankandondera, and H. Salihu. 2002. Voluntary counseling and testing for HIV among pregnant women presenting in labor in Kigali, Rwanda. *JAIDS* 31: 408–15.

Magongo, B., S. Magwaza, V. Mathambo, and N. Makhanya. 2002. *National report on the assessment of the public sector's voluntary counseling and testing programme.* Pretoria: Health Systems Trust.

Matovu, J., G. Kigozi, F. Nalugoda, F. Wabwire-Mangen, and R. Gray. 2002. The Rakai project counseling programme experience. *Tropical Medicine and International Health* 7: 1064–67.

Nuwaha, F., D. Kabatesi, M. Muganwa, and C. Whalen. 2002. Factors influencing acceptability of voluntary counseling and testing in Bushenyi district of Uganda. *East African Medical Journal* 79: 626–32.

Palmer, N., A. Mills, L. Gilson, H. Wadee, and H. Schneider. 2003. A new face for private providers in developing countries: What implications for public health? *Bulletin of the World Health Organization* 81: 292–97.

Pronyk, P., J. Kim, M. Makhubele, J. Hargreaves, R. Mohlala, and H. Hausler. 2002. Introduction of voluntary counseling and rapid testing for HIV in rural South Africa: From theory to practice. *AIDS Care* 14: 859–65.

Rispel, L., A. Beattie, M. Xaba, J. Cabral, N. Marawa, and S. Fonn. 1995. *A description and evaluation of primary health care services delivered by the Alexandra Health Centre and University Clinic.* Johannesburg: Centre for Health Policy.

Schneider, H., D. Blaauw, B. Magongo, and I. Khumalo. 1999. STD care in the private sector. *South African Health Review* 83–94. Durban: Health Systems Trust.

Shisana, O., and L. Simbayi, eds. 2002. *Nelson Mandela/HSRC study of HIV/AIDS: South African national HIV prevalence, behavioural risks and mass media; household survey 2002.* Cape Town: Human Sciences Research Council.

UNAIDS (Joint United Nations Programme on HIV/AIDS). 2002. *HIV voluntary counseling and testing: A gateway to prevention and care.* Geneva: UNAIDS.

Wilkinson, D., A. Connolly, A. Harrison, M. Lurie, and A. Abdool Karim. 1998. Sexually transmitted disease syndromes in rural South Africa: Results from health facility surveillance. *Sexually Transmitted Diseases* 25: 20–25.

World Bank. 2001. *World development report 2000/01: Attacking poverty.* New York: Oxford University Press.

Part III

Asia Studies

7

Bangladesh: Inequalities in Utilization of Maternal Health Care Services— Evidence from Matlab

A. T. M. Iqbal Anwar, Japhet Killewo,
Mahbub-E-Elahi K. Chowdhury, and Sushil Kanta Dasgupta

Bangladesh is one of the poorest countries in the world, with a maternal mortality ratio of 320 per 100,000 live births (NIPORT 2001). As part of its effort to promote safe motherhood and reduce maternal mortality, the government has been upgrading existing health facilities and services in order to make essential obstetric care (EOC) services available to all women. The target is to provide quality comprehensive EOC services in all 59 district hospitals, in 64 of the 90 maternal and child welfare centers (MCWCs), and in 120 of the 403 rural *thana* (subdistrict) health complexes (Bangladesh 1998).

Research Questions

Some progress has been made in the number of women receiving EOC services, but the question arises whether these are the women who really need such services. For example, the rise in caesarean section rates in Bangladesh from 0.7 percent in 1994 to 2.2 percent in 1999, may indicate some progress toward meeting the need for emergency obstetric care, but the fact that half of these procedures took place in private facilities may suggest that access is better for the urban elite than for the rural poor (Khan and others 1999).

Although inequity is a growing concern, few systematic studies of equity have been conducted in Bangladesh, particularly regarding maternal health care services. This study is an attempt to explore inequality in utilization of maternal health services provided by the International Centre for Diarrhoeal Diseases Research, Bangladesh (ICDDR,B) in its Matlab service area, a homogeneous rural area in Chandpur District. The following research questions are addressed:

- To what extent do women from the poorer segment of the population use the available essential obstetric care services in the Matlab ICDDR,B service area?
- What other sociodemographic factors influence utilization of maternal health care services?

Setting and Methodology

Matlab, a rural subdistrict in the Ganges-Meghna Delta with a population of 550,000, is situated about 55 kilometers southeast of Dhaka. As in most areas of flood-prone southern Bangladesh, rural people barely subsist on rice growing and fishing, use mostly water communication, and follow a male-dominated cultural pattern with such characteristics as seclusion of women in their compounds (Fauveau and others 1991). Since 1966, the ICDDR,B has maintained a Health and Demographic Surveillance System (HDSS) in the Matlab area that in 2001 covered a population of about 220,000. Information on births, deaths, marriages, and migration in the area is collected by community health research workers (CHRWs) through monthly house-to-house visits. In addition, the HDSS conducts periodic socioeconomic censuses, and data from them are available for 1974, 1982, and 1996.

The HDSS area is divided into two parts: an ICDDR,B service area, and a comparison (government service) area, each covering a population of about 110,000. The ICDDR,B service or "treatment" area is subdivided into four blocks (A, B, C, and D), each served by a health subcenter that provides maternal and child health services for its catchment population (figure 7.1). In addition, the ICDDR,B operates a 120-bed hospital in the town of Matlab (Matlab Hospital) that provides free services for the management of diarrheal diseases, as well as maternal and child health care.

Maternal Health Services Delivered

In 1987 the ICDDR,B initiated a community-based maternity care program in the northern half of the service area (blocks C and D), covering 48,000 people living in 39 villages (see figure 7.1). Two government-trained nurse-midwives were recruited and assigned to each subcenter in the program area to conduct home deliveries. Their duties were to work with CHRWs and traditional birth attendants and ensure that they were called in during

Figure 7.1. *Matlab ICDDR,B Health and Demographic Surveillance Area, Bangladesh*

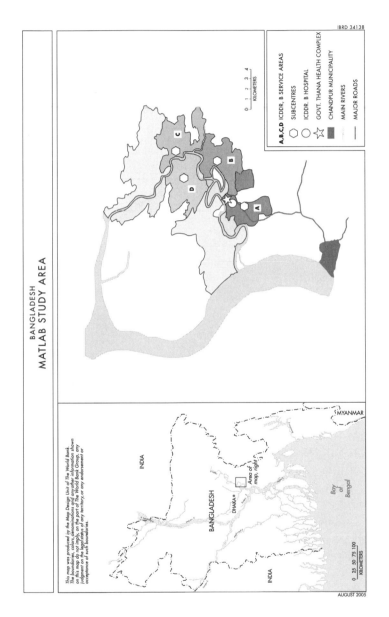

Source: Geographic information system, Health and Demographic Surveillance Unit, International Centre for Diarrhoeal Diseases Research, Bangladesh (ICDDR,B). Adapted.

labor; to pay antenatal visits to the pregnant women identified by CHRWs; to assess antenatal complication risks; to attend as many home deliveries as possible; to treat complications at the onset before they became severe; to organize referrals and accompany referred patients to the central clinic at Matlab, if judged necessary; and to visit as many new mothers as possible within 48 hours of delivery. (For details concerning the nurse-midwives' duties, the treatment guidelines, essential drugs, equipment, and the record-keeping system, see Fauveau and Chakraborty 1988.) Midwives were supported by two other program components: development of a referral chain, including a boatman and a helper to accompany patients day or night to the referral site, and installation of a maternity clinic at Matlab, where additional trained midwives and female physicians were always available for intensive surveillance, treatment, or further referral to the Chandpur District Hospital. The Matlab maternity clinic was not equipped with surgical, radiological, or modern laboratory facilities. The only items of obstetric equipment available were a vacuum extractor, a suction machine, and obstetric forceps. The emphasis was on immediate care of admitted patients and stabilization of patients for rapid transfer to higher-level comprehensive facilities, mostly in Chandpur, the district headquarters. In January 1990 the maternity care intervention was expanded to blocks A and B, following the same home-based strategy then practiced throughout the ICDDR,B service area and with similar referral linkages with the Matlab Hospital clinic and with comprehensive public and private EOC facilities in Chandpur.

In 1996 the strategy for providing maternity care services in the ICDDR,B service area began to shift from home-based to facility-based delivery of services. Community-based midwives and paramedics were withdrawn from the field and assigned to health subcenters to conduct normal deliveries. The block C subcenter was upgraded in November 1996 to provide basic EOC. Subsequently, all the other subcenters were upgraded as basic EOC facilities, and by 2001 the home-based strategy had been totally replaced by a facility-based strategy.

In addition to ICDDR,B services, maternity care services for the study population were available from the government thana health complex at Matlab, the government district hospital at Chandpur, and private clinics and hospitals located mostly in Chandpur.

Data and Methodology

This is a secondary data analysis study. It used the following existing surveillance and monitoring databases:

- the HDSS birth file (1997–2001)
- pictorial card data (1997–2001)
- the 1996 socioeconomic census data for the entire Matlab HDSS area

HDSS BIRTH FILE. The HDSS records all births in the ICDDR,B surveillance area, including stillbirths. During the reference period (1997–2001), 15,041 births occurred in the ICDDR,B service area. The limitation of birth files is that they contain no information on socioeconomic status or detailed service utilization. The HDSS, however, assigns to every individual and to every household in the surveillance area a unique identification number through which ICDDR,B surveillance and monitoring databases, including socioeconomic censuses, can be linked.

PICTORIAL CARDS. Pictorial cards are specially designed pregnancy-monitoring tools used to follow all mothers in the ICDDR,B service area throughout pregnancy, during delivery, and for 42 days (six weeks) after delivery. The CHRWs provide all new pregnant mothers with relevant background information and instruct them to preserve the cards carefully and submit them to the midwives during home visits or visits to the ICDDR,B facilities for maternity care services. Six weeks after childbirth, the CHRWs collect the cards from the mothers. The service providers (mostly midwives) use the cards as behavior change communication tools and to record mothers' relevant service uptake information. No economic information is collected through the cards, but they have room for recording a set of unique identification numbers for the women. For the reference period, during which 15,041 births in the ICDDR,B service area were recorded by the HDSS, 12,080 filled-in pictorial cards were available for analysis.

1996 SOCIOECONOMIC CENSUS. In the Matlab HDSS area, socioeconomic information is collected through periodic censuses, which were conducted in 1974, 1982, and 1996. For this study we used household-level socioeconomic information from the 1996 census to classify mothers into wealth quintiles.

MEASUREMENT OF SOCIOECONOMIC STATUS. In this study socioeconomic status is defined in terms of assets or wealth rather than income or consumption. We used principal component methods of data reduction to classify mothers into socioeconomic quintiles (Gwatkin and others 2000; Filmer and Pritchett 2001). Calculation of socioeconomic quintiles was based on the 14,306 mothers for whom household-level information on assets and other socioeconomic variables from the socioeconomic census of 1996 was available (see annex table 7.1).

DATA LINKING. Birth file data were linked with socioeconomic census data, using mothers' household identification numbers. Of 15,041 mothers in the birth file, socioeconomic information was recorded for 14,306 (95.1 percent). Pictorial cards were available for 12,080 (80.3 percent), and 11,555 (76.8 percent) had both pictorial cards and socioeconomic indicators.

Our current analysis covered 12,080 mothers who had a filled-in pictorial card; but for inequality analysis we could use only 11,555 of them. The number (N) therefore varies in different parts of the analysis.

The socioeconomic status of the 11,555 mothers who had both pictorial cards and socioeconomic information and who were included in the inequity analysis was quite similar to that of the 2,751 (14,306 minus 11,555) mothers with socioeconomic information but without pictorial cards. This suggests that any bias resulting from the incomplete coverage of pictorial cards was minimal.

TOOLS FOR DATA ANALYSIS. Data were entered and linked in Foxpro-2.6a software. For analysis, Excel 2000 and SPSS 10 were extensively used.

Findings

During the study period (1997–2001), of the 12,080 births monitored by pictorial cards, 19.0 percent took place in ICDDR,B facilities, 2.1 percent in government facilities, and 1.9 percent in private clinics and hospitals. Another 2.7 percent of births were attended by ICDDR,B midwives at home, and the remaining 74.4 percent were assisted by unskilled attendants at home (figure 7.2). So, in the ICDDR,B service area, a skilled birth attendant was present for 25.6 percent of deliveries during the reference period, which is much higher than the national average for Bangladesh. During the same period 83 percent of the mothers in the ICDDR,B service area made at least one antenatal visit; the mean number of visits for those who received antenatal care was 1.9 per pregnancy. Fifty-one percent of the mothers received postnatal care, and 1.7 percent underwent caesarean sections.

Bivariate Analysis

In bivariate analysis, socioeconomic status was found to be strongly associated with utilization of maternal health care services (table 7.1). In the ICDDR,B service area, poorer mothers used maternity care services less than did their better-off counterparts. A much smaller proportion of poor mothers (14.2 percent) had skilled attendants at delivery than did the least-poor mothers (45.8 percent). For deliveries, inequality was highest for use of pri-

Figure 7.2. *Obstetric Deliveries in ICDDR,B Service Area by Place of Delivery, 12,080 Births, Bangladesh, 1997–2001*

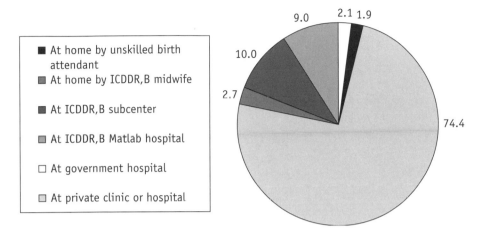

- ■ At home by unskilled birth attendant
- ■ At home by ICDDR,B midwife
- ■ At ICDDR,B subcenter
- ■ At ICDDR,B Matlab hospital
- ☐ At government hospital
- ☐ At private clinic or hospital

Source: ICDDR,B pictorial cards, 1997–2001.

vate sector facilities (rich-poor ratio, 12.0; concentration index, 0.46) and lowest for use of ICDDR,B resources (rich-poor ratio, 2.9; concentration index, 0.13–0.26). With respect to inequality, use of public facilities was intermediate (rich-poor ratio, 5.0; concentration index, 0.36). Among ICDDR,B services, facility-based care was more equitably distributed than home-based skilled delivery care. Among ICDDR,B facilities, services of the centrally located Matlab Hospital were found to be less pro-poor than services of peripheral subcenters. Disparities were found in access to antenatal care and postnatal care services as well, but the difference was less pronounced than for skilled attendance at deliveries. Inequality increased systematically for higher numbers of antenatal care visits. Among all indicators examined, inequality was highest for caesarean sections; the rate for poorest-quintile mothers was 0.5 percent, while that of mothers from the least poor quintile was 4.6 percent (rich-poor ratio, 9.2; concentration index, 0.47).

Although an increasing trend in use of maternity care services was observed in the study area, disparities stayed at about the same level throughout the reporting period (figure 7.3). In 1997, 18.5 percent of deliveries took place in facilities, while the population-based caesarean rate was 1.5 percent. By 2001, facility-based deliveries had increased to 28.9 percent and the caesarean rate to 2.6 percent (annex table 7.2). Over time, the increase in antenatal and postnatal care uptake was minimal, but the mean number of antenatal care visits increased significantly, from 1.66 in 1997 to 2.05 in 2001. In the bivariate analysis, other factors found to be significantly associated with uti-

Table 7.1. Utilization of Maternal Health Care Services, by Mother's Socioeconomic Status, 11,555 Cases, Bangladesh, 1997–2001 (Percent, unless otherwise indicated)

Indicator	Socioeconomic quintile					Total (N = 11,555)	Rich-poor ratio	Concentration index (CI)	CI standard error
	1 (poorest) (N = 2,335)	2 (N = 2,330)	3 (N = 2,306)	4 (N = 2,294)	5 (least poor) (N = 2,290)				
Delivery care									
At home by unskilled attendant	85.7	81.7	79.8	71.6	54.2	74.7	0.6	−0.0781	0.0316
At home by ICDDR,B midwives	1.5	2.1	1.6	2.6	5.7	2.7	3.8	0.2632	0.0716
At ICDDR,B subcenter	6.5	7.9	8.9	11.1	12.6	9.5	1.9	0.1312	0.0237
At ICDDR,B Matlab Hospital	4.8	6.8	7.4	10.1	17.8	9.3	3.7	0.2499	0.0535
At government hospital	1.0	0.8	1.3	2.0	5.0	2.0	5.0	0.3642	0.0559
At private clinics and hospitals	0.4	0.7	0.9	2.0	4.8	1.7	12.0	0.4599	0.0599
Total	100	100	100	100	100	100			

Socioeconomic quintile

Indicator	1 (poorest) (N = 2,335)	2 (N = 2,330)	3 (N = 2,306)	4 (N = 2,294)	5 (least poor) (N = 2,290)	Total (N = 11,555)	Rich-poor ratio	Concentration index (CI)	CI standard error
Number of antenatal visits									
None	22.4	19.8	17.0	14.3	12.8	17.3	0.6	−0.1144	0.0190
1	38.1	37.9	37.5	36.6	28.4	35.7	0.7	−0.0461	0.0272
2	24.8	26.7	27.5	28.9	29.3	27.4	1.2	0.0327	0.0079
3	10.7	10.7	12.3	13.3	18.9	13.2	1.8	0.1151	0.0353
4+	4.0	4.8	5.8	6.9	10.7	6.4	2.7	0.1925	0.0425
Total	100	100	100	100	100	100			
Received postnatal care	48.9	48.2	49.3	51.5	57.2	51.0	1.2	0.0311	0.0125
Delivered by caesarean section	0.5	0.5	0.7	1.7	4.6	1.6	9.2	0.4704	0.0429

Source: ICDDR,B pictorial cards, 1997–2001.

Note: The rich-poor ratio is the ratio between the figures for quintile 5 (least poor) and quintile 1 (poorest) for the same indicator. Percentages may not sum to total because of rounding.

Figure 7.3. *Trends in Access to Skilled Delivery Care by Wealth Quintile, 11,555 Cases, Bangladesh, 1997–2001*

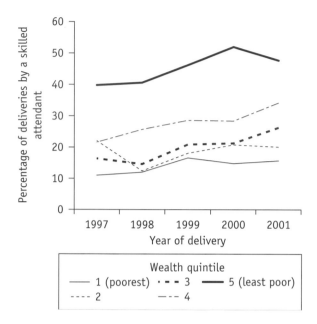

Source: ICDDR,B pictorial cards, 1997–2001.
Note: Summary inequality statistics, by year, are as follows:

	1997	1998	1999	2000	2001
Rich-poor ratio	3.6	3.4	2.8	3.5	3.0
Concentration index	0.21	0.21	0.21	0.21	0.21

lization of maternity services included mother's education, distance to the nearest subcenter, mother's age at delivery, religion, and parity (annex table 7.2). Distance to the nearest subcenter and mother's age and parity were found to have an inverse relationship to uptake of maternity services, while the relationship of other socioeconomic variables to utilization of maternity services was positive. Analysis also revealed that the higher the number of antenatal care visits, the higher were the figures for skilled attendance at delivery, caesarian section rates, and postnatal care uptake among the women.

Multivariate Analysis

From the bivariate analysis of the monitoring data, it is evident that poverty is a significant factor that indicates care-seeking behavior for maternal health services. In the subsequent analysis we developed a binary logistic regression model that had presence of a skilled attendant at birth (at a facility or at home) as the dependent variable and, as independent variables (regressors), socioeconomic status, mother's education, distance, mother's age, gravida, year of delivery, number of antenatal care visits, and religion. All the independent variables were recoded as categorical or ordinal categorical variables. In calculating the odds ratio for each category of independent variables, the first group was always taken as the reference category.

Table 7.2 shows the crude and adjusted odds ratios of utilization of skilled attendants at birth for various sociodemographic characteristics. Even after adjusting for the effects of all other covariates in the model, socioeconomic status maintained a significant relationship with the dependent variable; mothers from the least poor quintile were 3.4 times more likely to use a skilled birth attendant than poorest-quintile mothers.

The adjusted odds ratios for other independent variables also showed a clear relationship with attended delivery. For instance, a mother with one antenatal care visit was 2.04 times more likely to be delivered by a skilled birth attendant than a mother with no antenatal checkup. The odds ratios for skilled attendance at delivery were found to increase tremendously as the number of antenatal care visits rose. A mother with four antenatal care visits was 12.9 times more likely to be delivered by a skilled attendant than a mother with no antenatal care, after controlling for the effects of covariates.

Distance to the nearest subcenter was significantly associated with use of maternity care services. The probability of delivering at a facility decreased significantly with increasing distance. Mothers residing between 1 and 2 kilometers from subcenters were 55 percent less likely to use skilled delivery services than mothers residing less than 1 kilometer from subcenters.

Mother's education was independently a significant factor for skilled attendance at delivery. A mother with 10 or more years of schooling was 1.8 times more likely to be delivered by a skilled birth attendant than a mother with no formal education.

Gravidity was found to be inversely associated with uptake of services, but the effect of age on the dependent variable showed a contrasting result. In the bivariate analysis it was observed that with increasing age, the probability of using skilled care decreased (annex table 7.2). But when the effect of gravida was controlled for in multivariate analysis, age was positively associated with skilled attendance at birth (see table 7.2). Mothers age 35 years or more were 1.6 times more likely to be delivered at health facilities than mothers under age 20.

Mothers from minority religious groups were 1.8 times more likely to use a skilled attendant for delivering their babies than mothers from majority religious groups.

Table 7.2. Logistic Regression Results from Pictorial Card Data for Sociodemographic Correlates of Skilled Attendance at Birth in ICDDR,B Service Area, Bangladesh, 1997–2001

Independent variables (regressors)	Crude odds ratio	95 percent confidence intervals for crude odds ratio	Adjusted odds ratio[a]	95 percent confidence intervals for adjusted odds ratio
Socioeconomic status (wealth quintile)				
1 (poorest)	1.00	Reference category	1.00	Reference category
2	1.35	1.16–1.58	1.32	1.12–1.57
3	1.53	1.31–1.78	1.37	1.16–1.62
4	2.38	2.06–2.76	1.95	1.65–2.31
5 (least poor)	5.09	4.41–5.87	3.42	2.87–4.04
Education of mother				
No formal education	1.00	Reference category	1.00	Reference category
1–4 years	1.04	0.91–1.19	0.92	0.79–1.07
5–9 years	1.42	1.28–1.58	1.04	0.92–1.18
10+ years	3.75	3.32–4.23	1.82	1.56–2.13
Gravida				
1 (primigravida)	1.00	Reference category	1.00	Reference category
2	0.62	0.56–0.70	0.57	0.50–0.66
3	0.49	0.43–0.55	0.46	0.40–0.54
4	0.48	0.41–0.55	0.47	0.40–0.57
5+	0.39	0.32–0.44	0.42	0.34–0.51
Number of antenatal care visits				
None	1.00	Reference category	1.00	Reference category
1	2.03	1.72–2.4	2.04	1.69–2.46
2	4.39	3.72–5.18	4.14	3.44–4.99
3	7.33	6.13–8.76	6.43	5.25–7.87
4+	15.04	12.25–18.48	12.94	10.24–16.36

Independent variables (regressors)	Dependent variable: baby delivered by unskilled birth attendant (= 0); by skilled birth attendant (= 1)			
	Crude odds ratio	95 percent confidence intervals for crude odds ratio	Adjusted odds ratio[a]	95 percent confidence intervals for adjusted odds ratio
Age group of mother (years)				
10–19	1.00	Reference category	1.00	Reference category
20–34	0.80	0.71–0.91	1.10	0.93–1.28
35+	0.68	0.57–0.81	1.64	1.27–2.10
Distance of subcenter from home (kilometers)				
≤1	1.00	Reference category	1.00	Reference category
1.1–2	0.43	0.38–0.48	0.45	0.39–0.51
2.1–3	0.46	0.41–0.52	0.50	0.43–0.57
3.1–4	0.40	0.34–0.48	0.42	0.35–0.52
≥4	0.20	0.15–0.28	0.18	0.12–0.25
Religion of mother				
Muslim	1.00	Reference category	1.00	Reference category
Hindu or other	1.32	1.18–1.49	1.76	1.54–2.02
Year of delivery				
1997	1.00	Reference category	1.00	Reference category
1998	0.93	0.80–1.08	0.89	0.75–1.05
1999	1.27	1.09–1.47	1.07	0.90–1.26
2000	1.38	1.20–1.60	1.03	0.88–1.22
2001	1.49	1.29–1.71	1.08	0.92–1.27

Source: ICDDR,B pictorial cards, 1997–2001.
a. After controlling for the effects of all other covariates in the model.

Discussion

This study is an initial attempt to analyze inequalities in the use of maternal health care in Bangladesh, a country with low levels of and large socioeconomic differences in use of obstetric and other maternal health services. For example, the 2001 Bangladesh Maternal Health Services and Maternal Mortality Survey found that skilled professionals performed only 11.6 percent of all deliveries and that only 8.8 percent of deliveries took place in essential obstetric care facilities. Wide urban-rural and socioeconomic differentials were observed in that study. In urban areas skilled medical professionals attended 26.8 percent of births, but the figure was only 8.4 percent in rural areas. Only 3.4 percent of mothers from the poorest households had a skilled attendant at delivery, compared with 37.3 percent for the least-poor mothers. The rich-poor ratio for this indicator was 11.6.

Inequalities in Service Utilization

We examined variations by relative socioeconomic status (wealth quintile) in the utilization of maternal health care services among a seemingly homogenous group of poor mothers in a rural area of Bangladesh. In our study area, overall coverage of maternal health services was much better than the Bangladesh national averages. Nevertheless, inequality in utilization was still high for a population group with such seemingly limited economic disparities in an area where ICDDR,B services are provided free of charge. Study findings suggest that the ICDDR,B has succeeded in expanding use of maternal health care services, but not to all who need them. The equity goal has yet to be achieved.

Among different types of obstetric care provider in the study area, the disparity was highest for the for-profit private sector and lowest for ICDDR,B services, with the public sector in between. Private sector services are naturally less pro-poor because patients have to pay for them. Why services from public sector providers are less equitably distributed than ICDDR,B services is not clear, since both are provided free of charge. One reason may be that although public sector services are officially free, service recipients often have to pay unofficially for them.

Significant poor-rich differences in use were found even for the free ICDDR,B services. The likely reasons include indirect costs associated with use—for example, for transportation, referral, and lost time. Other factors that have to be considered are cultural barriers, lack of confidence in the health care system, lack of knowledge, and distance to the EOC facility in rural areas. Quality of care, both perceived and technical, could be another issue and is gaining the attention of program managers and policy planners. All these barriers affect the poorer segment of the community more than the better off.

Inequalities in caesarian sections appear particularly large. The World Health Organization and UNICEF have suggested that the population-based rate for caesarian sections should lie between 5 and 15 percent of all births (Maine, McCarthy, and Ward 1992). Anything below 5 percent indicates that a substantial proportion of women do not have access to potentially life-saving surgical obstetric care and may well die as a result. By this indicator, the maternal health situation in Matlab is still poor, as the estimated overall caesarian section rate is only 1.7 percent, slightly above the national average of 1.6 percent (NIPORT 2001). The rich-poor disparity for caesarian sections was highest in the ICDDR,B service area, as expected, since the intervention is costly and the ICDDR,B does not provide it. Women requiring caesarians are referred to public or private district-level facilities, which often charge far more than the poorer segments of the community can pay.

Role of Other Sociodemographic Factors

DISTANCE. According to the study findings, services from peripheral sub-centers are more equitably distributed than services from the centrally located Matlab Hospital. Distance was also shown to curtail service use. To ensure efficiency as well as equity, the decentralization of emergency obstetric care services—the approach chosen by the government of Bangladesh—should be strengthened.

ANTENATAL CARE. The low predictability of antenatal markers for adverse maternal outcomes has led some observers to rule out antenatal care as an efficient strategy in the fight against maternal and perinatal mortality. Few studies, however, have assessed the predictability of antenatal care screening for adverse maternal outcomes other than dystocia or perinatal death, and most of the studies have been hospital based (Vanneste and others 2000). Our study showed that the number of antenatal care visits is strongly associated with utilization of other maternal health care services such as skilled attendance at birth and postnatal care. Thus, antenatal care may not be an efficient strategy for identifying the women most in need of obstetric service delivery, but if promoted in conjunction with effective emergency obstetric care, it may become an effective instrument for improving use of those services.

MOTHERS' EDUCATION. The mother's education, even after controlling for the confounding effects of covariates, positively influences use of emergency obstetric services. To reduce maternal mortality, female education should be strengthened.

PARITY AND MATERNAL AGE. Parity and maternal age are mutually correlated, but parity affects utilization negatively and mother's age affects it positively, after controlling for the effects of covariates in logistic regression. Higher-parity mothers should therefore be targeted to improve indicator status for maternity services.

Conclusions

The high and rising overall utilization rates of maternal health care services in Matlab, compared with other areas of Bangladesh, and the persistent rich-poor gap indicate that ICDDR,B interventions through a program approach have managed to increase utilization but have not adequately addressed equity. Although maternity services are free in Matlab, inequality in utilization of EOC services is still unacceptably high. The reason may be that indirect costs such as transport, expense of referrals, and attendants' lost time adversely affect utilization. Quality of care, both perceived and technical, is gaining in importance among program managers and policy planners. The literature suggests that factors such as cultural barriers, lack of confidence in the health care system, and ignorance in rural areas need to be taken into account.

All these barriers affect mostly the poorer segment of the community. As a result, socioeconomic disparities in the use of maternal health care persist within the ICDDR,B service area, even as overall utilization of the services is improving. Study results suggest that providing free services does not ensure equity. To reduce maternal mortality rates to an acceptable level, we need to focus on programs that are efficient and effective. The persistence and the unacceptable levels of inequity in this sector are a cause for growing concern. Program managers and policy planners should make sure in the project planning and implementation phases that services are client focused and need based, high in quality, and within the reach of the neediest. Other access barriers also need to be explored and addressed to make maternal health care services equitable, efficient, and effective.

Annex Table 7.1. *Assets and Factor Scores in Matlab, Bangladesh*

	Unweighted			Household asset score	
Asset variable	Mean	Standard deviation	Asset factor score	If yes	If no
Has khat	0.27	0.44	0.10	0.18	−0.06
Has quilt	0.65	0.48	0.11	0.09	−0.15
Has mattress	0.51	0.50	0.12	0.13	−0.12
Has lamp	0.87	0.33	0.06	0.02	−0.16
Has watch/clock	0.60	0.49	0.11	0.10	−0.12
Has chair/table	0.61	0.49	0.11	0.10	−0.13
Has wardrobe	0.37	0.48	0.09	0.12	−0.06
Has radio	0.48	0.50	0.11	0.12	−0.10
Has television	0.06	0.24	0.07	0.28	−0.02

	Unweighted			Household asset score	
Asset variable	Mean	Standard deviation	Asset factor score	If yes	If no
Has bicycle	0.04	0.20	0.04	0.22	−0.01
Has boat	0.30	0.46	0.01	0.01	−0.01
Has cattle	0.34	0.48	0.04	0.06	−0.03
Has electricity	0.16	0.37	0.07	0.16	−0.03
Has solid wall	0.02	0.15	0.05	0.30	−0.01
Has tin wall	0.30	0.46	0.10	0.15	−0.06
Has tin and bamboo wall	0.13	0.34	0.02	0.04	−0.01
Has tin and other wall	0.06	0.24	−0.00	−0.01	0.00
Has bamboo wall	0.30	0.46	−0.05	−0.08	0.03
Has other wall	0.18	0.39	−0.08	−0.15	0.04
Has solid room	0.01	0.07	0.02	0.33	0.00
Has tin roof	0.96	0.21	0.04	0.01	−0.18
Has tin and bamboo roof	0.00	0.04	−0.00	−0.07	0.00
Has tin and other roof	0.01	0.07	−0.02	−0.23	0.00
Has bamboo roof	0.00	0.05	−0.01	−0.20	0.00
Has other roof	0.03	0.17	−0.05	−0.25	0.01
Female residents use septic tank	0.05	0.21	0.05	0.23	−0.01
Females residents use water-seal latrine	0.19	0.39	0.07	0.14	−0.03
Female residents use open latrine (solid/tin)	0.15	0.36	0.04	0.08	−0.01
Female residents use open latrine	0.60	0.49	−0.09	−0.07	0.12
Female residents use open place	0.00	0.06	−0.01	−0.09	0.00
Female residents use other latrine	0.01	0.10	−0.01	−0.09	0.00
Female residents use no latrine	0.00	0.06	−0.01	−0.13	0.00
Residents drink tubewell water	0.96	0.20	0.03	0.01	−0.01
Residents drink tank water	0.01	0.11	−0.01	−0.10	0.00
Residents drink river water	0.02	0.15	−0.03	−0.16	0.00
Residents drink canal water	0.00	0.06	−0.01	−0.16	0.00
Residents drink from other sources	0.00	0.03	−0.00	−0.03	0.00
Total land possessed by household head (decimals)	85.23	177.40	0.07	n.a.	n.a.
Total floor space (square feet)	309.86	199.60	0.11	n.a.	n.a.

Source: Bangladesh Socioeconomic Census, 1996.
n.a. Not applicable.

Annex Table 7.2. *Delivery, Antenatal Care, and Postnatal Care in Matlab, Bangladesh*
(Percent, except for total number of births)

Background characteristic	Delivery by skilled attendant (at home or at facility)	Received at least one antenatal care visit	Received postnatal care	Population-based caesarian section	Total number of births
Education of mother					
No formal education	21.0	80.6	48.7	1.3	6,718
1–4 years	21.6	83.7	52.6	1.0	1,548
5–9 years	27.4	85.3	53.0	1.2	2,472
10+ years	49.9	86.0	55.6	4.8	1,342
Total	*25.6*	*82.6*	*50.9*	*1.7*	*12,080*
Religion of mother					
Muslim	24.2	82.7	52.4	1.4	9,989
Hindu or other	29.7	82.4	42.1	2.4	1,655
Total	*24.9*	*82.6*	*50.9*	*1.6*	*11,644*
Year of delivery					
1997	22.0	81.0	52.5	1.5	1,661
1998	20.8	75.9	47.8	1.4	2,680
1999	26.3	83.7	50.7	1.3	2,444
2000	28.0	84.7	53.1	1.4	2,533
2001	29.5	87.1	51.1	2.6	2,762
Total	*25.6*	*82.6*	*50.9*	*1.7*	*12,080*
Distance of subcenter from house (kilometers)					
≤1	41.0	91.0	69.6	1.8	1,685
1.1–2	23.0	84.8	56.6	1.3	4,282
2.1–3	24.3	78.8	44.7	2.1	4,624
3.1–4	22.0	77.6	38.9	1.3	1,072
≥4	12.3	81.1	15.5	0.7	413
Total	*25.6*	*82.6*	*50.9*	*1.7*	*12,076*

Background characteristic	Delivery by skilled attendant (at home or at facility)	Received at least one antenatal care visit	Received postnatal care	Population-based caesarian section	Total number of births
Gravida					
1 (primigravida)	35.3	85.3	54.4	2.3	3,428
2	25.4	84.0	52.3	1.9	3,051
3	21.0	84.6	50.3	1.3	2,435
4	20.7	80.8	49.7	1.2	1,488
5+	17.0	73.5	43.2	0.8	1,651
Total	25.6	82.7	50.9	1.7	12,053
Number of antenatal care visits					
None	9.2	00.0	24.9	0.8	2,104
1	17.0	100.0	42.7	1.0	4,294
2	30.7	100.0	61.1	1.2	3,297
3	42.5	100.0	71.1	3.3	1,599
4+	60.3	100.0	80.9	6.4	786
Total	25.6	82.6	50.9	1.7	12,080
Age group of mother (years)					
10–19	29.8	84.0	51.4	1.1	1,442
20–34	25.3	83.1	51.1	1.7	9,485
35+	22.4	76.4	48.1	1.6	1,153
Total	25.6	82.6	50.9	1.7	12,080

Source: ICDDR,B pictorial cards, 1997–2001.

Note

This study was supported by the International Centre for Diarrhoeal Diseases Research, Bangladesh (ICDDR,B) and the Reaching the Poor Program. We thank all the staff of the Matlab Maternity Care Programme and the Health and Demographic Surveillance Unit (HDSU). We appreciate the assistance of the project funded by the U.S. Agency for International Development (USAID) to assess "the acceptability, effectiveness and cost of strategies designed to improve access to basic obstetric care in rural Bangladesh," which provided data files. We also thank the geographical information system (GIS) staff of the ICDDR,B, which designed the map. We are grateful to Abbas Uddin Bhuiya and Kim Streatfield of the Public Health Sciences Division of ICDDR,B for their valuable contributions.

References

Bangladesh, Ministry of Health and Family Welfare. 1998. Programme implementation plan: Health and population sector programme (1998–2003), pt. 1. Dhaka.

Fauveau, V., and J. Chakraborty. 1988. Maternity care in Matlab: Present status and possible interventions. Special publication 26, International Centre for Diarrhoeal Disease Research, Bangladesh, Dhaka.

Fauveau, V., K. Stewart, S. A. Khan, and J. Chakraborty. 1991. Effect on mortality of community-based maternity-care programme in rural Bangladesh. *Lancet* 338(8776): 1183–86.

Filmer, Deon, and Lant H. Pritchett. 2001. Estimating wealth effects without expenditure data—or tears: An application to educational enrollments in states of India. *Demography* 38(1): 115–32.

Gwatkin, Davidson. 2002. Who would gain most from efforts to reach the Millennium Development Goals for health? World Bank, Washington, DC.

Gwatkin, Davidson R., Shea Rutstein, Kiersten Johnson, Rohini Pande, and Adam Wagstaff. 2000. Socioeconomic differences in health, nutrition, and population—45 countries. Health, Nutrition, and Population Department, World Bank, Washington, DC. http://web.worldbank.org/WBSITE/EXTERNAL/TOPICS/EXTHEALTHNUTRITIONANDPOPULATION/EXTPAH/0,,contentMDK:20216957~menuPK:400482~pagePK:148956~piPK:216618~theSitePK:400476,00.html.

Khan, M. S. H., S. T. Khanam, S. Nahar, T. Nasreen, and A. P. M. S. Raham. 1999. Review of availability and use of emergency obstetric care (EOC) services in Bangladesh. Associates for Community and Population Research (ACPR), Dhaka.

Maine, D., J. McCarthy, and V. M. Ward. 1992. Guidelines for monitoring progress in the reduction of maternal mortality. Statistics and Monitoring Section, United Nations Children's Fund, New York.

NIPORT (National Institute of Population Research and Training). 2001. Bangladesh maternal health services and maternal mortality survey. Final report. ORC Macro, Calverton, MD.

Vanneste, A. M., C. Ronsman, J. Chakraborty, and A. D. Francisco. 2000. Prenatal screening in rural Bangladesh: From prediction to care. *Health Policy and Planning* 15(1): 1–10.

8

Cambodia: Using Contracting to Reduce Inequity in Primary Health Care Delivery

J. Brad Schwartz and Indu Bhushan

In the mid-1990s, war and political upheaval had left Cambodia with limited health care infrastructure, especially in rural areas. The numbers of paramedical and management staff were adequate, but training and quality of care were inconsistent, and morale was low (Bhushan, Keller, and Schwartz 2002). The primary health care system was unable to deliver an adequate level of services. For example, only 39 percent of children between 12 and 23 months of age were fully immunized (NIS and ORC Macro 2000).

To address these issues, the Cambodian government obtained a loan from the Asian Development Bank (ADB) for the restructuring and broadening of the primary health care system through the development and implementation by the Ministry of Health of a coverage plan modeled on World Health Organization (WHO) guidelines. The plan included the construction or rehabilitation of health centers, each designed to serve about 10,000 people, and the merger of small administrative districts into operational districts with an average population of about 150,000. It also defined a minimum package of activities for health centers. This consisted of basic preventive and curative services, including immunization, birth spacing, antenatal care, provision of micronutrients, and simple curative care for diarrhea, acute respiratory tract infections, and tuberculosis.

Design of the Contracting Test

As part of the overall implementation plan funded by the ADB loan, the Ministry of Health conducted a large-scale test of contracting with nongovernmental organizations (NGOs) for the delivery of primary health care services. In 1997, prior to the construction of health facilities and the procurement of equipment, a precontract baseline household survey was carried out in candidate rural districts. The ministry awarded NGO contracts in five districts; for comparison, four districts where health services were provided by the government were included in the trial. The contracting test started at the beginning of 1999. A follow-up household survey was conducted two and a half years later, in the summer of 2001. The information from the baseline and follow-up surveys comprises a unique data set for comparing the distributional equity of primary health care services provided by contractors and by government.[1]

To make the test districts as comparable as possible, the following were excluded as candidate districts: districts included in the Ministry of Health Accelerated District Development program, which were to receive additional support; districts already receiving significant donor assistance; and districts that contained provincial capitals, which receive more government funding than other districts because of their provincial hospitals.

The districts were randomly assigned to one of three health care delivery models:

- *Contracting-out.* The contractors had complete line responsibility for service delivery, including hiring, firing, and setting wages; procuring and distributing essential drugs and supplies; and organizing and staffing health facilities.
- *Contracting-in.* The contractors worked within the Ministry of Health system to strengthen the existing district administrative structure. The contractors could not hire or fire health workers, although they could request their transfer. Drugs and supplies were provided through normal Ministry of Health channels. In addition, the contractor received a nominal budget supplement for staff incentives and operating expenses.
- *Government provision.* The government district health management team (DHMT) continued to manage the services. Drugs and supplies were provided through normal Ministry of Health channels. As in contracted-in districts, the DHMT received the nominal budget supplement for staff incentives and operating expenses.

An international competitive bidding process was used to select contractors for the contracted-out and contracted-in districts. Precisely defined and objectively verifiable health care service indicators were measured for all contracted and government districts, using the data collected from the baseline survey, and well-defined goals for improvement in service coverage and coverage of the poor were set. Precontract performance goals were established for child immunization and vitamin A provision, antenatal care, delivery by a trained birth attendant, delivery in a health facility, and knowledge and use of birth spacing in each district. More important for this study, an equity goal of targeting services to the poorest half of the population was mandated for all districts.

At the time of the precontract survey, in all candidate districts less than 20 percent of planned health facilities were functional, and health service coverage was poor. Prior to bidding, all potential contractors and the managers of the government districts were given the precontract indicators for each district and the coverage and equity targets to be achieved by the end of the four-year test.

Contract awards were based on the quality of the technical proposal and on price. The nine operational districts included in the contracting test consisted of two contracted-out, three contracted-in, and four government districts. The test districts were spatially separated, in three different provinces. Each had a population of between 100,000 and nearly 200,000, for a total of over 1.25 million people (table 8.1).

NGOs were awarded four-year contracts at a fixed annual price per capita for administering and providing specific primary health care ser-

Table 8.1. *Districts Selected for Cambodia's Health Care Contracting Test*

Health care model and district	Province	Population (2001)
Contracted-out		
Ang Rokar	Takeo	109,459
Memut	Kampong Cham	109,321
Contracted-in		
Cheung Prey	Kampong Cham	167,725
Kirivong	Takeo	197,623
Pearaing	Prey Veng	188,854
Government		
Bati	Takeo	164,006
Kamchay Mear	Prey Veng	112,403
Kruoch Chmar	Kampong Cham	102,639
Preah Sdach	Prey Veng	110,013

Source: Ministry of Health, Cambodia.

vices. All winning bidders were international NGOs with previous experience working in Cambodia. Contracted-out districts were responsible for
purchasing their own supplies and materials and for paying labor costs.
These expenses were included in the Ministry of Health budget for contracted-in and government districts. Construction and renovation of health
centers, referral (district) hospitals, and district health offices, as well as fur-
niture and equipment, were provided for all nine test districts and were not
included as expenditures under the contracts. The Ministry of Health
retains ownership of these assets.

Average annual recurrent expenditure per capita during the two-and-a-
half year period was $3.88 for the contracted-out districts; $2.40 for the contracted-in districts; and $1.65 for the government districts (table 8.2). The
difference in expenditure levels between the contracted and government
districts is largely accounted for by NGO technical assistance provided by
district managers. Net of district management technical assistance, expenditure per capita for contracted-in districts ($1.63) was nearly the same as for
government districts ($1.65); the higher expenditure level for contracted-out
districts ($2.60) is largely attributable to higher staff salaries.

Research Questions

This study addresses the following questions:

1. Were primary health care services equally distributed before and
   after the contracting test? Which type of district made the largest

Table 8.2. *Average Annual Recurrent Expenditure Per Capita for Health Care Models in Contracting Test, Cambodia*
(U.S. dollars)

Expenditure category	Contracted-out	Contracted-in	Government provision
NGO technical assistance	1.28	0.77	0.0
Staff salaries[a]	1.32	0.55	0.53
Drugs, supplies, and operating expenses[b]	1.28	1.08	1.12
Total	*3.88*	*2.40*	*1.65*

Source: Schwartz 2001.
a. Salaries, bonuses, and other allowances.
b. Drugs, medical supplies, travel, fuel, per diem, office supplies, communications, building and vehicle maintenance and repair, and utilities.

gains in reaching the poor between the pre- and postcontracting surveys?

As is often the case in developing countries, we would expect an unequal distribution of health care services prior to the contracting test. Using bivariate analysis we examine the equity of the distribution of health care services before and after the trial in each test district, as well as the direction and magnitude of change during the trial, and compare contracted districts with government districts.

2. What factors other than wealth are related to an equitable distribution of primary health care services? When these factors are controlled, did the poor receive more health care services than the nonpoor in contracted or in government districts? What are the policy implications of these findings?

District managers faced different budget constraints, different baseline values for coverage and distribution of services, and possible differences in population demographics, all of which may have influenced resource allocation decisions. Recognizing these differences, we use multivariate methods to isolate the effect of contracting on distribution of services to the poor while controlling for these other related factors.

Methodology

To identify the poor, principal component analysis (PCA) is used to construct a wealth index of households. Concentration indexes and multivariate regressions are employed to test whether the distribution of health services to the poor improved under contracting.

Wealth Index

In the absence of income or consumption data from the household surveys, household ownership of assets, which serves as a proxy for household wealth, is used as the basis for constructing a wealth index for the study. To enable comparisons between the baseline and follow-up surveys, the types of household asset used to construct the index were restricted to those covered by questions asked in both household surveys: whether there was a permanent type of roof on the house (brick, cement, metal, or a combination of these materials) and whether anyone in the household owned a bicycle, radio, motorcycle, television, oxcart, motorboat, or at least one cow.

The wealth index was constructed by coding each asset as equal to one if the household had the asset and equal to zero if it did not. Principal component analysis, which searches for the linear combination of the assets that yields the maximum possible variance in the data, was conducted, and the first principal component was retained (Filmer and Pritchett 1999; Wagstaff 2002). The PCA wealth index was used to rank households (and thereby the individuals in each household) in the sample as a whole for each of the two surveys and was constructed separately for each of the nine districts for each survey.[2]

We follow the approach used by Wagstaff and Watanabe (2002), using artificial convenient regressions to test for any statistically significant differences between the equity results from ranking individuals within each district and those obtained by ranking individuals in the nine districts taken as a whole. The results of the tests indicate no statistically significant differences. That is, differences in the concentration indexes for the nine districts based on comparison of a wealth ranking of households from all districts with a wealth ranking of the households within each district are not statistically significant. In absolute terms, an individual ranked as poor in one district would be ranked as poor in all other districts. This suggests that observed differences in the equity of health care services between districts are not attributable to differences in wealth across districts and implies that at the time of the two surveys the populations in the districts made up a fairly homogeneous group of rural households as measured by asset ownership.[3]

Concentration Indexes

Bivariate concentration indexes were calculated to quantify the degree of economic inequality for health care service indicators across districts and across surveys. The Newey-West regression estimator, which corrects the standard error of the estimated concentration index for serial correlation of the fractional rank variable, as well as any heteroscedasticity, was used (Wagstaff, Paci, and van Doorslaer 1991; Newey and West 1994; Kakwani, Wagstaff, and van Doorslaer 1997).

Need-Standardized Use of Public Health Facilities

Assessment of the use of public health facilities for treatment of illness requires standardization to correct for differences in the need to seek health care at a public health facility. We assume that need for other health care services (child immunization, antenatal care, birth delivery by a trained professional, and so on) is the same for all individuals targeted for each of these types of care. For the use of public health facilities for treatment of illness, we follow the procedure developed by Wagstaff and van Doorslaer (2000) to take into account individuals' need for medical care. This procedure uses a two-step indirect standardization, with the estimation of a nonlinear prediction equation in the first step, to generate values of need-expected curative health care at a public facility.

To proxy the need for medical care, we include demographic dummy variables for gender and age categories in the estimation of a first-stage probit model for all individuals in each survey in order to obtain predictions of the probability that an individual will choose a public health facility for treatment of an illness.[4] The Newey-West regression estimator is used in the second step to obtain (a) the estimated concentration index and its standard error of the need-expected probability of seeking health care at a public health facility and (b) the indirectly standardized concentration index.[5]

Multivariate Method

We examine the relative weight of factors that may be related to the receipt of health services, using descriptive probit regressions. In this analysis, no attempt is made to model all the factors that predict the receipt of services in each survey. Rather, we use the multivariate analysis as an extension to confirm the bivariate analysis and to test whether the simple correlations between wealth and receipt of services and between contracted and noncontracted districts hold when controlling for other related factors such as district expenditures, initial coverage levels, and population demographics. A probit regression is estimated for the pooled precontract (1997) and evaluation (2001) surveys for each health service indicator.

Nature and Source of Data

The baseline household survey was carried out in May–June 1997; the follow-up survey was conducted in June–August 2001, two and a half years after the contractors were in place in the first quarter of 1998.[6] The follow-up household survey used the same baseline survey instrument, with a few exceptions.

The Sample

A standard cluster survey methodology was used for the household surveys. The sample size was calculated so as to allow each district to be compared with its own performance statistics at the time of the follow-up survey. In each district, 30 villages (clusters) were selected randomly, stratified by health center catchment area with a probability proportionate to population size. The total population of each district was divided by 30 (clusters), giving a sampling interval of k, where each kth village was selected as a survey cluster. The probability of a village's being selected was thus proportional to the size of the population of that village.[7] The same villages sampled in the baseline survey were resurveyed in the 2001 follow-up survey.

Sample sizes were calculated to yield reliable estimates of the immunization status of children age 12–23 months, antenatal care provision, and type of birth attendant. For immunization, 7 children age 12–23 months were required from each cluster to provide 210 children per district for estimates ±10 percent, with a 95 percent confidence interval. For antenatal and birth provider information, 7 women who had given birth within the prior 12 months (including stillbirths but excluding miscarriages) were required from each cluster, yielding 210 women in each district for estimates ±10 percent, with a 95 percent confidence interval.[8] Thus, in each district about 420 households were sampled, consisting of about 210 households with a child between 12 and 23 months old and about 210 households with a woman who had given birth in the previous year. There was some overlapping of households where both conditions were met.

In addition to information on child immunization, antenatal care, and birth provider, data were collected from all sampled households on socioeconomic and demographic characteristics, as well as on use of curative health care services by all individuals in each household. Because the average household size in both surveys is between five and six individuals, sample sizes, depending on the health care indicator, range from about 210 children, 210 women, and 420 households to more than 2,000 individuals in each district. In all, more than 20,000 individuals are included in each household survey (table 8.3).

Health Care Indicators

The contractual indicators used for service coverage are consistent with the priority topics that have a prominent place in the United Nations Millennium Development Goals (MDGs) and that appear frequently in World Bank poverty reduction strategy papers (PRSPs). These focus on preventive child and maternal health care—for example, child immunization and vitamin A provision, antenatal care, delivery by a trained birth attendant, delivery in a health facility, and use and knowledge of modern birth-spacing

Table 8.3. Sample Sizes, Cambodia Study

Health care model and district	Child age 12–23 months		Child age 6–59 months		Women with birth in prior 12 months		Women with child age 6–23 months		Individuals reported sick in past 4 weeks		Total individuals		Total households	
	1997	2001	1997	2001	1997	2001	1997	2001	1997	2001	1997	2001	1997	2001
Contracted-out														
Ang Rokar	203	208	329	346	211	210	418	408	496	616	2,245	2,275	418	408
Memut	197	208	361	351	199	209	399	414	523	529	2,235	2,403	399	414
Contracted-in														
Cheung Prey	196	209	371	353	212	210	409	410	510	558	2,352	2,267	409	410
Kirivong	196	207	333	342	205	210	407	409	404	543	2,291	2,388	407	409
Pearaing	209	203	343	333	205	210	415	413	569	471	2,408	2,248	415	413
Government provision														
Bati	206	209	367	348	211	210	417	412	549	591	2,369	2,331	417	412
Kamchay Mear	206	207	341	328	202	210	411	416	533	428	2,223	2,019	411	416
Kruoch Chmar	218	205	380	345	201	209	419	415	267	605	2,325	2,323	419	415
Preah Sdach	194	204	306	342	220	210	418	414	606	512	2,589	2,130	418	414
Total	1,825	1,860	3,131	3,088	1,866	1,888	3,713	3,711	4,457	4,853	21,037	20,384	3,713	3,711

Source: Keller and Schwartz 2001.

methods. No specific coverage goal was given for the use of public health care facilities for curative care—only that the poor be targeted for services. Table 8.4 provides definitions of the health care indicators included in the contracts and goals.

Baseline and follow-up values for the health care service indicators are given in table 8.5. At the time of the follow-up survey in mid-2001, well before completion of the contracting test at the end of 2002, most districts had already achieved several of the predefined contractual goals, which many people had thought overambitious at the time the contracts were awarded. Initial large investments of capital and labor were likely responsible for much of this early success, but returns to these investments were increasingly marginal. Still, the increases in indicators achieved by mid-2001 were impressive (figure 8.1; tables 8.5 and 8.6). The overall average in

Table 8.4. *Health Service Indicators: Definitions and Coverage Goals, Contracting-Out Test, Cambodia*

Indicator	Definition	Goal (percent)
Fully immunized child (FIC)	Children age 12–23 months fully immunized.	70
Vitamin A (VITA)	High-dose vitamin A received twice in the past 12 months by children age 6–59 months.	70
Antenatal care (ANC)	At least two antenatal care visits, with blood pressure measurement at least once, for women who gave birth in the prior year.	50
Delivery by trained professional (TDEL)	Birth attendant was a qualified nurse, midwife, doctor, or medical assistant for women with a delivery in the past year.	50
Delivery in a health facility (FDEL)	Birth was in a private or public health facility for women with a delivery in the past year.	10
Use of modern birth-spacing method (MBS)	Women with a live child age 6–23 months currently using a modern method of birth spacing.	30
Knowledge of modern birth spacing (KBS)	Women who gave birth in the prior 24 months know four or more modern birth-spacing methods and where to obtain them.	70
Use of public health care facilities (USE)	Use of district public health care facilities (district hospital or primary health care center) for illness in the prior four weeks.	Increase[a]

Source: Ministry of Health, Cambodia.
a. Percentage goal not specified.

Table 8.5. Health Care Service Coverage by District and Indicator, Cambodia, 1997 and 2001 Surveys (percent)

Health care model and district	Fully immunized child (FIC)		Vitamin A (VITA)		Antenatal care (ANC)		Delivery by trained professional (TDEL)		Delivery in health facility (FDEL)		Use of modern birth-spacing method (MBS)		Knowledge of modern birth spacing (KBS)		Use of public health care facilities (USE)	
	1997	2001	1997	2001	1997	2001	1997	2001	1997	2001	1997	2001	1997	2001	1997	2001
Contracted-out																
Ang Rokar	27.1	57.2	28.5	53.8	20.4	65.2	43.6	42.4	9.9	16.2	8.9	29.3	11.7	90.7	0.4	15.3
Memut	23.3	73.6	47.1	57.8	6.1	42.1	18.9	25.7	2.0	11.0	17.3	37.1	19.5	58.9	0.9	7.1
Contracted-in																
Cheung Prey	26.5	49.8	50.1	38.5	22.2	53.9	28.8	21.4	2.4	7.6	17.8	29.9	22.0	57.8	1.7	3.5
Kirivong	40.8	61.8	46.5	62.9	10.7	36.7	13.2	24.8	4.8	8.6	15.3	35.2	17.9	80.9	0.7	5.2
Pearaing	23.4	53.7	33.2	64.0	4.3	25.2	39.7	52.6	2.9	19.5	12.9	33.0	21.2	66.3	0.4	5.3
Government provision																
Bati	64.5	76.6	46.5	56.9	17.1	42.4	43.6	49.5	5.2	12.4	15.6	27.2	16.4	85.4	0.8	5.1
Kamchay Mear	24.3	40.6	36.4	34.1	3.5	16.2	14.9	24.8	0.5	4.8	10.7	23.7	20.0	77.6	1.1	1.4
Kruoch Chmar	31.7	68.8	50.5	24.4	16.4	21.5	28.9	31.9	4.9	9.0	13.8	24.6	27.7	64.3	0.9	3.2
Preah Sdach	15.5	27.9	32.7	38.9	5.0	10.5	10.5	13.8	2.3	1.9	16.5	29.2	12.9	68.6	1.1	1.9

Source: Cambodia contracting test, baseline and follow-up household surveys.
Note: See table 8.4 for full definitions of terms.

Figure 8.1. *Changes in Health Care Coverage Rates, Cambodia Study, 1997–2001*

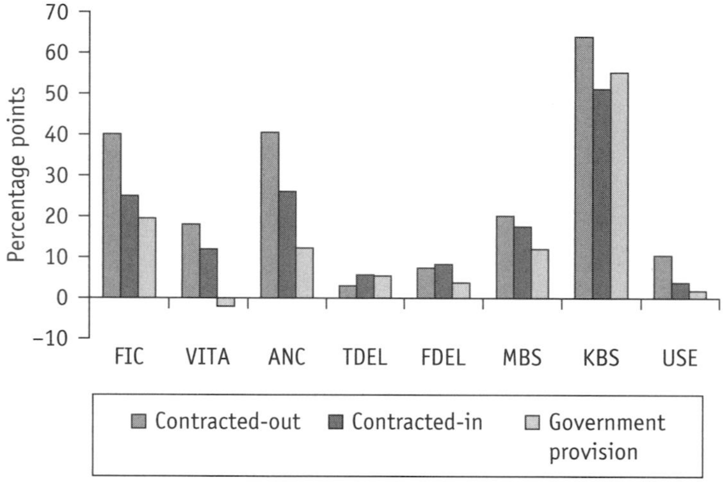

Source: Cambodia contracting test, baseline and follow-up household surveys.

Note: FIC, fully immunized child; VITA, vitamin A; ANC, antenatal care; TDEL, delivery by trained professional; FDEL, delivery in a health facility; MBS, use of modern birth-spacing method; KBS, knowledge of modern birth spacing; USE, use of public health care facilities. For full definitions of terms, see table 8.4.

the nine districts for fully immunized children, for example, increased from 30.9 to 56.7 percent, almost doubling in two and a half years.

Findings about Distribution

Contracted districts outperformed the government districts with respect to changes in the distribution of health care services from an initial distribution favoring the nonpoor toward a more equitable or pro-poor distribution.

Baseline Distribution

As expected, the 1997 baseline distribution of health care services in the nine test districts is found to be inequitable in all districts, largely to the disadvantage of the poor. Concentration indexes for health care services before and after the contracting test began are given in table 8.7.[9] Negative values indicate a pro-poor distribution, and positive values indicate a distribution favoring the nonpoor.

Table 8.6. Changes in Health Care Service Coverage by District and Indicator, Cambodia, 1997–2001 (percentage points)

Health care model and district	Fully immunized child (FIC)	Vitamin A (VITA)	Antenatal care (ANC)	Delivery by trained professional (TDEL)	Delivery in health facility (FDEL)	Use of modern birth-spacing method (MBS)	Knowledge of modern birth spacing (KBS)	Use of public health care facility (USE)
Contracted-out								
Ang Rokar	30.1	25.2	44.7	-1.2	6.2	20.4	79.0	14.9
Memut	50.2	10.7	36.0	6.8	9.0	19.8	49.4	6.2
Contracted-in								
Cheung Prey	23.3	-11.5	31.7	-7.8	5.2	12.0	35.8	1.8
Kirivong	21.0	16.4	26.0	11.6	3.7	19.9	73.0	4.5
Pearaing	30.3	30.8	20.8	12.9	16.6	20.1	45.1	4.9
Government provision								
Bati	12.0	10.3	25.3	5.9	7.2	11.6	70.5	4.3
Kamchay Mear	16.3	-2.3	12.7	9.9	4.3	13.0	57.6	0.3
Kruoch Chmar	37.1	-26.2	5.1	3.0	4.1	10.8	36.6	2.3
Preah Sdach	12.4	6.2	5.5	3.3	-0.4	12.7	55.7	0.8

Source: Cambodia contracting test, baseline and follow-up household surveys.
Note: See table 8.4 for full definitions of terms.

Table 8.7. Concentration Indexes, Cambodia, 1997 and 2001 Surveys

Health care model and district	Fully immunized child (FIC)		Vitamin A (VITA)		Antenatal care (ANC)		Delivery by trained professional (TDEL)		Delivery in health facility (FDEL)		Use of modern birth-spacing method (MBS)		Knowledge of modern birth spacing (KBS)		Use of public health care facilities (USE)	
	1997	2001	1997	2001	1997	2001	1997	2001	1997	2001	1997	2001	1997	2001	1997	2001
Contracted-out																
Ang Rokar	0.131*	−0.028	−0.030	−0.028	0.011	−0.020	0.100*	−0.099*	0.371*	0.187	−0.003	0.004	−0.017	−0.007	0.051	−0.091*
Memut	0.178*	0.022	0.007	0.013	0.439*	0.136*	0.293*	0.189*	0.332	0.399*	0.197*	0.023	0.444*	0.026	0.236	−0.096*
Contracted-in																
Cheung Prey	0.159*	0.006	0.052	0.029	0.057	0.032	0.020	0.132	0.228	0.175	−0.112	−0.009	0.074	−0.010	0.065	0.127*
Kirivong	0.066	0.026	−0.055	0.001	−0.136	−0.348	−0.105	−0.310	−0.234	−0.439	0.118	0.011	0.024	0.009	0.004	−0.058
Pearaing	0.172	−0.015	0.094*	0.003	0.230	0.189*	0.118*	0.131*	0.049	0.185*	−0.077	−0.070	0.110*	−0.006	0.072	0.075
Government provision																
Bati	0.040	−0.004	0.059	0.003	0.017	0.042	0.031	0.429	−0.140	0.129	0.174	0.162	0.091	0.010	−0.103	−0.051
Kamchay Mear	−0.021	0.058	0.038	−0.029	−0.112	0.316*	0.022	0.273*	−0.333	0.205	0.251*	0.164*	0.229*	0.210*	−0.287*	0.134
Kruoch Chmar	0.182*	0.081*	0.017	0.113*	0.152	0.291*	0.066	0.269*	0.172	0.359*	0.180*	0.298	0.077	0.040	−0.154	0.094
Preah Sdach	0.021	−0.031	0.042	0.059	0.225	0.508*	0.186	0.297*	0.229	0.024	0.175*	0.021	0.001	0.009	0.247	0.296*

Source: Cambodia contracting test, baseline and follow-up household surveys.
Note: See table 8.4 for full definitions of the terms.
* Statistically significant at the 0.05 level.

Only one indicator, the use of public facilities for illness in Kamchay Mear, shows a statistically significant distribution in favor of the poor before the contracting test began. Immunization, use of a trained birth practitioner, and use and knowledge of modern birth spacing account for most of the remaining statistically significant indexes that have relatively large inequality levels in favor of the nonpoor. Eight of these concentration indexes are in the two districts selected for contracting-out, Ang Rokar and Memut, and these show the highest level of inequality for five of the eight health care indicators.

Of the three districts chosen for contracting-in, Pearaing has three statistically significant and positive health service indexes (vitamin A, trained birth delivery, and knowledge of modern birth spacing), and Cheung Prey has one (fully immunized child). Four of the eight health care services in the districts to be contracted-in do not have statistically significant indexes, suggesting that the concentration index is not different from zero, or a wealth-neutral distribution of these services at the baseline. The remaining six statistically significant indexes are spread over the four government districts selected for comparisons in the contracting test. These indexes show that three of the government districts have distributions favoring the nonpoor for the use of modern birth spacing. Four of the health care services in these districts—vitamin A, antenatal care, trained birth practitioner, and facility delivery—do not have statistically significant indexes, suggesting an equitable distribution of these services.

Follow-Up Distribution

Two and a half years into the contracting test, the distribution of health care services overall appears to have shifted toward a more equitable distribution that is less favorable to the nonpoor across the nine districts, but with few exceptions the distribution is not pro-poor. In 2001 contracted-out districts show pro-poor use of public facilities. Half of the concentration indexes found for three of the four government districts favor the nonpoor, and these are spread across all health care services. The remaining government district (Bati) appears to be an exception, with no statistically significant concentration indexes in 2001, indicating an equal distribution of services across poor and nonpoor groups.

Changes between the Baseline and Follow-Up Surveys

Perhaps more important than the static results found for the baseline and midterm surveys are the direction and magnitude of changes in concentra-

Figure 8.2. *Changes in Concentration Index by Health Care Indicator and Model, Cambodia Study*

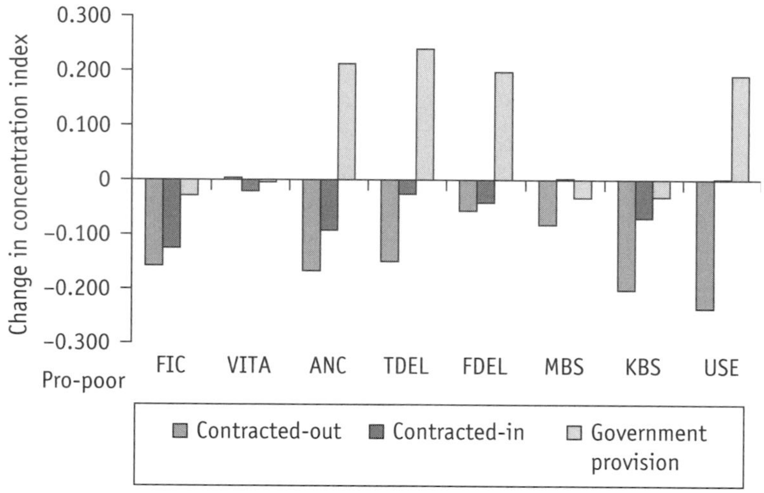

Source: Cambodia contracting test, baseline and follow-up household surveys.

Note: FIC, fully immunized child; VITA, vitamin A; ANC, antenatal care; TDEL, delivery by trained professional; FDEL, delivery in a health facility; MBS, use of modern birth-spacing method; KBS, knowledge of modern birth spacing; USE, use of public health care facilities. For full definitions of terms, see table 8.4.

tion indexes. These suggest that the provision of health care services in contracted districts has become more equitable or more pro-poor during the time that the contracting test has been in place (figure 8.2). The direction, magnitude, and statistical significance of changes in the concentration indexes between the baseline and midterm surveys are given in table 8.8.

Of the statistically significant changes in concentration indexes, all those for the contracted-out districts show movement toward improving equity in the provision of health care services. Negative values, indicating an increase in a pro-poor distribution (or a decrease in a distribution favoring the nonpoor) are found for immunization, trained birth delivery, knowledge of birth-spacing methods, and use of public facilities in contracted-out districts. Similarly, for contracted-in districts, all the statistically significant changes in concentration indexes show movement toward a more pro-poor distribution of health care services, including immunization and knowledge of modern birth spacing. By contrast, all but one statistically significant change in concentration indexes for the government districts show movement toward a nonpoor distribution of services. All are in the same three government districts found to have distributions favoring the nonpoor in the 2001 survey.

Table 8.8. Change in Concentration Indexes by District and Health Care Indicator, Cambodia, 1997–2001

Health care model and district	Fully immunized child (FIC)	Vitamin A (VITA)	Antenatal care (ANC)	Delivery by trained professional (TDEL)	Delivery in health facility (FDEL)	Use of modern birth-spacing method (MBS)	Knowledge of modern birth spacing (KBS)	Use of public health care facility (USE)
Contracted-out								
Ang Rokar	-0.159*	0.003	-0.031	-0.199*	-0.184	0.006	0.010	-0.142*
Memut	-0.156*	0.006	-0.303	-0.104	0.067	-0.173	-0.419*	-0.333 *
Contracted-in								
Cheung Prey	-0.154*	-0.024	-0.026	0.112	-0.054	0.104	-0.084	0.062
Kirivong	-0.039	0.056	-0.212	-0.205	-0.206	-0.107	-0.015	-0.061
Pearaing	-0.187*	-0.092	-0.041	0.013	0.136	0.007	-0.116*	0.004
Government provision								
Bati	-0.044	-0.056	0.25	0.398	0.269	-0.012	-0.082	0.052
Kamchay Mear	0.079	-0.067	0.427*	0.251*	0.538	-0.088	-0.019*	0.421*
Kruoch Chmar	-0.101	0.096	0.139	0.203*	0.187	0.118	-0.038	0.247
Preah Sdach	-0.052	0.018	0.282	0.111	-0.205	-0.155	0.008	0.049

Source: Cambodia contracting baseline and followup household surveys.
* Statistically significant at the 0.05 level.

Multivariate Results

The multivariate results are consistent with the findings of the bivariate concentration indexes. When differences in district expenditures and demographic characteristics are controlled for, the contracted districts perform better in targeting the poorer half of the population than do the government districts. District managers in contracted districts appear to be more responsive and more effective in organizing, managing, and monitoring service delivery to reach the poor than district managers in government districts, all else being equal.

For each of the health care services, we include time (2001 survey), membership in the poorest half of households, district location (collinear with district expenditures), and mother and child characteristics as categorical (dummy) variables in probit regressions to examine the relative weight of each factor on the likelihood of an individual's receiving the health care service. In addition, we include interaction terms for membership in the poorest half of the households, location in a contracted district, and time (2001 survey) to examine more systematically the effect of contracting on the distribution of services.

The probit results for the pooled baseline and follow-up survey data are given in table 8.9. They include estimated (transformed) coefficients, which show the effect on the probability of receiving each service of a discrete change in each dummy variable (omitted category noted) from zero to one (dF/dx) while holding all else constant.[10] Underlying coefficients found to be statistically significant at the 0.01 level are noted. The regression coefficients were obtained using Stata statistical software, with a *probit* estimation, and the transformed coefficients (dF/dx), or marginal effects, were obtained using the *dprobit* Stata command. The transformed coefficients indicate the independent effect on the predicted probability of changing each categorical variable relative to the omitted variable. The standard errors of coefficient estimates are corrected for multiple observations in villages using the cluster option.

The most striking results are found for the independent effect of the interaction term for household wealth, location in a contracted district, and time (2001 survey). The statistically significant and positive results suggest that individuals from the poorest half of households in contracted districts in 2001 were more likely to receive health care services.[11]

Because the district location variable is perfectly collinear with per capita expenditure in each district, the independent effect of district location captures differences in expenditure levels, as well as other district-specific differences in health delivery system management, implementation methods, and supervision. The district location variables are found to be positive and statistically significant independent factors of the likelihood of receiving services relative to the omitted low-performing government district, when controlling for other factors included in the estimation. A child living in Memut, for example, is estimated to have a 0.285 higher probability of being fully immunized than one living in Preah Sdach, the omitted government district. Residence in any of the three government districts included is also found to be a statistically significant and positive factor in the probability of full immunization relative to the omitted government district, and these effects are seen to be large. A child living in Bati, for example, had a 0.445 higher probability of being fully immunized than one living in Preah Sdach. While the coverage statistics indicated increased full immunization coverage in all districts, the multivariate results for the pooled sample, controlling for other factors, appear to give added weight for large increases in full immunization (Memut and Krouch Chmar), and for sustained, relatively high full immunization coverage (Bati and Kirivong).

The independent effect of time (that is, of an observation's being from the 2001 follow-up survey) on the likelihood of receiving each of the health care services is positive and statistically significant and suggests that all individuals, regardless of location and other factors, were more likely to receive these health care services in 2001 than at the time of the baseline survey. These results are consistent with the increases in health care service coverage rates shown in table 8.6.

The results for the independent effect of wealth in the pooled baseline and follow-up sample suggest that individuals from the poorest half of the population are less likely to receive child immunization, to be delivered by a trained birth attendant, and to know and use modern birth-spacing methods but are more likely to use public facilities for illness. In addition, the results found for the interaction term for being an individual from the poorest half of households at the time of the follow-up survey in 2001 suggest that these individuals were less likely to receive vitamin A and antenatal care and to use public facilities. Together, these results suggest that in all districts, being poor was and still is associated with a lower likelihood of receiving health care services. The results are consistent with the bivariate concentration indexes in table 8.7, which indicate that few health care services are well targeted to the poor in any of the districts, contracted or not.

The results found for the control variables for mother and child characteristics suggest that mothers' education is positively associated with a higher likelihood of a child's receiving health care services. This is a common finding in the literature.

Table 8.9. *Probit Results, Marginal Effects (dF/dx) on the Probability of Health Services Received in the Pooled Baseline and Follow-Up Surveys, Cambodia*

Variable	Fully immunized child (FIC)	Vitamin A (VITA)	Antenatal care (ANC)	Delivery by trained professional (TDEL)	Delivery in health facility (FDEL)	Use of modern birth-spacing method (MBS)	Knowledge of modern birth spacing (KBS)	Use of public health care facility (USE)
2001 follow-up survey	0.249*	0.073*	0.263*	0.066*	0.057*	0.140*	0.558*	0.198*
Household wealth								
Poorest one-half	−0.072*	−0.011	−0.009	−0.049*	−0.019	−0.050*	−0.063*	0.038*
Interaction terms								
Poorest one-half, contracted district, 2001 survey	0.085*	0.107*	0.145*	0.066*	0.013	0.066*	0.059*	0.124*
Poorest one-half, 2001 survey	0.009	−0.068*	−0.132*	−0.054	−0.015	−0.005	0.007	−0.106*
District (Preah Sdach omitted)								
Contracted-out (highest expenditures)								
Ang Rokar	0.165*	0.008	0.367*	0.305*	0.114*	0.005	0.077*	0.223*
Memut	0.285*	0.135*	0.207*	0.156*	0.071*	0.016*	0.104*	0.089*
Contracted-in (medium expenditures)								
Cheung Prey	0.149*	0.055	0.353*	0.158*	0.039*	−0.016	−0.039	0.020
Kirivong	0.274*	0.150*	0.153*	0.055	0.054*	−0.014	−0.005	0.041*
Pearaing	0.129*	0.083*	0.023	0.349*	0.101	−0.040	−0.011	0.038*
Government provision (lowest expenditures)								
Bati	0.445*	0.136*	0.258*	0.352*	0.078*	−0.037	0.077*	0.050*
Kamchay Mear	0.108*	−0.014	0.009	0.088*	−0.001	−0.070*	0.090*	0.015
Krouch Chmar	0.279*	0.007	0.156*	0.212*	0.065*	−0.053*	0.043	0.029

	(1)	(2)	(3)	(4)	(5)	(6)	(7)	(8)
Mother's education (omitted variable, no education)								
1–3 years	0.069*	-0.020	0.073*	0.060*		-0.010	-0.006	0.075*
4–6 years	0.118*	0.040*	0.108*	0.122*		0.025*	0.030*	0.104*
7+ years	0.185*	0.063*	0.187*	0.258*		0.089*	0.070*	0.186*
Mother's age (years) (omitted variable, <20)								
20–24	0.019	0.086	0.053	-0.033		-0.006	0.116*	0.077*
25–29	0.031	0.115*	0.059*	-0.057		-0.024	0.115*	0.083*
30–34	0.056	0.156*	0.041	-0.078*		-0.013	0.126*	0.096*
35–39	0.037	0.113*	0.030	-0.095*		-0.022*	0.079	0.057
40+	0.001	0.099*	-0.022	-0.050		-0.010	0.061	0.025
Child's sex = male								
Sex = male	0.032*	0.008	—	—		—	—	-0.009
Age (months) (omitted variable, <5)								
5–19								-0.001
20–29								0.005
30–39								0.004
40+								0.002
Predicted probability	0.439	0.447	0.210	0.274	0.061	0.202	0.422	0.110
Number of observations	3,619	6,219	3,754	3,754	3,754	5,290	7,424	9,310
LR χ^2	578.3	205.8	710.7	441.9	211.9	169.4	2,727.1	1,059.7
Prob > χ^2	0.000	0.000	0.000	0.000	0.000	0.000	0.000	0.000
Pseudo R^2	0.116	0.124	0.174	0.097	0.111	0.108	0.267	0.141
Log likelihood	-2,196.4	-2,174.1	-1,685.7	-2,052.8	-849.4	-1,695.6	-3,738.6	-3,271.7

Note: See table 8.4 for fuller definitions of terms.

* Statistically significant at the 0.01 level.

Limitations

The study is limited by inability to identify differences in underlying motivations, resource allocation decisions, incentives, and district managers' service delivery and monitoring methods. These shortcomings may have led to the observed differences in the distribution of health care services in contracted districts compared with government districts.

Until further research is conducted, we can only speculate about the reasons for the varied outcomes. Perhaps the international NGO managers were better trained than their local counterparts in management, implementation, supervision, and monitoring methods for targeting the poor. Perhaps the NGO district managers expected future personal rewards if they achieved all the goals set for them. This was the first large-scale contracting experience for the NGOs, and it may be that proven managers were assigned to Cambodia to increase the chances of success and enable the NGOs to maintain a good reputation for providing health care services in developing countries and possibly to win follow-on contracts or contracts in other countries. Perhaps higher guaranteed wages and bonuses paid to health care workers in contracted districts provided more effective motivation to attain contractual goals—and more than compensated for unofficial fees and bonuses collected by government health care workers. These types of questions need further investigation, in general and in other large-scale contracting projects such as those in Afghanistan, Bangladesh, and Pakistan.

Implications

The Cambodia contracting test is the first known large-scale test with baseline and follow-up survey data suitable for systematic examination of whether NGO contracts are an effective means of providing health care services that reach the poor. This chapter compares contracted districts with noncontracted government districts, using data from the 1997 baseline and 2001 follow-up household surveys, to determine which districts were successful in targeting health care services to the poorest half of households—an equity goal for all districts included in the test. Bivariate concentration indexes and multivariate analysis results are consistent. They suggest that although all districts increased health care service coverage, the contracted districts outperformed the government districts in targeting services to the poor, even when controlling for other factors, including differences in expenditure levels, starting values, and demographics.

It is difficult to generalize to other countries Cambodia's experience with reaching the poor through contracting services. The dearth of physical infrastructure and the large numbers of entrenched government health care workers in rural areas of Cambodia at the start of the contracting test were conditions conducive to innovative approaches such as rational redelineation of operational districts and testing of new service delivery methods to rapidly rebuild the primary health care system. Circumstances are similar in densely populated urban areas in the four largest cities of Bangladesh and the rural areas of Afghanistan and Pakistan. The results of large-scale contracting projects in those areas could help shed light on the question of whether the experience in Cambodia offers an effective model for other developing countries.

Notes

We are indebted to the Ministry of Health of the Royal Government of Cambodia for permission to conduct the study. We also thank Davidson Gwatkin, Benjamin Loevinsohn, Adam Wagstaff, Abdo Yazbek, and two anonymous reviewers for helpful comments and suggestions. Any remaining errors are our own.

1. A similar contracting experiment in Guatemala to improve service delivery to indigenous people did not collect precontract baseline data that would have enabled pre- and postcontract comparisons (Loevinsohn 2000).

2. An alternative index that weighted household assets by the scarcity of the assets was also tested and produced similar results.

3. The index constructed for each district is arbitrarily chosen to present the remaining results of the study.

4. Use of public health facilities only for those who reported an illness, standardized for choosing a public health facility, was also tested and produced nearly identical results.

5. Details of the method may be found in World Bank (2002).

6. No significant change in service coverage was experienced between the baseline survey in mid-1997 and the beginning of the contracting test in 1999. The intervening period was taken up by preparatory steps: the international bidding process, construction and rehabilitation of health facilities, and procurement of equipment.

7. Further details of village mapping, randomized selection of eligible households, sample sizes, within-district statistical confidence intervals, and survey instruments for household and health facility surveys are given in Keller and Schwartz (2001).

8. The sample sizes include an adjustment of 2x for the clustering effect. It was assumed initially that 30 percent of women received antenatal care.

9. A complete listing of concentration indexes, standard errors, *t*-values, and sample sizes for each indicator is available from the authors on request.

10. The results shown for child immunization are reported in Schwartz and Bhushan (forthcoming).

11. An exception is birth delivery in a health facility, which was found to be positive but not statistically significant.

References

Bhushan, Indu, Sheryl Keller, and J. Brad Schwartz. 2002. Achieving the twin objectives of efficiency and equity: Contracting health services in Cambodia. ERD Policy Brief 6, Economics and Research Department, Asian Development Bank, Manila.

Filmer, Deon, and Lant Pritchett. 1999. The effect of household wealth on educational attainment: Evidence from 35 countries. *Population and Development Review* 25(1): 85–120.

Kakwani, Nanak, Adam Wagstaff, and Eddy van Doorslaer. 1997. Socioeconomic inequalities in health: Measurement, computation, and statistical inference. *Journal of Econometrics* 77(1): 87–104.

Keller, Sheryl, and J. Brad Schwartz. 2001. Evaluation report: Contracting for health services pilot project. Social Sectors Division, Mekong Department, Asian Development Bank, Manila.

Loevinsohn, Benjamin. 2000. Contracting for the delivery of primary health care in Cambodia: Design and initial experience of a large pilot-test. WBI Online Journal. World Bank, Washington, DC. http://info.worldbank.org/etools/docs/library/48616/oj_cambodia.pdf.

NIS (National Institute of Statistics), Directorate General for Health, Cambodia, and ORC Macro. 2000. *National Health Survey 1998*. Phnom Penh.

Newey, W. K., and K. D. West. 1994. Automatic lag selection in covariance matrix estimation. *Review of Economic Studies* 61(4): 631–53.

Schwartz, J. Brad. 2001. Cost-effectiveness of contracting health care services in Cambodia. Social Sectors Division, Mekong Department, Asian Development Bank, Manila.

Schwartz, J. Brad, and Indu Bhushan. Forthcoming. Improving equity in immunization through public-private partnership in Cambodia. University of North Carolina at Chapel Hill and Asian Development Bank.

Wagstaff, Adam. 2002. Inequalities in health in developing countries: Swimming against the tide? Policy Research Working Paper 2795, World Bank, Washington, DC.

Wagstaff, Adam, and Eddy van Doorslaer. 2000. Measuring and testing for inequity in the delivery of health care. *Journal of Human Resources* 35(4): 716–33.

Wagstaff, Adam, and Naoko Watanabe. 2002. What difference does the choice of SES make in health inequality measurement? Technical note, World Bank, Washington, DC.

Wagstaff, Adam, Pierella Paci, and Eddy van Doorslaer. 1991. On the measurement of inequalities in health. *Social Science and Medicine* 33: 545–57.

World Bank. 2002. Quantitative techniques for health equity analysis: Technical notes. Technical note 13, World Bank, Washington, DC.

9

India: Assessing the Reach of Three SEWA Health Services among the Poor

M. Kent Ranson, Palak Joshi, Mittal Shah, and Yasmin Shaikh

The Self-Employed Women's Association (SEWA), a trade union of informal women workers, was founded in 1972 by Ela Bhatt in Ahmedabad, Gujarat State, India, and is headquartered there. It has more than 469,000 members in 9 of the state's 19 districts.[1] SEWA "is an organization of poor, self-employed women workers. These are women who earn a living through their own labor or small businesses. They do not obtain regular salaried employment with welfare benefits like workers in the organized sector. They are the unprotected labor force of [India]" (SEWA 1999, 83). The organization has two main goals: to organize women workers to achieve full employment and to make them individually and collectively self-reliant, economically independent, and capable of making their own decisions.

Illness, disability, and death are major threats to the overall security of SEWA members. Almost since its inception, SEWA has provided preventive and primary health care in one form or another. Unlike many other SEWA services, such as savings and credit through SEWA Bank and insurance through Vimo SEWA, the services provided by SEWA Health are available to nonmembers as well as to SEWA members. Providing health services to the very poor, particularly those living in areas not otherwise served by government or by nongovernmental organizations (NGOs), has been one of SEWA's primary objectives. Providing health care services to this poor, largely illiterate, and geographically dispersed population poses many challenges.

In India, as elsewhere, the poor die earlier and have higher levels of morbidity than the better off (World Bank 2003). One reason is the difficulty they face in obtaining health care services. In theory, government provision of health care should cover the poor, but in practice it often does not. This leaves health policy makers and donors with the vexing problem of identifying and overcoming constraints faced by the poor in accessing health care. Health care provision through NGOs—or member-based organizations, or community-based organizations, or people's organizations—has been suggested as one means of "reaching the poor" (Pachauri 1994).

Research Questions and Background

District-specific data on the availability and utilization of health services are limited, especially with respect to the activities of private and unqualified practitioners. Gujarat, in comparison with India as a whole, has a thriving private for-profit health care sector. The problems with publicly and privately provided care are the same in Gujarat as elsewhere in India: a large but underfunded public sector, a fast-growing but unregulated private sector, and high out-of-pocket expenditures by patients (Peters and others 2002).

Most people in both urban and rural Gujarat use the private sector for outpatient and inpatient services. According to the 1995–96 National Sample Survey Organization (NSSO) survey, 81.8 percent of outpatient treatments among rural residents and 76.3 percent of treatments in urban areas were received from private sector providers. The private sector accounted for 71.0 percent of hospitalizations in urban Gujarat and for 67.4 percent in rural Gujarat (Mahal and others 2000). Among the areas included in this study, the public health care system is strong only in Ahmedabad City, where four large government hospitals provide outpatient and inpatient care.

Distance and lack of financial resources are major barriers to access to health care among the poor in Gujarat. In the districts covered in this study, health care, particularly expensive curative inpatient care, is widely available in urban centers. But for those who live in villages far from an urban center, the closest source of allopathic care may be many hours away. "Twelve percent of rural women have to travel at least 5 km to reach the nearest health facility" (IIPS and ORC Macro 2001, 33).

SEWA's Health Services

SEWA first became actively involved in the public health field in the early 1970s with health education and provision of maternity benefits. In the early

1980s SEWA negotiated with the government of India to help distribute maternity benefits to poor women. (Ghee, a dairy product similar to butter, was provided in kind.) A focus of SEWA Health has always been to build capacity among local women, especially traditional midwives (*dais*), so that they become the barefoot doctors of their communities. Today, SEWA's health-related activities are many and diverse. They include primary health care, delivered through 60 stationary health centers and mobile health camps; health education and training; capacity building among local SEWA leaders and dais; provision of high-quality, low-cost drugs through drug shops; occupational and mental health activities; and production and marketing of traditional medicines.

Equity has always been a key concern at SEWA Health. SEWA Union targets the poorest women workers—those who work in the informal sector. SEWA Health aims to provide services to the poorest among SEWA Union's members, particularly those who are living below the poverty line (less than $1 per day). Administrators at SEWA Health were particularly interested in this study because of their desire to assess the extent to which their services reach the poorest and to learn how the services might be better targeted. The study deals with three specific activities: reproductive health mobile camps, tuberculosis detection and treatment, and women's health education, as described in table 9.1.

The size of SEWA Health's target population varies somewhat by type of service. For example, tuberculosis detection and treatment services are delivered to men and women of all ages in two of Ahmedabad City's five zones. The reproductive health mobile camps and the women's health education sessions target women of reproductive age, particularly those who are SEWA Union members. SEWA Union's total membership in Gujarat State is 469,306. In the areas covered by this study, membership is 153,813 in Ahmedabad City, 30,219 in Ahmedabad District (excluding Ahmedabad City), and 100,316 in Anand and Kheda Districts. (Anand District was formed from Kheda District in 2001; because the data cover Kheda District before the division, we refer to Anand-Kheda as a single district in the study.)

REPRODUCTIVE HEALTH (RH) MOBILE CAMPS. In response to demand from people in remote and underserviced areas, SEWA Health began organizing mobile health camps in 1999. The camps typically address a certain set of illnesses—for example, general eye health, male reproductive tract infections, and female reproductive and child health.[2] The RH mobile camps are the most frequently conducted and are the focus of this study. RH mobile camps

Table 9.1. *Summary of the Three SEWA Health Services Covered by the Reaching the Poor Study, India*

Variable	Reproductive health mobile camps	Tuberculosis detection and treatment	Women's health education
Target population	Women of reproductive age	Men and women, all ages	Women of reproductive age
Geographic coverage	Mainly Ahmedabad, Kheda, and Patan Districts	North and East Zones of Ahmedabad City (population roughly 375,000)	Mainly Ahmedabad, Kheda, and Patan Districts but also the other districts where SEWA Union has members
Annual rate of utilization	About 12,500 women a year	575 patients under treatment at the DOTS center; 23 served by barefoot DOTS workers	Approximately 6,000 women per year
Cost to user	5 rupee consultation fee; medicines sold at wholesale price (approximately one-third market price)	Services free; indirect costs only	5 rupee SEWA Union membership fee
External donor	UNFPA and government of India	WHO, government of India, and Ahmedabad Municipal Corporation	Government of India, UNFPA, Ford Foundation, and MacArthur Foundation
Human resources currently devoted to activity	6 part-time physicians; 50 barefoot doctors and managers	5 stationary centers (each with 2 to 3 staff); 11 grassroots DOTS providers	35 grassroots workers and full-time staff

Source: Authors' compilation.
Note: DOTS, directly observed treatment, short course; SEWA, Self-Employed Women's Association; UNFPA, United Nations Population Fund; WHO, World Health Organization. All the programs listed began in 1999. In 2001 Kheda District was divided into Kheda and Anand Districts; SEWA operates in both.

operate mainly in Ahmedabad City, Ahmedabad District, and Anand-Kheda and Patan Districts. They are largely funded by the United Nations Population Fund (UNFPA) and the government of India. More than 35 camps are held each month, and the average attendance per camp is 60, with roughly equal numbers of women and children. The camps serve more than 12,500 adult patients a year. Health care at the camps is provided by impaneled physicians and 50 barefoot doctors and managers. The camps are repeated in each area, on average, once a year.

Activities at the RH mobile camps include education and training, examination and diagnostic tests (including cervical examination and Pap smears), treatment, referral and follow-up. Camps are usually held during the afternoon and last three to four hours. Those attending the camps are asked to pay a contribution of 5 rupees (Rs) and one-third of the total cost of medicines provided, although even these fees may be waived for those who are very poor.

Increasingly, particularly in rural areas, SEWA Health conducts the camps in collaboration with the government of Gujarat State at primary health centers (PHCs), which are usually located in or near small villages. These camps differ from the standard "area" camps described above in that medicines are given free of charge and are restricted to those in the government's formulary, and health care is provided by public doctors and nurses. SEWA provides free transportation to women living in neighboring villages.

TUBERCULOSIS DETECTION AND TREATMENT. Since 1999, SEWA Health has collaborated with the World Health Organization (WHO), the government of India, and the Ahmedabad Municipal Corporation to provide tuberculosis treatment (directly observed treatment, short course, or DOTS) to residents of Ahmedabad's North and East Zones, which have a total population of roughly 375,000. These zones were assigned to SEWA under the Revised National Tuberculosis Control Programme (RNTCP). Services are currently provided through five stationary centers, two of which include laboratory facilities, and 11 barefoot doctors. Patients are identified through local education and information meetings or are referred from the government hospital in the area. Diagnostic services and medicines, which would otherwise cost from 7,000 to 9,000 rupees per full course of treatment, are provided free of charge. To date, almost 4,500 people have received treatment for tuberculosis (4,135 through the stationary centers, and 230 from the barefoot DOTS workers). Among those overseen by the barefoot doctors, the dropout rate is almost nil, while the dropout rate at stationary centers is 7 percent. The sputum conversion rate among those who complete treatment is 97 percent.

WOMEN'S HEALTH EDUCATION. Apart from the education provided at health centers and health camps, SEWA Health organizes many health education sessions in the nine districts where SEWA is active, primarily in Ahmedabad, Anand-Kheda, and Patan. In 2000/01 approximately 6,000 adult women participated in these sessions, which are organized on demand by barefoot doctors and managers. Each education session lasts two days, and six different packages are offered: SEWA orientation; first aid; general disease and HIV/AIDS; immunization and child care; airborne and waterborne diseases and tuberculosis; and "Know Your Body," which focuses on sexual and reproductive health. Each woman's name and address is recorded, and the woman obtains a certificate of participation for attending all six sessions. In all, 35 grassroots trainers and full-time staff provide education. These efforts are supported by the government of India, the UNFPA, the Ford Foundation, and the MacArthur Foundation.

Potential Constraints on Utilization of SEWA Health's Services

Table 9.2 provides an overview of the conceptual framework that guided this study. It divides the constraints that may prevent SEWA Health from

Table 9.2. *Potential Demand- and Supply-Side Constraints on Utilization of SEWA Health's Services by the Poor*

Demand side	Supply side
Time constraints (work, domestic chores, child-care commitments, and the like)	Inappropriate timing (for example, conflicts with working hours)
Lack of transportation to or from the service	Inaccessible location
Lack of information or knowledge about the service (not knowing about the service; not understanding the potential benefit of the service)	Problems with service quality (for example, not user friendly)
Perceived cost (direct costs of the service; indirect costs of transportation)	Failure to adequately advertise and promote the services (for example, among those who are homebound because of a disability and those who do not leave the home for work)
Fear (for example, of high costs, condescending doctors, or being asked to read something)	Fees or medicine costs too high
Lack of trust in SEWA Health	Indirect costs, such as time lost from work, too high
Belief that health is not important	Infrequent visits by mobile camps
Lack of positive self-concept; for example, women may seek care for husbands and children but not for themselves	
Perceived poor quality of services	

Source: Authors' compilation.

reaching the poorest women into demand-side factors (characteristics of individuals or groups in the target population) and supply-side factors (characteristics of SEWA Health).

Methodology

The research was carried out in the two districts where SEWA Health was functioning most intensively: Ahmedabad District (population 5.8 million, including Ahmedabad City, 2001 census) and Anand-Kheda District (3.8 million).

Data for the study were gathered in three phases. In the first phase, qualitative data were collected to identify possible constraints on utilization of SEWA Health services by those of low socioeconomic status (SES) and the nature of any such constraints. In the second phase, quantitative exit survey data were collected to assess the socioeconomic status of SEWA Health service users for comparison with that of nonusers and the population as a whole. In the third and final phase, in-depth interviews were conducted with SEWA Health workers to explore the factors underlying the success of the urban health services.

Phase 1

Six focus group discussions among SEWA Health's target population and six in-depth interviews with SEWA Health functionaries were undertaken. Two interviews of each type were conducted for each of the three SEWA Health services being studied.

The focus group discussions were held in poor areas—either slums in Ahmedabad City or poor rural areas. For each group discussion, we purposefully selected two women of reproductive age who had recently used SEWA Health services and two women living in adjacent or nearly adjacent homes who had not used the services, for a total of four. To be eligible to participate, women had to be willing to spend at least one hour in the focus group discussion at the assigned time, at a place within their residential area. No attempt was made to select the poorest women living in these poor areas. Any attempt to exclude the "nonpoor" from the interviews would have been entirely subjective because we had not developed any objective indicators of socioeconomic status. In fact, that was one of the objectives of the focus group discussions. Each session began with a participatory wealth-ranking exercise. Women then discussed whether and why the poorest women or households in their area had difficulty in accessing SEWA Health services.

In-depth interviews were conducted with SEWA Health grassroots service providers. These women were asked to describe their work with SEWA Health and to discuss problems faced by the poor in accessing the services.

Focus group discussions and in-depth interviews were conducted in Gujarati. With the permission of respondents, they were videotaped. They were later translated into English and transcribed by the interviewer. The transcribed interviews were coded, applying predefined codes and using N-Vivo software.

Phase 2

SAMPLE SIZE. The aim was to interview 500 users of each of the three SEWA Health services, for a total of 1,500 interviews. We estimated the necessary sample size using proportions. For this calculation, we decided to look at whether the proportion of SEWA Health users falling below the 30th decile, which roughly approximates the poverty line in Gujarat, was significantly different from 30 percent. The standard error for the proportion of SEWA Health users below the 30th decile would be highest for a value of 50 percent. To achieve a 95 percent confidence interval of <5 percent—that is, of 47.5 to 52.5 percent—a total of 385 observations per service would be required. Our sample sizes were well above this figure.

QUESTIONNAIRE. The questionnaire included items about the service user, family characteristics, household assets, utilities, dwelling, and land ownership, as well as several questions about respondents' perceptions of the SEWA Health service used.[3] We were careful to include all questions about household assets, utilities, dwelling, and land ownership that were in the 1998–99 Demographic and Health Survey (DHS) in Gujarat State. The wording of the questions asked was identical to that in the DHS, and our interviewers were trained using the DHS instruction manuals.

The questionnaires were administered by six female grassroots researchers who received more than two weeks of training. Pilot testing was conducted for one week, with each researcher administering between 8 and 10 questionnaires. Throughout the survey, all questionnaires were carefully checked by two field supervisors.

SAMPLING. Methods of sampling varied slightly between the three SEWA Health services in order to capture as random a set of respondents as possible.

In the case of the reproductive health mobile camps, a list of camps planned for a one-month period was compiled. (The camps operate Monday through Saturday.) The number of camps ranged from one to three per day. For each day, one camp was randomly selected (if only one camp was planned, that one was automatically selected), and all users at the selected camps were interviewed. After completing the 500th interview, we continued until all respondents at the final camp had been interviewed; thus, we ended up with a sample greater than 500.

For the women's education sessions, we received the schedule one week at a time. The number of camps ranged from three to four per day. Each day, two sessions were randomly selected, and all users at the selected sessions were interviewed. Again, this resulted in a sample slightly larger than 500.

For the tuberculosis detection and treatment services, the interview team was divided to cover the five DOTS centers. The list of patients kept by the centers was found to include many people who had discontinued or completed their course of medication, and these lists were deemed inappropriate for sampling. Over approximately four weeks, all people presenting to these centers were interviewed, resulting in a sample size substantially greater than 500.

REINTERVIEWS. To check the reliability of responses, we reinterviewed approximately 10 percent of all respondents in both urban and rural areas. The reinterviews were generally conducted within 72 hours of the first interview, at the respondent's home and by a different interviewer from the one who conducted the first interview.

DATA ENTRY AND ANALYSIS. Questionnaire data were double-entered into a custom-made EpiInfo database. Data were analyzed using Stata statistical software.

Socioeconomic status indexes were constructed on the basis of factor analysis of a reference standard database. These indexes were then applied to the users surveyed in our study. Urban and rural data were analyzed separately, on the assumption that wealth indicators vary markedly between urban and rural Gujarat.

For the urban sample, we chose from three reference databases: DHS 1998–99, all urban Gujarat State (N = 1,709); DHS 1998–99, Ahmedabad City (N = 476); and a Vimo SEWA 2003 database for Ahmedabad City (N = 746). After comparing these databases, we chose to use Vimo SEWA 2003 as the reference standard. A small number of variables that were available both in the Vimo SEWA database and from our exit surveys were dropped from the analyses on the basis of comparisons between the DHS and Vimo SEWA databases. It was believed that differences between the databases with respect to these specific indicators were attributable to the limited reliability of the indicator rather than to changes in socioeconomic conditions in Ahmedabad City during the five-year period.

For our rural sample, we chose from three reference databases: DHS 1998–99, all rural Gujarat State (households from 19 districts, N = 2,223); DHS 1998–99 for only the two districts where our exit surveys were conducted (N = 309); and a Vimo SEWA 2003 database for nine rural Gujarati districts, including the two districts where we conducted exit surveys (N = 784). Ultimately, it was impossible to choose between the DHS 1998–99 database for all rural districts and the Vimo SEWA 2003 database, so we used both in turn as reference databases and tested the sensitivity of results to choice of database.

Phase 3

Six in-depth interviews were conducted with SEWA Health grassroots managers. These women were asked to describe their work with SEWA Health and to discuss whether they thought SEWA Health services reached poorer residents of Ahmedabad City and why they thought so.

The interviews were conducted in Gujarati and were audiotaped. They were later translated into English and transcribed by the interviewer. The transcribed interviews were coded, applying predefined codes and using N-Vivo software.

Nature and Sources of Data

This section briefly describes the two reference databases—DHS 1998–99 and the 2003 Vimo SEWA (SEWA Insurance)—that provided information on the socioeconomic status (SES) of the general population.

DHS Database

The SES indexes were derived from DHS 1998–99, also known as the National Family Health Survey–2 (NFHS–2). Data were collected by the International Institute for Population Sciences (IIPS), Mumbai. The NFHS–2 (IIPS and ORC Macro 2001) was a follow-up to the first National Family Health Survey (NFHS–1), conducted in 1992–93. The primary aim of the NFHS–2 was to provide state- and national-level information on fertility, family planning, infant and child mortality, reproductive health, child health, nutrition of women and children, and the quality of health and family welfare services and to examine this information in the context of related socioeconomic and cultural factors.

In all, 4,153 households were selected in Gujarat. Rural and urban areas were sampled separately. The rural sample was constructed in two stages: the selection of 87 villages (or groups of villages, in the case of small, linked villages) with probability proportional to population size (PPS), followed by the selection of 15 to 60 households within each village. In urban areas a three-stage sampling procedure was followed. First, 46 wards were selected with PPS. Next, from each selected ward, one census enumeration block was selected with PPS. Finally, households were selected using systematic sampling in each selected enumeration block.

Vimo SEWA Data

The Vimo SEWA data were collected from May through August 2003 under a joint project carried out by Vimo SEWA (SEWA Insurance) and the London School of Hygiene and Tropical Medicine and funded by the Wellcome Trust. This survey was part of baseline work intended to assess the socioeconomic status of Vimo SEWA members (in comparison with the general population) prior to implementation of interventions intended to optimize the equity impact of the insurance scheme. The Vimo SEWA questionnaire was based on a standardized tool developed by the International Food Policy Research Institute (IFPRI) to measure the poverty of microfinance institution clients (Henry and others 2000). The questionnaire included sections on dwelling-related indicators (size and condition of dwelling and facilities available), family structure, food-related indicators, and other asset-based indicators.

This survey was administered to 800 households in Ahmedabad City and 800 households in the nine rural districts of Gujarat where Vimo SEWA has members. Two-stage random cluster sampling was used. In Ahmedabad City 50 enumeration blocks (out of 10,385) were first randomly sampled. Within each enumeration block, 16 households were randomly selected from the enumeration block maps (2001 census). In rural Gujarat 50 towns or villages were randomly sampled with PPS (1991 census) of the town or village. As in Ahmedabad, 16 households within each town or village were randomly sampled from enumeration block maps.

Findings about Distribution

The socioeconomic status of SEWA Health service users is compared here with that of the general population, first for urban and then for rural areas.

Urban Findings

For all three services in urban areas, the mean SES scores of the users are significantly lower than the mean SES score (by definition, 0) of the general population (reference population: Ahmedabadis in the Vimo SEWA survey, 2003). The mean SES scores are –0.42 for RH camp users (95 percent confidence interval = –0.51 to –0.34), –0.36 for tuberculosis detection and treatment users (95 percent confidence interval = –0.43 to –0.29), and –0.61 for women's education participants (95 percent confidence interval = –0.88 to –0.35).

As can be seen in figure 9.1, the percentage of users falling below the 30th decile of the SES score—which roughly approximates the poverty line in India—was about 50 percent for all of the services. The percentage of users falling below the 30th decile was 51.9 percent for RH camp users (95 percent confidence interval = 46.7 to 57.0 percent), 47.4 percent for tuberculosis detection and treatment users (95 percent confidence interval = 43.5 to 51.2 percent), and 47.5 percent for women's education participants (95 percent confidence interval = 36.2 to 59.0 percent).

The concentration curves for all three services suggest that SEWA Health services are equitably distributed in Ahmedabad City and that they are predominantly used by people from poorer households (figure 9.2). All three concentration curves lie well above the line of equality. The concentration indexes are –0.37 for RH mobile camps, –0.33 for tuberculosis detection and treatment, and –0.37 for women's education sessions.

Of the urban users, 104 were reinterviewed at their homes. The index scores for these reinterviews correlate highly with scores based on the original interviews. A paired t-test shows no significant difference; first interview to reinterview, $p = 0.25$.

Rural Findings

The mean SES scores of RH camp users do not differ significantly from the mean score for the general population, regardless of which reference standard database is used. The women's education participants have a significantly higher mean SES score relative to the Vimo SEWA 2003 database but not the DHS 1998–99 database. Using the Vimo SEWA 2003 database as reference standard, the mean SES scores are 0.024 for RH camp users (95 percent confidence interval = –0.054 to 0.10) and 0.19 for women's education participants (95 percent confidence interval = 0.12 to 0.27). Using the DHS 1998–99 database (all 19 rural districts) as reference standard, the mean SES scores are –0.068 for RH camp users (95 percent confidence interval = –0.14

Figure 9.1. *Frequency Distribution of Urban SEWA Health Users by Deciles of the Socioeconomic Status Index Score*

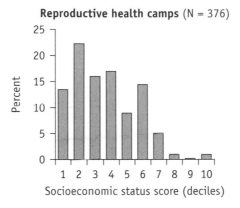

Reproductive health camps (N = 376)

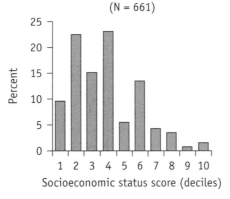

Tuberculosis detection and treatment (N = 661)

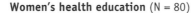

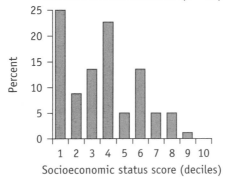

Women's health education (N = 80)

Source: Authors' calculations.

Figure 9.2. *SEWA Health Service Utilization Concentration Curves, Ahmedabad City*

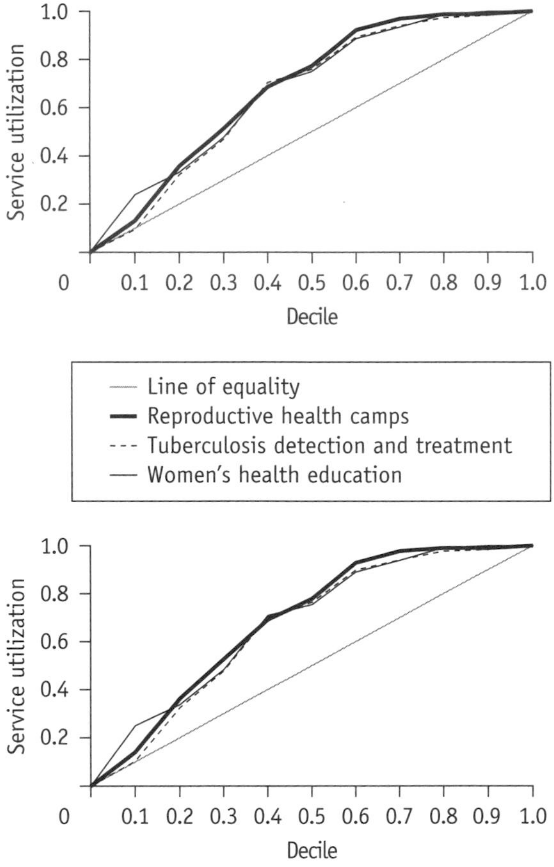

Source: Authors' calculations.

to 0.0082) and 0.068 for women's education participants (95 percent confidence interval = –0.0086 to 0.15).

Figure 9.3 shows the frequency distribution of rural SEWA Health users by deciles of SES index score for both reference standards. Users of both the RH camps and the women's education sessions are significantly less likely to fall below the 30th percentile than are households in the general population. Using Vimo SEWA 2003 as the reference standard, only 5.7 percent of RH camp users (95 percent confidence interval = 2.6 to 10.5 percent) and 8.5 percent of women's education participants (95 percent confidence interval = 6.0 to 11.6 percent) fall below the 30th percentile. Similarly, with DHS 1998–99 as the reference standard, 8.2 percent of RH camp users (95 percent

Figure 9.3. *Frequency Distribution of Rural SEWA Health Users, by Deciles of the Socioeconomic Status Index Score*

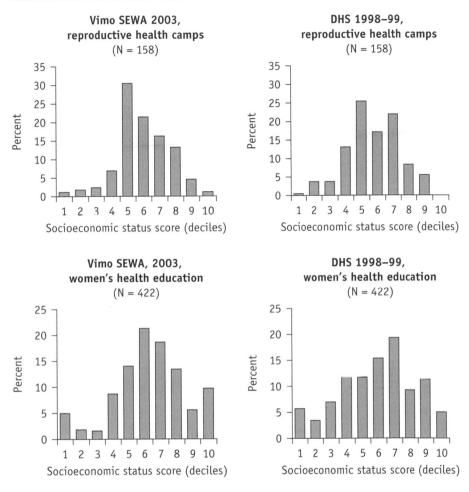

Vimo SEWA 2003,
reproductive health camps
(N = 158)

DHS 1998–99,
reproductive health camps
(N = 158)

Vimo SEWA, 2003,
women's health education
(N = 422)

DHS 1998–99,
women's health education
(N = 422)

Source: Authors' calculations.

confidence interval = 4.5 to 13.7 percent) and 16.4 percent of women's education participants (95 percent confidence interval = 13.0 to 20.2 percent) fall below the 30th percentile.

The concentration curves for both services, like the frequency distributions above, suggest that SEWA Health's rural services do not effectively target the very poorest (figure 9.4). The concentration indexes (using Vimo SEWA 2003 as the reference standard) are 0.091 for RH mobile camps and 0.16 for women's education sessions. (Concentration curves and indexes

Figure 9.4. *SEWA Health Service Utilization Concentration Curves, Rural Areas (Vimo SEWA 2003 as Reference Standard)*

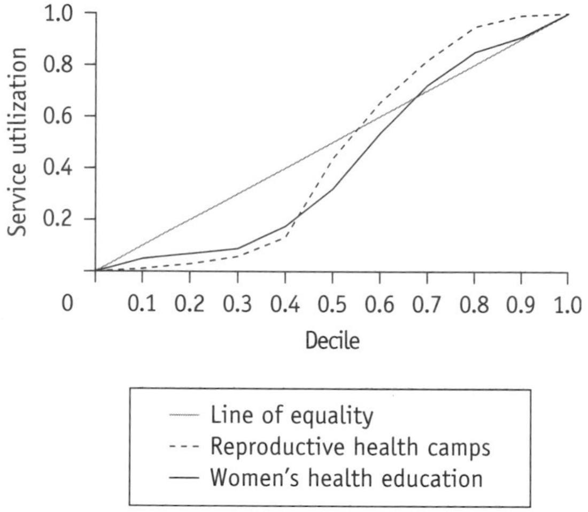

Source: Authors' calculations.

using DHS 1998–99 as the reference standard are very similar and are not presented here.)

Of the rural users, 60 were reinterviewed at their homes. The index scores for these reinterviews correlate highly with scores based on the original interviews. A paired *t*-test shows no significant difference; first interview to reinterview, $p = 0.286$.

Reasons for the Distribution

Drawing on focus group discussions with SEWA Health users and nonusers and on in-depth interviews with SEWA Health functionaries, this section explores factors that underlie SEWA Health's success in reaching the poor of Ahmedabad City and the nature of constraints on utilization of SEWA Health services by people of low socioeconomic status, particularly in rural areas.

Success Factors in Reaching the Poor

Several grassroots workers attributed SEWA Health's success in reaching the poor to the fact that it treats poor people with respect and "warmth":

The patients say that, "at other places, people don't listen to us, and respond to us, like you do." Since this is SEWA's center, they choose to come here. (*SEWA Health tuberculosis grassroots worker, Amraiwadi, Ahmedabad City*)

Other organizations do not give out detailed information the way the SEWA workers do. We treat the women like they are our family members. The members say that, "Compared to other organizations, you work closely and warmly with us." They say, "We need warmth, and the rich people can not give us that." (*SEWA Health grassroots worker, Dholka, Ahmedabad District*)

The fact that the services are generally free or low cost makes them more accessible to the poor:

When we made home visits, we saw that the patients did not even have money for food. Then we explained to the patients that, "It is okay if you don't have money. You don't have to spend any money at the [tuberculosis DOTS] center. If you take medicines and get cured, then you will be able to earn money." (*SEWA Health tuberculosis grassroots worker, Amraiwadi, Ahmedabad City*)

. . . and the medicines [at RH mobile camps] are also good and low cost. The same medicines are available for Rs 200 to Rs 250 outside [in private drug shops] but we give them for Rs 20 or Rs 25 in our health camps. (*SEWA Health grassroots worker, Daskroi Taluka, Ahmedabad District*)

Convenient timing was cited as a factor in utilization of the tuberculosis detection and treatment services:

The hours of the center are good, since the patients have to go to work early, and our center operates from 7:30 in the morning to 4 in the afternoon. (*SEWA Health tuberculosis grassroots worker, Amraiwadi, Ahmedabad City*)

Physical location was seen as contributing to the success of SEWA Health services:

. . . another reason being that we go right to their doorsteps, and we discuss their problems and the positive happenings in their lives. (*SEWA Health grassroots worker, Daskroi Taluka, Ahmedabad District*)

We provide a convenient location to the patient, telling them that, "This is an easy location for you to come and take the medicines." (*SEWA Health tuberculosis grassroots worker, Amraiwadi, Ahmedabad City*)

Finally, the fact that SEWA Health's services are delivered largely by women was also perceived as increasing their reach among poor women:

> We give our introduction as a union of self-employed women, which means poor women. So the women think that, "Since this is a women's organization, wherever we go we will be dealing with women," and so they feel secure. (*SEWA Health grassroots worker, Daskroi Taluka, Ahmedabad District*)

> For area [RH mobile] camps we get female doctors for the women, which is very good, and more and more women attend because of this. Since there is a female doctor, they feel secure. (*SEWA Health grassroots worker, Daskroi Taluka, Ahmedabad District*)

Constraints

The cost, or perceived cost, of services is at times a barrier to using the RH mobile camps. In one interview women explained that on hearing that some charge is being levied for the medicines, the poorest would simply not come:

> *Participant 1:* Since it is an issue of money they don't come . . . Some people would like to come to get the medicines. But then they would wonder as to whether it would cost them. Then they would not come.

> *Interviewer:* But then you would have the information that the medicines are at low cost?

> *Participant 1:* That they [the health workers] would inform, but then it would cost at least something . . . So when they hear this some people would not come. (*focus group discussion 6, Varna Village, Dholka Taluka, Ahmedabad District*)

For some, even the Rs 5 registration fee is enough to prevent utilization:

> *Interviewer:* There were other women in the area who said they wanted a checkup [as mentioned earlier by one woman]. What happened to them?

> *Participant 2:* I had five or six other women with me. But then they all left. They said that "they ask for money over here" so they all left.

> *Interviewer:* But then it was Rs 5?

> *Participant 1:* The situation is not good.

Participant 2: Where to get Rs 5 from? (*focus group discussion 5, Chamanpura Area, Ahmedabad City*)

Even SEWA Health grassroots workers acknowledged that the fees charged at the RH mobile camps prevent some from using them:

Grassroots worker: No we cannot provide free medicines for half of these people. Only around two to three women [per camp] are able to get it for free.

Interviewer: So what about the rest?

Grassroots worker: They don't come!

Interviewer: They would not visit at all?

Grassroots worker: No, they would not come to the camp. We cannot tell everyone that we will get them medicines for free! (*in-depth interview 4, Gangad Village, Bawla Taluka, Ahmedabad District*)

Women also reported that the RH mobile camps are difficult for women to attend, as they often coincide with working hours:

Interviewer: What are the reasons why people who should ideally visit the camp are not able to do so?

Grassroots worker: At times there is a season in the village [presumably referring to seasons when there is work in the fields]. Then these women go to do work. Because of which they cannot come [to the camps]. If the work is going on, and the women have gone for that, can they come [to the camps]? (*in-depth interview 3, Vanoti Village, Thasra Taluka, Kheda District*)

Grassroots worker: Mostly the poorest of women would go out and do work [for daily wages]. They would say that "I will have to lose my wages [to be able to attend the camp]." (*in-depth interview 4, Gangad Village, Bawla Taluka, Ahmedabad District*)

For the health education sessions, the fact that the timing may coincide with work was reported as a major barrier to access:

Interviewer: What are the reasons why some women would not sit in the training?

Grassroots worker: If the woman has gone to work. She would come for the first and the second session, but then if she starts working after that she is not able to sit for the training. She would tell us that, "since I have started working I cannot sit." (*in-depth interview 1, Shankarbhuvan, Ahmedabad City*)

Interviewer: So are the women of very poor category [as classified in the focus group discussion] also able to take advantage [of the training sessions]?

Grassroots worker: When we went to give this training they [the women] told us that you should keep it for two days only, because if we have to go and work outside then how can we sit in your training? (*in-depth interview 3, Vanoti Village, Thasra Taluka, Kheda District*)

Interviewer: In our women's education program, are the very poor women able to come?

Grassroots worker: The very poor women are not able to sit. But if we do the training at night, only then they are able to sit with us. Because during the day, they have to go to do work. Hence the very poor women are not able to sit in our trainings . . . So they would say, "Please come at night." (*in-depth interview 4, Gangad Village, Bawla Taluka, Ahmedabad District*)

The health education sessions are unique among the services studied in that a full course consists of 12 days of training (2 days per month) spread over six months. Any barrier to access may prevent women from attending the training sessions entirely or may prevent them from attending the full 12 days of training.

Limitations

This section highlights some of the key methodological weaknesses (and strengths) of the study.

Reference Standard Databases

When our draft questionnaire was conceived, it was assumed that our sole reference standard database would be DHS 1998–99. Thus, we were restricted by the contents of the DHS questionnaire and database as to the kinds of assets and household characteristics that could be included in the SES index. For example, it was noted during our fieldwork that the wealth of rural households in Gujarat can be measured by their possession of kitchen utensils such as brass and steel plates (*thalis*) and water vessels, but because this category of asset was not included in the DHS questionnaire, it could not be examined as an indicator in our study. Similarly, variables relating to food security and household spending on clothing and footwear—which are found in other studies to be reliable indicators of socioeconomic status—were not available in the DHS database.

Our analyses comparing the DHS 1998–99 survey data with Vimo SEWA 2003 data suggest that urban (or, more specifically, Ahmedabadi) households have grown significantly wealthier, while rural households have grown significantly poorer. We cannot completely rule out the possibility that these changes stem from methodological differences. (For example, the Vimo SEWA surveyors may have been more persistent in revisiting rural households where nobody was present on the first visit, and these might have been the poorer households.) We were able to overcome limitations in the older DHS data by relying more heavily on comparisons with the Vimo SEWA reference standard. (This raises an important methodological question for future studies: when should a reference standard be considered too old to be useful?)

Sample Size

When we calculated our sample size, we assumed that urban and rural areas would be treated as one. But when we started analyzing the qualitative and quantitative data, we realized that urban and rural data would have to be analyzed separately. Thus, we ended up with sample sizes for rural RH mobile camps (N = 158), urban RH mobile camps (N = 376), and urban women's education (N = 80) that are well below the desired sample size of 500. For the urban results, this is somewhat irrelevant, given that even with these small sample sizes, all three urban services were found to be used by people who were significantly more likely than the general population to fall below the 30th decile.

Exit Survey Data

Since the exit survey was conducted at the same site where the SEWA Health service was delivered, respondents may have misrepresented their wealth. We reinterviewed approximately 10 percent of all respondents, however, in both urban and rural areas. The SES index scores generated, based on the reinterviews, were consistent with scores based on the original interviews. This suggests that there were no large, systematic errors in responses given during the exit survey.

Comparability between Reference Standard and Exit Survey Data

The rural DHS data were collected from rural areas throughout the state of Gujarat (19 districts), while our exit survey data were collected in only two rural districts. Similarly, the rural Vimo SEWA data represent 9 districts. Rural RH camp users and women's education recipients were found not to be among the poorest. It might be asked whether the two districts where the study was carried out, Ahmedabad and Anand-Kheda, are wealthier than other rural districts in the state. But our comparison of the study districts with the whole state (the 19 districts covered in DHS 1998–99) showed no significant difference in the mean SES score and very few significant differences on the basis of individual variables.

Implications

The study found that in Ahmedabad City, SEWA Health's services are used disproportionately by the poor (table 9.3). Differences between the three urban health services studied were not statistically significant. In rural areas SEWA Health's services are used by people who do not differ significantly in socioeconomic status from the general population. The rural health services do not effectively target those below the 30th percentile. In the case of rural RH mobile camps, reaching the poorest may be hindered by the cost (or perceived cost) of services at the health camps. In addition, the rural poor may have difficulty attending the rural health camps and the women's education sessions because the schedules of these services coincide with working hours.

For the most part, the urban services seem to be effectively targeting the poor. Some likely reasons for this success can be identified:

- Services, especially RH mobile camps and women's education sessions, are offered "right at people's doorsteps." In other words, SEWA Health takes the services to the poor rather than trying to bring the poor to the services.

Table 9.3. *Percentage of All Service Users in Poorest Three Deciles*

Service	Urban	Rural
Reproductive health camps	51.9	5.7–8.2
Tuberculosis detection and treatment	47.4	8.5–16.4
Women's health education	47.5	

Source: Authors' calculations.

- The services arc delivered by (or at least in part by) the poor themselves.
- The services are generally combined with efforts to educate and mobilize the community. For example, in advance of the RH mobile camps, SEWA Health workers go door to door, educating people about the service and motivating them to use it.
- Costs are low—certainly, relative to the private for-profit sector.
- SEWA is an entity that people know and trust.

As SEWA Health grows and evolves, efforts should be made not to alter or disturb the characteristics that are likely to have contributed to success in reaching the poor.

The study suggests several changes that can be made by SEWA Health to better reach the poorest in the target population, particularly in rural areas. The first is to hold RH mobile camps and adult health education sessions outside normal working hours. The second is to ensure that the cost of seeking care (registration fees and payments for medicines) at the RH mobile camps does not pose an impediment to access among the poorest. Already, SEWA Health waives the registration fee and the medicine fee for those who appear to be particularly poor—typically, a few women at each camp. Perhaps these exemptions could be granted more liberally and in a more objective manner—for example, by exempting all who possess a below-poverty-line card.

There are likely to be other, broader reasons underlying the difficulties in delivering services to the rural poor. Studies in other SEWA departments have documented similar discrepancies in the equity of utilization of rural versus urban services. For example, the poorest rural members of SEWA's insurance scheme, Vimo SEWA, have lower rates of claims than the less poor. Reasons for this differential include:

- Problems of geographic access, both to inpatient facilities and to Vimo SEWA's grassroots workers
- Weaker links (less frequent and less intensive contact) between members and local Vimo SEWA representatives in rural areas
- Weaker capacity among Vimo SEWA grassroots workers in rural areas.

It must be remembered that failure of a service to reach the poorest of the rural poor does not necessarily mean that the service has failed in reaching the poor. Even households that fall in the higher deciles of the SES index in rural areas should be considered "less poor" rather than "wealthy." Compared with their urban counterparts, these rural households have less in the way of cash reserves, material wealth, and, thus, economic security.

More generally, our findings suggest that delivery of services through a broad-based, development-oriented union can facilitate equitable delivery of health care services. Government and donors can help ensure that established NGOs with an interest in providing health services have the capacity and the resources to do so.

Notes

This chapter is a condensed version of a study prepared for the World Bank's Reaching the Poor Program. The full study is available from the authors on request.

Guidance and supervision for the study were provided by Mirai Chatterjee, coordinator, SEWA Social Security. The authors thank the many SEWA staff and members who contributed to the study. The following SEWA staff were directly involved in data collection, analysis, or entry: supervisor, Jayshree Shinde; grassroot researchers, Bhartiben Parmar, Chandrikaben Solanki, Niruben Makwana, Padmaben Anjaria, Rajeshwariben Bhatt, and Roshan Bhayani; data entry, Kinnari Shah, Smita Panchal; SEWA Academy team, Bijalben Rawal, Mitaben Parikh; Video SEWA team, Arunaben Parmar, Dakshaben Mehta, Darshanaben Parmar, Leelaben Dantani, Manjulaben Raval, and Neelamben Shah; and the entire SEWA Health team.

1. In 2001 several districts in the state were divided, and the number of districts increased from 19 to 25. Today, SEWA works in 11 (before the split, 9) of these districts. To facilitate comparison with DHS 1998–99, we refer to the 19 districts as they existed prior to 2001. The redistricting most important for our report is the division of Kheda District into Anand and Kheda Districts.

2. The focus of this chapter is on adult women users of the reproductive and child health camps. For this reason, these camps are referred to as reproductive health (RH) mobile camps throughout the chapter.

3. The full questionnaire and the detailed technical appendixes are included in the longer version of this chapter, which can be obtained from the authors.

References

Henry, C., M. Sharma, C. Lapenu, and M. Zeller. 2000. *Assessing the relative poverty of microfinance clients: A CGAP operational tool.* Washington, DC: International Food Policy Research Institute.

IIPS (International Institute for Population Sciences) and ORC Macro. 2001. *National family health survey, 1998–99 (NFHS-2): Gujarat.* Mumbai, IIPS.

Mahal, A., J. Singh, F. Afridi, V. Lamba, A. Gumber, and V. Selvaraju. 2000. Who benefits from public health spending in India? National Council of Applied Economic Research, New Delhi.

Pachauri, S. 1994. Introduction and overview. In *Reaching India's poor: Nongovernmental approaches to community health,* ed. S. Pachauri, 13–30. New Delhi: SAGE Publications.

Peters, D. H., A. S. Yazbeck, R. R. Sharma, G. N. V. Ramana, L. H. Pritchett, and A. Wagstaff. 2002. Better health systems for India's poor: Findings, analysis, and options. World Bank, Washington, DC.

SEWA (Self-Employed Women's Association). 1999. *Self-Employed Women's Association: Annual report 1999.* Ahmedabad, India: SEWA.

World Bank. 2003. Multi country reports by HNP indicators on socioeconomic inequalities. Washington, DC. http://www.worldbank.org/poverty/health/data/statusind.htm

10

India: Equity Effects of Quality Improvements on Health Service Utilization and Patient Satisfaction in Uttar Pradesh State

David Peters, Krishna Rao, and G. N. V. Ramana

During the past half century, India has made substantial improvements in health outcomes (Ramana, Sastry, and Peters 2002). Yet health conditions for India's billion people are still comparable to those in other low-income countries. India's infant mortality rate, for instance, is 68 deaths per 1,000 live births, compared with 76 for the low-income group (World Bank 2002). Uttar Pradesh, which, with its population of 170 million people, is India's most populous state, has benefited little from the advances that have been made.[1] With an infant mortality rate of 83 per 1,000 live births, Uttar Pradesh is worse off than the average low-income country and is India's lowest-ranked state in terms of human development.[2]

Socioeconomic inequalities in utilization of health care and in health outcomes are large in India and are even more pronounced in Uttar Pradesh and neighboring states. This suggests that the poor have benefited less than the better off from publicly provided health services (Gwatkin and others 2000; Mahal and others 2001; Peters and others 2002). According to the analyses, poorer Indians use health services much less than do the better off. The distribution of inpatient days, outpatient treatments, and obstetric care at public facilities favors the higher expenditure quintiles, although immunizations and antenatal and postnatal care at public facilities and outreach programs are much more evenly distributed. Financial barriers and user dissatisfaction are suggested as important reasons why the poor eschew health services.

A major policy response to this undesirable situation has been to improve the quality of health services offered at public facilities. Yet it is not known whether these efforts will benefit the poor or whether the nonpoor will capture better services. Experience in testing the hypothesis that quality improvements will benefit the poor is limited, and one well-documented case suggests that the testing process is far from simple. Victora and others (2000) found that targeting child health services to the poor dramatically increased their utilization levels and reduced inequalities. The effect of these interventions on mortality and nutritional status, however, was first felt by those of higher socioeconomic status and helped the poor only after health outcomes in the better-off groups had reached a threshold level. This result led the authors to postulate the "inverse equity hypothesis": new interventions lead to initial increases in health inequalities, and declines occur only in later periods, when health outcomes among lower socioeconomic groups begin to improve.

Another strategy for raising utilization rates is to make health services more responsive to the public by seeking to improve the public's perception of them. Various determinants of user perceptions of health service quality have been highlighted in the literature. They include provider behavior (Haddad and Fournier 1995; Aldana, Piechulek, and Al-Sabir 2001); respect for privacy (Aldana, Piechulek, and Al-Sabir 2001); waiting times (Aldana, Piechulek, and Al-Sabir 2001); availability of drugs (Haddad and Fournier 1995); and staff competence (Haddad and Fournier 1995). Evidence from Bangladesh (Andaleeb 2000), the Democratic Republic of Congo, then called Zaire (Haddad and Fournier 1995), and Niger (Chawla and Ellis 2000) indicate that user perception of quality is an important determinant of utilization when user fees are increased. Little is known, however, about how user perceptions vary with socioeconomic status or whether improvements in technical quality improve quality perceptions across all or only some socioeconomic groups. This study addresses these issues by testing the effect of a health reform intervention in Uttar Pradesh on patient satisfaction and utilization among different socioeconomic groups.

The Intervention

The Uttar Pradesh Health Systems Development Project (UPHSDP) is a $110 million World Bank–assisted project designed to improve the quality of and access to health services in the state. The project components include policy reform, management development, institutional strengthening, and improvements in access to and quality of health services. Since the project began in July 2000, a series of activities has been launched, including management training, new staffing patterns and placement procedures, initiation of a fee exemption policy and other financing reforms, provision of essential drugs, and rehabilitation and repair of equipment and facilities (table 10.1). The management and financing reforms were implemented across the state; the interventions in physical and human resources were implemented at project sites located in poorer regions of the state. The selection of project sites was based on scoring criteria that included the condition of public health infrastructure and area socioeconomic indicators.

Research Questions

The primary objective of this study is to evaluate the impact of the quality improvements initiated under the UPHSDP on patient satisfaction and uti-

Table 10.1. *Activities Implemented under the Uttar Pradesh Health Systems Development Project, 2000–2002*

Areas of intervention	Specific activities
Management development	• Motivational exercises for all management staff, emphasizing personal mastery in leadership and excellence in service delivery. • Management training of all management staff.
Human resources strengthening	• Placement of staff according to new manpower norms to reduce overstaffing in major cities and understaffing in rural areas. • "Fixed day approach" to rotation of medical staff to ensure that underserved project sites receive the services of specialists.
Physical inputs	• Repairs, renovation, and equipping of block-level primary health centers (PHCs, 6-bed facilities that provide outpatient services), community health centers (CHCs, 30-bed hospitals), district hospitals (DHs, hospitals with 100 or more beds), and female district hospitals associated with DHs. (Most of the female hospitals are on separate campuses but in the same city as the district hospital.) • Increased supply of essential drugs to project sites.
Financing reforms	• Initiation of new exemption policy for user charges for ration cardholders (those below the poverty line) and for selected public health services; upward revision of rates; and permitted retention of up to 50 percent of revenues at the facility.

Source: UPHSDP project documents.

lization levels. Of particular interest is whether the project interventions led to increased service utilization and satisfaction on the part of disadvantaged groups—the poor and the lower castes—and how these groups fared relative to better-off groups.

Methodology

This study uses a quasi-experimental design to investigate the impact of the UPHSDP on utilization and patient satisfaction. The design and sampling timelines are illustrated in figure 10.1. Prior to the start of the project, all district hospitals (DHs), female district hospitals (FDHs), community health centers (CHCs), and primary health centers (PHCs) in Uttar Pradesh were rated according to the condition of their physical infrastructure, staff positions, availability of drugs and equipment, and utilization rates and on the economic characteristics of the community. Facilities with low scores were eligible for project interventions. For eligible district hospitals, the associated female district hospitals were first selected. From a selected DH district, one eligible community health center and at least one eligible primary health center from the selected CHC catchment area were assigned to the project interventions. Thus, the project female district hospitals, community health centers, and primary health centers were from the same districts as the selected district hospitals, but not all the community and primary health centers in a selected district were covered by the project. In all, 117 facilities in 28 districts were brought under the UPHSDP: 28 district hospitals, 25 female district hospitals, 28 community health centers, and 36 primary health centers. Most project facilities were in the poorer eastern and central regions of Uttar Pradesh.

In 1999, before the project began, a baseline study of service utilization and patient satisfaction was conducted at these 117 project facilities and at an equal number of controls. The control district hospitals were randomly selected from nonproject districts. The control community and primary health centers were randomly selected from within the same districts as the project community health centers and primary health centers in the sample.

For the follow-up survey in 2003, a subset of 47 baseline project and control facilities was resampled. Project facilities sampled at the baseline were stratified into one of the four regions of Uttar Pradesh. From each, one project district hospital and its associated female district hospital were randomly selected. In the eastern and central regions, where most of the project district hospitals and female district hospitals are located, two project district hospitals and their associated female district hospitals were randomly selected. Similar numbers of control district hospitals and their associated

Figure 10.1. *Study Design and Sample, Uttar Pradesh*

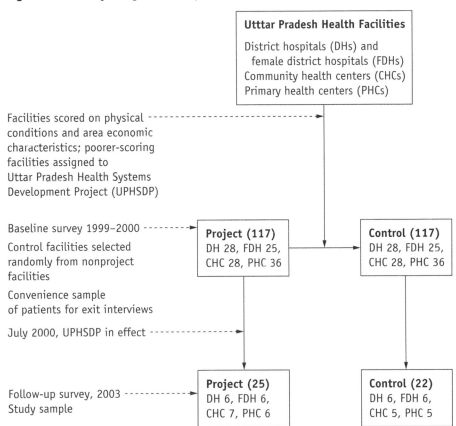

Source: UPHSDP project documents.

female district hospitals were randomly selected in each region from the pool of facilities sampled at the baseline. The final samples include 12 district hospitals (6 project and 6 control), 12 female district hospitals (6 project and 6 control), 12 community health centers (7 project and 5 control), and 11 primary health centers (6 project and 5 control). The analysis used in this paper is based on these 47 facilities for which there are observations both at baseline and for the follow-up period.

Nature and Sources of the Data

Data for this study are drawn from a variety of sources. The two most important are the project evaluation surveys, which include a baseline survey in 1999 and a follow-up survey in 2003. These were supplemented with information from the National Family Health Surveys (NFHS) of 1992–93 and 1998–99 for Uttar Pradesh conducted by the International Institute of Population Sciences (IIPS), Mumbai. Details of the analytical methods used are described below.

Data Collection

Baseline information was collected in 1999–2000; the follow-up survey was carried out between April and September 2003. Different survey organizations conducted each round of the study, leading to some inconsistencies in methods. For the baseline survey, interviewers were given targets of 40 new outpatients at district hospitals, 30 at community health centers, and 20 at primary health centers. For the follow-up survey, the targets were 60 outpatients at district hospitals, 30 at community health centers, and 20 at primary health centers. In both surveys outpatients were sampled as they left the health facility on the basis of convenience sampling; the interviewer selected successive patients on finishing the previous interview. The total number of sampled patients is 1,660; the breakdown by facility type is shown in annex table 10.1. The exit interviews provided data on patients' socioeconomic and demographic status and on their satisfaction with health services. Data from facility records collected by the interviewers included information on the number of new outpatient visits to the facility in the preceding months. (Returning patients were excluded from this analysis.) The facility data were endorsed by a facility official.

Different questionnaires were used to assess patient satisfaction at baseline and follow-up surveys. Each survey had high internal reliability (α = 0.87 at baseline and 0.84 at follow-up). In this chapter, an item common to the surveys on overall satisfaction with the care is used to compare responses from the baseline with those in the follow-up period. Patients were asked to respond to the statement "You are very satisfied with the medical care you are receiving," and their answers were recorded on a five-point scale: (1) strongly disagree, (2) disagree, (3) neutral, (4) agree, or (5) strongly agree.

Analytical Methods

Two indicators of socioeconomic status were used: the population wealth quintile of the patient, and caste status. Patients were assigned to population wealth quintiles on the basis of their asset ownership as recorded in the exit interview questionnaire. First, patient household assets from the baseline and follow-up surveys were made comparable with assets used in

NFHS 1998–99 for Uttar Pradesh, which is derived from a representative sample of the state's population. Separate sets of assets were used in the baseline and follow-up surveys, although there is some overlap between assets (annex table 10.2). Second, a principal component analysis from the NFHS asset data was used to assign standardized asset scores and population quintile cutoffs separately for the baseline and follow-up surveys, following the methods described by Gwatkin and others (2000) and Filmer and Pritchett (2001). These scores were then applied to the patient's asset information from the baseline and follow-up surveys. Total asset scores for each patient were calculated by summing across assets, and the totals were compared with their respective quintile cutoffs from the Uttar Pradesh NFHS. Because of extreme lumping of scores in the baseline survey, the bottom two quintiles were combined into one group comprising the lowest 40 percent, which was used as the reference group for comparison. The bottom two quintiles of the population correspond roughly to the population below the poverty line. The facility records do not contain any information on the socioeconomic background of the patients. We therefore indirectly estimated utilization levels by wealth group by using the distribution of new outpatients sampled in the baseline and follow-up exit interviews and applying it to the average number of new outpatients seen at the facility over comparable six-month periods (July to December) in 2000 and 2002.

Caste is an important indicator of social position in India, where there has been much evidence of discrimination toward lower castes. In this study, lower-caste groups include scheduled castes, scheduled tribes, and other backward castes. Anyone not belonging to these three groups was classified as higher caste. In the analysis, we compare the outcomes of interest for the combined lower-caste group of patients and the higher-caste patients.

To estimate the project's net effect, we conducted a difference-of-differences (DOD) analysis. We subtracted the change from baseline to follow-up in control facilities from the change between surveys in project facilities for both utilization numbers and satisfaction scores. Subtracting this change observed in control sites from the change in project sites gives an estimate of change in utilization (or satisfaction) attributable to the project and to other time-variant nonproject factors specific to project facilities. To examine the project's effect on distribution, we compared the results for lower and higher wealth groups, as well as for lower-caste and higher-caste groups. In addition, we stratified the analysis by level of facility because distribution of resources is often different at hospitals and clinics. The satisfaction score was also evaluated using multiple linear regression to assess the effects of the project on wealth and caste while controlling for the age and sex of the patient and the type of facility. Ordinal logistic regression models gave similar results. The linear regression model used the following equation:

$$Y_i = \beta_0 + \beta_1 R_i + \beta_2 P_i + \beta_3 RP_i + \beta_Q Q_i + \beta_{Q1} QR_i + \beta_{Q2} QP_i + \beta_{Q3} QRP_i + \beta_I I_i$$
$$+ \beta_F F_i + \varepsilon_i$$

where Y is the overall satisfaction score, ranging from 1 to 5; R is an indicator variable for the survey round (1 = follow-up, 0 = baseline); P is an indicator variable for project group (1 = project, 0 = control); RP is the interaction of R and P; and Q is a vector of indicator variables showing the population quintile to which the patient belongs. There are two indicator variables in this vector indexing: patients in the middle quintile, and those in the highest two quintiles. The reference category is the lowest two quintiles; QR is the interaction between Q and R; QP is the interaction between Q and P; QRP is a vector containing three-way interactions between RP and Q; I is a vector of individual characteristics (age, gender, and caste status); and F is a vector of the facility assessment score before the project.

Of interest are the coefficient β_3 and the coefficient vector β_{Q3} of RP and vector QRP; β_3 gives the difference-of-differences estimate of patient satisfaction for those in the two poorest quintiles. The linear combination of β_3 and the coefficients in β_{Q3} gives the difference of differences for those in the middle quintile and the two least poor quintiles. The coefficients in β_{Q3} estimate the difference in the difference-of-differences estimates between the middle quintile, the two least poor quintiles, and the two poorest quintiles.

Findings

There were two important findings:

- *Utilization and distribution.* The project increased utilization at all types of health facilities and for both the poor and the better off, but the wealthier groups had the largest gains.
- *Patient satisfaction and distribution.* Patient satisfaction overall improved only at lower-level project facilities, not at hospitals. The wealthiest group showed gains in satisfaction with every type of facility, and the improvements were significantly higher than for the poorest group, which showed positive gains only at the community health centers.

Utilization and Distribution

Background characteristics of the patients interviewed are similar with respect to the distribution of age and gender at the baseline; relatively small changes were recorded in the follow-up period (annex table 10.3). The background characteristics of the samples in both surveys are generally similar to those of the state population.

Table 10.2 shows mean monthly new outpatient visits per facility for each type of health facility. Mean monthly visits per facility were estimated by dividing mean new outpatient visits in the last six months of 2000 and 2002 by the number of facilities in each group. The data indicate a consistent increase in mean monthly outpatient visits at every project site level. Meanwhile, mean outpatient visits declined between baseline and follow-up in all control facilities. The last column in table 10.2 shows that between the baseline and follow-up surveys, the increase in mean outpatient visits was higher in project than in control sites across all facility types. This suggests that overall utilization at every type of facility improved as a result of the project.

Table 10.3 shows the estimated mean monthly number of new outpatient visits per facility at each survey round by wealth and caste group, based on the distribution of the sampled outpatients interviewed (see annex table 10.4). The estimated number of new outpatient visits for the bottom two quintiles (the poorest 40 percent) increased between the baseline and follow-up periods across all project and control facility types. A similar trend is seen for the highest 40 percent in project facilities, with the exception of project commu-

Table 10.2. Mean Monthly New Outpatient Visits Per Facility at Project and Control Facilities, Baseline and Follow-Up Rounds, Uttar Pradesh

Facility type	Baseline (July–Dec. 2000)		Follow-up (July–Dec. 2002)		Difference between follow-up and baseline		Difference of differences (project minus control)
	Project	Control	Project	Control	Project	Control	
District hospital	9,486	7,534	9,795	7,202	309	−332	641
Female district hospital	2,525	2,489	2,555	2,183	30	−306	336
Community health center	1,401	1,626	1,480	1,111	79	−515	594
Primary health center	801	729	1200	628	399	−101	500
All facilities (mean)	3,467	3,630	3,672	3,066	205	−564	769

Source: UPHSDP 2003 evaluation survey.

Table 10.3. Distribution of Mean Monthly Number of New Outpatient Visits Per Facility by Wealth and Caste Group, Uttar Pradesh

| Facility type and year | Group | Wealth quintile | | | Caste status | | |
		Lowest 40 percent	Middle 20 percent	Highest 40 percent	Lower caste	Higher caste	Total
All facilities							
2002	Project	1,104	661	1,908	2,023	1,649	3,672
2000	Project	575	982	1,910	1,652	1,815	3,467
2002	Control	1,002	542	1,521	1,588	1,478	3,066
2000	Control	575	804	2,251	1,800	1,830	3,630
District hospital							
2002	Project	2,144	1,270	6,380	4,712	5,083	9,795
2000	Project	973	2,432	6,081	3,892	5,594	9,486
2002	Control	1,806	1,349	4,048	3,467	3,736	7,203
2000	Control	973	1,694	4,866	3,713	3,821	7,534
Female district hospital							
2002	Project	475	363	1,717	1,201	1,354	2,555
2000	Project	472	407	1,645	1,010	1,515	2,525
2002	Control	528	348	1,308	1,056	1,128	2,184
2000	Control	243	213	2,034	941	1,548	2,489
Community health center							
2002	Project	672	394	414	971	509	1,480
2000	Project	274	480	647	746	655	1,401
2002	Control	541	188	383	653	458	1,111
2000	Control	368	476	782	798	828	1,626
Primary health center							
2002	Project	532	281	387	832	368	1,200
2000	Project	156	313	332	475	326	801
2002	Control	317	116	195	378	250	628
2000	Control	175	257	297	500	230	729

Source: UPHSDP 2003 evaluation survey.
Note: Mean monthly outpatient visits are average new outpatient visits per month per facility between July and December of the indicated year.

nity health centers. For the control facilities in this group, the number of new outpatient visits declined consistently between the two survey rounds.

The results for lower-caste members show an increase in new outpatient visits at project sites at each type of facility. At control facilities, visits declined at every facility level except female hospitals. For upper-caste members, new outpatient visits declined between survey rounds at all project facility levels except primary health centers. Similar trends are observed for control facilities.

Figure 10.2 highlights the difference-of-differences effects, showing that over time new outpatient visits at project sites increased more than at control sites at all facility types for the two least poor quintiles. This suggests that the UPHSDP had a positive impact on number of visits among the better off. For those in the two poorest quintiles, increases over time in new outpatient visits at project sites have been greater than at control sites for district hospitals, community health centers, and primary health centers. For female district hospitals, the increase was greater for control sites. This suggests that the UPHSDP has had an impact on increasing new outpatient visits at all types of facilities except the female hospitals. For every type of facility, however, the difference of differences in new outpatient visits for the highest 40 percent is higher than for the lowest 40 percent, indicating that wealthier groups benefited more from the project than did poorer groups.

Figure 10.2. *Difference of Differences in Average New Monthly Visits at Project and Control Health Facilities for Patients from Lowest and Highest Wealth Groups, Uttar Pradesh*

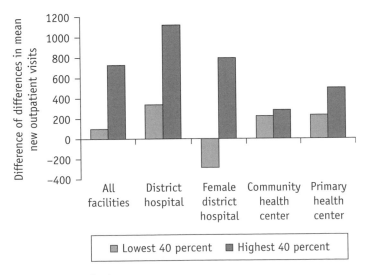

Source: UPHSDP 2003 evaluation survey.

Patient Satisfaction Levels and Distribution

Table 10.4 shows that the project had a significant effect in raising patient satisfaction scores at community and primary health centers but not at hospitals. The direction of change for control site facilities was negative at all levels.

Disaggregation of satisfaction levels according to wealth group and caste (table 10.5) shows that the largest negative changes were among patients from the lowest 40 percent and at district hospitals. The changes among lower-caste members appear to be less pronounced.

Multiple linear regression was used to examine the difference of differences between project and control sites for the different wealth groups. The highlights are shown in figure 10.3; detailed results are presented in annex table 10.5. The DOD results indicate that for patients in the wealthiest 40 percent of the population, the project had a significant impact on improving satisfaction overall (p-value = 0.01), in particular at community health centers (p-value = 0.001) and primary health centers (p-value = 0.01). Among patients in the poorest 40 percent of the population, the DOD change was positive only at the community health centers, although it was not significantly different from zero at any type of facility. Contrasting the relative DOD changes for patients in the wealthiest 40 percent and the poorest 40 percent, there were significantly greater improvements in satisfaction overall (DOD = 0.40, p-value = 0.04), as well as at the primary health centers (DOD = 0.93, p-value = 0.03). In these models, caste did not have a significant effect, suggesting that wealth influences satisfaction more than does caste.

Table 10.4. Mean Patient Satisfaction Scores by Survey Round and Facility Type, Uttar Pradesh

			Facility type			
Survey round	Group	All	District hospital	Female district hospital	Community health center	Primary health center
2003	Project	3.92	3.76	3.89	4.08	4.22
1999	Project	4.01	3.94	4.15	3.85	4.20
2003	Control	3.88	3.88	3.97	3.81	3.79
1999	Control	4.10	3.94	4.20	4.22	4.17
Difference of differences		0.13	−0.12	−0.03	0.64**	0.40*

Source: UPHSDP baseline survey and 2003 evaluation survey.
* Significant at $p < 0.05$.
** Significant at $p < 0.01$.

Table 10.5. Mean Satisfaction Scores by Wealth Group and Caste for Project and Control Sites at Baseline and Follow-Up, Uttar Pradesh

Facility type and round	Group	Wealth quintile			Caste status		
		Lowest 40 percent	Middle 20 percent	Highest 40 percent	Lower caste	Higher caste	Total
All facilities							
2003	Project	3.98	3.88	3.90	3.94	3.90	3.92
1999	Project	4.23	4.04	3.93	4.02	4.01	4.01
2003	Control	3.98	3.77	3.85	3.89	3.86	3.88
1999	Control	4.08	4.06	4.13	4.09	4.12	4.10
District hospital							
2003	Project	3.86	3.52	3.77	3.72	3.79	3.76
1999	Project	4.45	4.04	3.82	3.99	3.91	3.94
2003	Control	3.94	3.89	3.86	3.87	3.89	3.88
1999	Control	3.93	3.98	3.93	3.94	3.93	3.94
Female district hospital							
2003	Project	4.24	3.88	3.79	4.00	3.78	3.89
1999	Project	4.17	4.20	4.13	4.13	4.16	4.15
2003	Control	4.23	3.97	3.86	4.06	3.88	3.97
1999	Control	4.06	4.07	4.23	4.06	4.28	4.20
Community health center							
2003	Project	4.00	3.93	4.34	4.08	4.08	4.08
1999	Project	4.08	3.92	3.69	3.82	3.88	3.85
2003	Control	3.86	3.44	3.92	3.80	3.82	3.81
1999	Control	4.33	4.00	4.29	4.27	4.17	4.22
Primary health center							
2003	Project	3.98	4.50	4.35	4.11	4.42	4.22
1999	Project	4.33	4.13	4.20	4.22	4.16	4.20
2003	Control	4.00	3.47	3.63	3.82	3.73	3.79
1999	Control	4.00	4.21	4.23	4.19	4.12	4.17

Source: UPHSDP baseline survey and 2003 evaluation survey.

Figure 10.3. *Difference of Differences in Mean Patient Satisfaction Scores from Project to Control Health Facilities by Wealth Group, Uttar Pradesh*

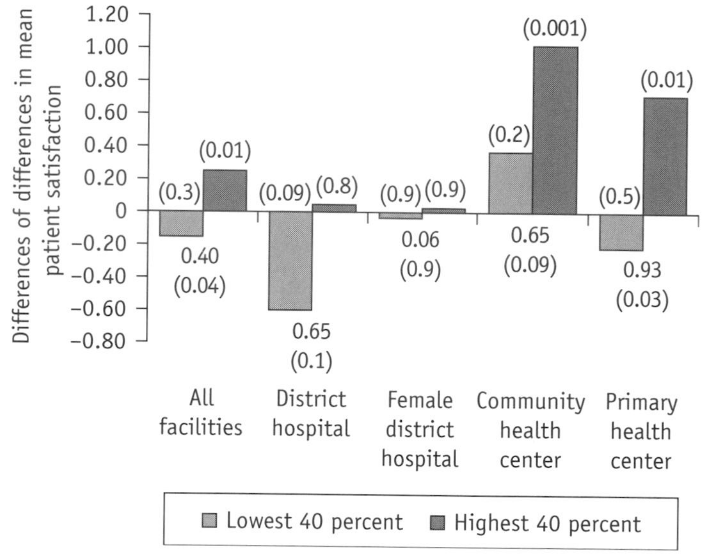

Source: UPHSDP baseline survey and 2003 evaluation survey.

Note: Figures in parenthesis are *p*-values of the difference-of-difference (DOD) estimates. Figures above the bars test whether the DOD estimates are different from zero. Figures below the bars show the point estimate of the difference of the DOD estimate between the lowest and highest 40 percent wealth groups.

Study Limitations

A number of limitations arose from sampling and measurement methods. The study was not a pure experiment because the intervention facilities were not randomly assigned and the same patients were not interviewed at baseline and follow-up. The best way to limit any potential bias was to select control facilities randomly, make concurrent before-and-after measurements, and control for potential systematic differences in facility and patient characteristics in the multivariate analysis. The assessment of the socioeconomic distribution of utilization was based on the assets of patients sampled in the baseline and follow-up rounds, which, again, were not random samples. There is, however, no reason to believe that patients were sampled differently at project sites and control sites, limiting any bias that might have been introduced. Another potential bias is that in both rounds patients were interviewed for satisfaction at the facilities (although after completing the visit), which may bias results upward. But the effect should not be different between project and control sites at baseline and follow-up, so the difference-of-differences measures should still be valid. The estimates of monthly averages for outpatient visits contained data that were incomplete, particularly for the primary health centers. Although the project and control sites for outpatient visits were matched by district, this thin sample might not produce robust estimates.

Inconsistencies between the baseline and follow-up surveys added to the constraints by (a) reducing the number of facilities that could be compared and the number of assets that could be used for assessing wealth groups and (b) changing the instrument used to assess patient satisfaction. We could not find a systematic bias in the data, but we believe that the net effect of these changes is a random increase in the amount of error in our measurements. This increases the likelihood of being unable to detect additional effects of the project on satisfaction at the higher-level facilities and for the lower wealth groups. It does not change the main findings that utilization increased for all, especially the wealthier groups, and that satisfaction with services increased at the community and primary health centers and more consistently for the wealthier groups than for the poor.

Finally, caution must be used in interpreting the patient satisfaction ratings. Differences in perceptions may not reflect actual differences in quality. For example, it is not clear whether poorer socioeconomic groups express higher levels of satisfaction because the quality of services they receive is better or because they have lower expectations.

Implications

These results suggest that a project to improve quality of care can have positive impacts on utilization and on patient satisfaction. The project effects on both were greater at lower-level facilities than at district hospitals. This could be because project implementation was more rapid and less disruptive at lower levels or because targeting (that is, the selection of sites to be improved) is more effective at peripheral levels. The lower-level facilities could have been more dysfunctional for several years, so that any small improvement had a significant effect on user perceptions.

The project improved absolute levels of utilization among the poorest 40 percent of the population. The gains were largest at lower levels of care (community and primary health centers), although absolute changes in utilization were greater at the district hospitals. Utilization by the wealthier group, however, increased by even larger numbers at all types of facilities and most notably at the higher-level facilities (district hospitals and female district hospitals). This supports the hypothesis that wealthier groups are the first to benefit when general improvements are made.

The patient satisfaction results were similar to the utilization results in that wealthier groups consistently benefited more than the lower wealth groups. But the relationships between satisfaction and utilization were not parallel, as patient satisfaction actually decreased for the lowest group, particularly at district hospitals. The decline may be explained by the disruption often involved in implementing physical improvements, but it points to another caution: more attention should be paid to patients' perceptions, or the increases in utilization may not be sustained. The gains in satisfaction in the top two quintiles may partly explain why they had higher utilization increases than patients from the poorest 40 percent of the population. Although further study on the role of patient satisfaction is warranted, the findings suggest that more emphasis should be placed on explicitly trying to satisfy the demands of poor patients. Organizing health care around patients' concerns, particularly those of patients who have least access to care, may be necessary for bringing health services to the poor.

In conclusion, the study demonstrates that broad-based projects to improve the quality of care can have a positive impact on utilization and patient satisfaction. The relationship between utilization, satisfaction, and vulnerable groups is complex, suggesting that general reform projects may have less predictable effects on the poor. Although the poor did benefit from the project, the gains were greater for the wealthier groups, supporting the inverse equity hypothesis (Victora and others 2000) that interventions tend to initially increase health inequalities.

Annex Table 10.1. Distribution of New Outpatients Sampled for Baseline and Follow-Up Surveys, Uttar Pradesh
(Number of patients)

Type of facility	Baseline			Follow-up		
	Project	Control	Total	Project	Control	Total
District hospital	195	209	404	369	347	716
Female district hospital	155	164	319	183	182	365
Community health center	184	106	290	218	148	366
Primary health center	123	108	231	110	103	213
All facilities	657	587	1,244	880	780	1,660

Source: UPHSDP baseline survey and 2003 evaluation survey.

Annex Table 10.2. *Percentage Distribution of Household Assets, Uttar Pradesh Samples*
(percent)

Asset	1999 baseline			2003 follow-up			Uttar Pradesh 1998–99[a]
	Project	Control	Total	Project	Control	Total	
Any toilet	40	43	41	38	38	38	26
Electricity	29	35	32	50	48	49	36
Cook with gas	17	21	19	27	24	25	12
House pucca	36	44	40	31	32	32	24
House semipucca	30	29	29	32	30	31	31
Television	19	25	22	39	37	38	21
Agricultural land	61	56	59	—	—	—	65
Livestock	54	61	57	—	—	—	64
Private water pipe	—	—	—	20	17	18	10
Public water pipe	—	—	—	5	7	6	2
Handpump, private	—	—	—	35	35	35	46
Handpump, public	—	—	—	27	28	27	29
Well, private.	—	—	—	3	3	3	4
Well, public	—	—	—	10	10	10	10
Lighting, electric	—	—	—	50	48	49	36
Lighting, kerosene	—	—	—	49	52	50	64
Lighting, oil	—	—	—	0	0	0	0
Motorcycle	—	—	—	24	22	23	8
Bicycle	—	—	—	86	82	84	65
Radio	—	—	—	47	46	47	31
Fan	—	—	—	46	44	45	33
Sewing machine	—	—	—	29	27	28	23

Sources: UPHSDP baseline survey and 2003 evaluation survey; IIPS and ORC Macro (2000).
a. Data from National Family Health Survey 1998–99 (NFHS-2).

Annex Table 10.3. *Background Characteristics of All Outpatients in Baseline and Follow-Up Surveys, Uttar Pradesh*

Variable	Baseline (1999)			Follow-up (2003)			Uttar Pradesh[a]
	Project	*Control*	*All*	*Project*	*Control*	*All*	
Number of facilities	25	22	47	25	22	47	n.a.
Number of patients	657	587	1,244	880	780	1660	n.a.
Age (years)	25.24 (17.61)	26.24 (17.35)	25.71 (17.48)	28.46 (16.89)	29.12 (17.44)	28.77 (17.15)	n.a.
Male (percent)	50	47	48	50	47	49	51
Urban (percent)	—	—	—	34	36	35	20
Scheduled caste (percent)	19	18	19	22	19	21	21
Scheduled tribe (percent)	2	2	2	0	0.38	0.18	2
Other backward caste (percent)	27	30	28	33	32	33	30
High caste (percent)	52	50	52	46	48	47	41
Patient asset score	0.37 (1.64)	0.63 (1.84)	0.49 (1.74)	1.15 (2.80)	0.96 (2.79)	1.06 (2.79)	n.a.
Baseline facility rating score	11.27 (1.32)	9.18 (2.70)	10.34 (2.30)				

Sources: UPHSDP baseline survey and 2003 evaluation survey; IIPS and ORC Macro (2000).
Note: Numbers in parentheses are standard deviations.
n.a. Not applicable.
a. Data from National Family Health Survey 1998–99 (NFHS-2).

Annex Table 10.4. *Distribution of Sampled New Outpatients by Wealth Group and Caste at Project and Control Facilities at Baseline (1999) and Follow-Up (2003), Uttar Pradesh*
(percent)

Facility type and year	Group	Wealth quintile[a]				Caste status			Sample size
		Lowest 40 percent	Middle 20 percent	Highest 40 percent	Total	Lower	Higher	Total	
All facilities									
2003	Project	30	18	52	100	55	45	100	895
1999	Project	17	28	55	100	48	52	100	657
2003	Control	33	18	50	100	52	48	100	780
1999	Control	16	22	62	100	50	50	100	587
District hospital									
2003	Project	22	13	65	100	48	52	100	370
1999	Project	10	26	64	100	41	59	100	195
2003	Control	25	19	56	100	48	52	100	347
1999	Control	13	22	65	100	49	51	100	209
Female district hospital									
2003	Project	19	14	67	100	47	53	100	183
1999	Project	19	16	65	100	40	60	100	155
2003	Control	24	16	60	100	48	52	100	182
1999	Control	10	9	82	100	38	62	100	164
Community health center									
2003	Project	45	27	28	100	66	34	100	218
1999	Project	20	34	46	100	53	47	100	184
2003	Control	49	17	34	100	59	41	100	148
1999	Control	23	29	48	100	49	51	100	106
Primary health center									
2003	Project	44	23	32	100	69	31	100	124
1999	Project	20	39	41	100	59	41	100	123
2003	Control	50	18	31	100	60	40	100	103
1999	Control	24	35	41	100	69	31	100	108

Source: UPHSDP baseline survey and 2003 evaluation survey, annex 4.
a. Quintiles based on population-level estimates (IIPS and ORC Macro 2000).

Annex Table 10.5. *Multiple Linear Regression Models for Satisfaction Scores, Uttar Pradesh*

	Reference category	All facilities			District hospitals			Female district hospitals			Community health centers			Primary health centers		
		Coef	se	t	Coef	se	t	Coef	se	t	Coef	se	t	Coef	se	t
Project (P)	Control	0.13	0.141	0.96	0.49	0.320	1.54	-0.02	0.278	-0.08	-0.18	0.255	-0.69	0.82	0.306	2.70**
Round (R)	Baseline	-0.09	0.120	-0.75	0.04	0.238	0.18	0.13	0.257	0.52	-0.44	0.223	-1.99*	-0.05	0.217	-0.25
R * P		-0.16	0.164	-0.95	-0.60	0.359	-1.68	-0.04	0.339	-0.11	0.37	0.289	1.28	-0.22	0.315	-0.69
Wealth quintile 3 (W3)	Wealth quintiles 1-2	-0.02	0.134	-0.14	0.07	0.261	0.26	-0.03	0.322	-0.08	-0.31	0.256	-1.22	0.13	0.231	0.58
Wealth quintiles 4-5 (W4-5)	Wealth quintiles 1-2	0.06	0.115	0.53	0.06	0.229	0.25	0.14	0.232	0.60	-0.01	0.234	-0.03	0.18	0.224	0.80
P * W3		-0.17	0.179	-0.94	-0.43	0.387	-1.12	0.07	0.400	0.18	0.15	0.323	0.46	-0.30	0.325	-0.92
R * W3		-0.20	0.170	-1.18	-0.12	0.315	-0.39	-0.24	0.384	-0.62	-0.10	0.337	-0.29	-0.60	0.336	-1.78
P * W4-5		-0.36	0.158	-2.30*	-0.65	0.346	-1.88	-0.17	0.296	-0.59	-0.36	0.300	-1.20	-0.33	0.316	-1.04
R * W4-5		-0.19	0.140	-1.38	-0.14	0.268	-0.52	-0.49	0.281	-1.76	0.06	0.292	0.20	-0.51	0.303	-1.69
R * P * W3		0.29	0.230	1.24	0.13	0.469	0.29	-0.18	0.507	-0.35	0.17	0.420	0.41	1.19	0.468	2.55*
R * P * W4-5		0.40	0.192	2.09*	0.65	0.398	1.63	0.06	0.376	0.17	0.65	0.379	1.71	0.93	0.428	2.16*
Age	—	0.00	0.001	0.23	0.00	0.002	1.56	0.00	0.003	-0.96	0.00	0.002	-0.41	0.00	0.002	-0.60
Sex	Female	0.05	0.037	1.36	0.08	0.067	1.14	-0.04	0.116	-0.36	0.11	0.076	1.48	0.12	0.088	1.40
Caste	Low caste	0.00	0.038	0.06	0.03	0.067	0.49	-0.01	0.073	-0.17	-0.03	0.078	-0.34	0.04	0.091	0.41
Facility score	—	0.01	0.009	1.34	0.01	0.015	0.99	0.03	0.015	2.19*	-0.03	0.048	-0.72	-0.23	0.077	-2.99**
Constant		3.93	0.138	28.36**	3.61	0.270	13.39**	3.86	0.274	14.07**	4.55	0.437	10.42**	6.07	0.726	8.36**

Source: UPHSDP baseline and 2003 evaluation survey.
* Significant at $p < 0.05$.
** Significant at $p < 0.01$.

Notes

We thank Davidson Gwatkin, Abdo Yazbeck, and Adam Wagstaff for their invaluable help and advice. We would also like to acknowledge the assistance of the Academy of Management Studies (AMS), Lucknow, India, which facilitated data collection. Our thanks also go to the project management unit of the Uttar Pradesh Health Systems Development Project, Lucknow, for all their assistance during data collection.

1. In November 2000 Uttar Pradesh was divided into two states, Uttar Pradesh and Uttaranchal. This analysis focuses only on data from the current Uttar Pradesh state.

2. Other Uttar Pradesh statistics illustrate this lag. 42 percent of the rural population lives below the poverty line, 70 percent of the women are illiterate, and, according to the 1995/96 National Sample Survey (1998), utilization of public health services is very low. Only 6 percent of deliveries took place in a public health facility; 0.4 percent of Uttar Pradesh residents were hospitalized at a public hospital in one year (44 percent of all hospitalizations); and only 60 outpatient visits per 1,000 population were made at a public facility (6 percent of all outpatient visits).

References

Andaleeb, S. S. 2000. Public and private hospitals in Bangladesh: Service quality and predictors of hospital choice. *Health Policy and Planning* 15(1): 95–102.

Aldana, J. M., H. Piechulek, and A. Al-Sabir. 2001. Client satisfaction and quality of care in rural Bangladesh. *Bulletin of the World Health Organization* 79(6): 512–17.

Chawla, M., and R. P. Ellis. 2000. The impact of financing and quality changes on health care demand in Niger. *Health Policy and Planning* 15(1): 76–84.

Filmer, Deon, and Lant H. Pritchett. 2001. Estimating wealth effects without expenditure data—or tears: An application to educational enrollments in states of India. *Demography* 38(1): 115–32.

Gwatkin, Davidson, Shea Rutstein, Kiersten Johnson, Rohini Pande, and Adam Wagstaff. 2000. Socio-economic differences in health, nutrition and population—45 countries. Health, Nutrition and Population Department, World Bank, Washington, DC. http://web.worldbank.org/WBSITE/EXTERNAL/TOPICS/EXTHEALTHNUTRITIONANDPOPULATION/EXTPAH/0,,contentMDK:20216957~menuPK:400482~pagePK:148956~piPK:216618~theSitePK:400476,00.html.

Haddad, S., and P. Fournier. 1995. Quality, cost and utilization of health services in developing countries: A longitudinal study in Zaire. *Social Science and Medicine* 40(6): 743–53.

IIPS (International Institute for Population Sciences) and ORC Macro. 2000. *National Family Health Survey (NFHS-2) 1998–99: India.* Mumbai: IIPS; Calverton, MD: ORC Macro.

Mahal, A., J. Singh, F. Afridi, V. Lamba, A. Gumber, and V. Selvaraju. 2001. Who benefits from public spending in India? National Council of Applied Economic Research, New Delhi.

Peters, D. H., A. S. Yazbeck, R. R. Sharma, G. N. V. Ramana, L. H. Pritchett, and A. Wagstaff. 2002. Better health systems for India's poor: Findings, analysis, and options. World Bank, Washington, DC.

Ramana, G. N. V., J. G. Sastry, and D. H. Peters. 2002. Health transition in India: Issues and challenges. *National Medical Journal of India* 15: 37–42.

Victora, G. C., J. P. Vaughan, F. C. Barros, A. C. Silva, and E. Tomasi. 2000. Explaining trends in inequalities: Evidence from Brazilian child health studies. *Lancet* 356(9235): 1093–98.

World Bank. 2002. *World development indicators 2002.* Washington, DC: World Bank.

11

Nepal: The Distributional Impact of Participatory Approaches on Reproductive Health for Disadvantaged Youths

Anju Malhotra, Sanyukta Mathur, Rohini Pande, and Eva Roca

This chapter presents findings from a community-based study testing the effectiveness of participatory approaches in improving services and outcomes for youth reproductive health in Nepal. The study was motivated by the desire to test the impact of participatory approaches in improving youth reproductive health. Nepal was chosen because youth reproductive health needs are especially acute there and little is being done to meet them.

Context and Research Questions

The findings are based on microlevel analysis from primary quantitative and qualitative data collected to evaluate an intervention study conducted from 2001 to 2003. In this study we test whether key principles advocated by development practitioners for making services work for poor people can be effectively operationalized through small, community-based programmatic interventions. In particular, our study seeks to establish whether participatory intervention programs can increase empowerment of and accountability to poor and disadvantaged populations. By amplifying client voice and widening choice, do such programs act as critical mechanisms for improving service accessibility and health outcomes for the disadvantaged?

The study targeted youth reproductive health as the outcome of interest for a number of important reasons. For reproductive health policy and programming, a focus on youth is critical because adolescence is when most men and women experience the key transitions of initiating sexuality, entering marriage, and starting childbearing. Yet most young people embark on this life stage with insufficient information about sexual and reproductive health, inadequate support and guidance from adults, and limited access to health care resources. Youth itself is a disadvantage in accessing reproductive health information and services. In most countries young people are denied reproductive health services in critical ways that do not apply to older age groups, most often because of social and moral assumptions and judgments concerning youth sexuality and service needs (Mathur, Malhotra, and Mehta 2001). This tends to hold true even in countries where many adolescents are married or in unions and therefore at high risk of unwanted pregnancies or disease (Senderowitz 1999).

Lack of access to reproductive health services among young people is an issue of some urgency. Demographically, the world now has the largest-ever youth generation—more than a billion young people between the ages of 10 and 19—and 84 percent of them live in developing countries (UNFPA 2004). More than at any other time in history, the health, capabilities, and actions of adolescents will define not only their own life outcomes but also the future of their societies.

Our study was motivated by the desire to test the impact of participatory approaches in improving youth reproductive health. In the field of development programming, community-based and participatory programs have been advocated as more effective than traditional approaches. They involve the beneficiaries in program design, implementation, and evaluation, thus serving as means of empowering communities, creating ownership of the interventions, and fostering accountability to poor clients (World Bank 2004). Empowerment and accountability can improve service delivery by amplifying clients' voice and broadening their choices. At a macro level, increased client power can strengthen accountability in the relationship between poor people and providers, between poor people and policy makers, and between policy makers and providers (World Bank 2004).

This process should also work at a micro, community level. For example, well-informed, mobilized, and organized community members can exert power by contributing financial resources and coproducing health services. With regard to youth reproductive health, self-care is a particularly vital type of service coproduction because information and social support are important means of promoting practices such as safe sex, contraceptive use, and prenatal care. Participatory processes increase awareness and information sharing. Better information, in turn, can lead to change in self-care behaviors, to expanded consumer power, and to the use of complaint and redress mechanisms. For youth reproductive health in particular, information sharing is critical for raising community awareness of key demand-side barriers, including attitudinal, normative, and institutional constraints such as early marriage, son preference, and sexual double standards (Mensch, Bruce, and Greene 1998; Norman 2001).

Participatory programs may strengthen clients' power in their dealings with clinical service providers. Availability of, access to, and quality of services may improve because clients who actively participate in decision making are more likely than those who do not to be motivated and able to monitor services and exert leverage on providers for better services. Community-based participatory programs may empower disadvantaged citizens by providing access to information and to decision-making bodies and by increasing their ability to build coalitions, influence the political process and the allocation of resources, and establish monitoring and accountability mechanisms (Cornwall and Gaventa 2001). In addition to the coproduction issues raised above, adolescents approached in a consultative, inclusive manner are more likely to increase their knowledge base, critical thinking, and decision-making abilities on intimate issues related to sexual and reproductive health (McCauley and Salter 1995; Senderowitz 1998).

For all these reasons, microlevel, community-based participatory programs have enormous potential for influencing the relationship between disadvantaged youths and service providers, as well as the relationship between disadvantaged youths and policy makers. To date, however, no comprehensive evaluations have been conducted on the effectiveness of a participatory process at the community level in implementing programs for adolescent reproductive health in developing countries and, in particular, in reaching poor and otherwise disadvantaged youths. Our study offers such an evaluation, focusing on a program in Nepal.

We chose Nepal for our study because youth reproductive health needs there are especially acute. Despite a large youth population and chronically poor outcomes on a number of reproductive health indicators among young people, this issue has received limited programmatic and policy attention.

Early marriage, a strong predictor of reproductive risk, is nearly universal in Nepal: girls marry at an average age of 16, and 52 percent begin childbearing by the age of 20. Only 55 percent of the women under age 20 who had given birth reported receiving antenatal care, 14 percent of the births were attended by trained personnel, and only 9 percent of deliveries took place in a health facility. Less than 7 percent of married women in the 15–19 age group reported using any method of contraception, and only 4 percent reported a modern method. Rural women in Nepal, who are typically poorer than their urban counterparts, marry and initiate childbearing two to three years earlier, on average, than urban women and are eight times less likely to use antenatal services and to deliver in a health facility (Nepal, Ministry of Health, and others 2002).

Study Design

In the Nepal Adolescent Project (NAP) we employed a quasi-experimental case-control study design to implement and test the effectiveness of a community-based, client-centered participatory approach aimed at improving the sexual and reproductive health of adolescents in rural and urban Nepal. The five-year project was conducted from 1998 to 2003 as a collaboration between an international service delivery organization (EngenderHealth), an international research organization (International Center for Research on Women), and two local Nepali nongovernmental organizations (NGOs), New ERA Ltd., and BP Memorial Health Foundation. The project was conducted in two study sites, one urban and one rural, and two control sites, one urban and one rural. Participatory methodologies and techniques were utilized during the research, needs assessment, intervention design, implementation, and monitoring and evaluation phases in the two study sites. More traditional reproductive health research, design, and intervention elements were implemented in the two control sites. The overall intervention period ranged from 12 to 24 months; the first set of interventions began in November 2000, and the last set ended in March 2003.

The rural and urban areas were chosen to permit a clear differentiation in infrastructure, service options, levels of economic development, and standard of living.[1] In other words, the rural-urban difference in site selection itself was intended to capture structural disadvantages, as well as wealth differentials. Because of the requirements of intervention design, we also needed to select communities that were readily accessible by road and already had institutions such as a secondary school and a health post. Thus, the communities included in this study are more developed than the typical Nepali rural or urban setting. The communities selected were randomly assigned to study or control.

The study and control sites were differentiated by implementation methods and by the elements included. In comparison with the control sites, the overall design and implementation efforts in the study sites were more comprehensive, inclusive, and interactive, with a great deal of attention to building community ownership and involvement at every step. This was achieved by setting up mechanisms and structures such as advisory and coordination teams and consultative committees that engaged youths and adult community members, especially the disadvantaged. At the intervention design stage, an action planning process was conducted in which the needs assessment results were shared and analyzed with the community, and community task forces were created to set priorities and design feasible interventions. Program implementation structures were more inclusive in the study sites, with community-level committees that allowed both adults and youths to increase their authority and decision-making power in the project. With its mandate for a participatory approach, the project staff used strategies to ensure the active involvement of disempowered groups—the poor, women, and ethnic minorities—in these structures and processes (for example, by setting up rotating representation). The control sites had no such participatory processes or structures.

Intervention components were very different for study and control sites. Study site interventions attempted to address structural, normative, and systemic barriers to youth reproductive health, while the control sites addressed only the most immediate risk factors such as sexually transmitted diseases (STDs) and unwanted pregnancies. Thus, interventions in the study site linked youth reproductive health programs with other programs deemed to influence the environment where youths live; such programs included adult education programs, activities to address social norms, and economic livelihoods interventions. Eight such linked interventions, developed and prioritized by community members, were implemented in the study sites. For comparison, the project staff designed and implemented in the control sites three standard reproductive health interventions that focused on basic risk factors. Socioeconomic disadvantages based on gender, rural-urban residence, wealth, ethnicity, schooling status, and marital status were a specific focus of the intervention design and approach in the study sites but not in the control sites. The difference in focus is especially relevant to this analysis.

In the context of this intervention research design, we examine here whether the participatory or the nonparticipatory intervention approach is more successful in reducing the gaps between the disadvantaged and the advantaged in access to youth reproductive health services and in outcomes.

Data and Methodology

In our analysis, we use cross-sectional quantitative household and adolescent survey data collected at baseline and endline for the Nepal Adolescent Project, as well as relevant qualitative and participatory data (see annex 11.1). For the quantitative surveys, a 100 percent census of households was taken in the rural areas at the baseline and endline. Because the population base in the urban area is larger, a 50 percent random sampling was considered sufficient. This resulted in a sample size of 965 households at baseline and 1,003 households at endline.

The age group sampled for the adolescent survey at baseline was 14 to 21 years old. Since most of the service-related interventions were targeted at that age group, for the endline we tracked this cohort which was by then 18 to 25 years old. The study design allowed us to track the cohort, but not specific individuals, within each community. Since the intervention design was at the community level, interventions to increase knowledge and information covered a broader population. To ensure capture of the impact of such interventions on younger adolescents, we included the age 14–17 group in the endline sample (see table 11.1).[2] Although the full sample covering married and unmarried males and females age 14–21 at baseline and age 14–25 at endline is fairly large, the subsamples for each site are relatively small. These small subsample sizes pose limitations for multivariate analysis, especially where the analysis requires a focus on further subcategories such as married females who have had a pregnancy.

Dependent Variables

The survey data offer a number of interesting outcome variables, including knowledge, behavior, attitudes, and service use, for several factors relevant to youth reproductive health. Here we focus on three dependent variables

Table 11.1. *Adolescent Survey Samples and Subsamples, Nepal*

Sample and subsample base	Adolescent survey sample sizes (married and unmarried, males and females)	
	Baseline (age 14–21)	*Endline (age 14–25)*
Urban study	184	260
Urban control	164	260
Rural study	175	205
Rural control	198	254
Total	721[a]	979

Source: Nepal Adolescent Project, 1999 baseline adolescent and household surveys and 2003 endline adolescent and household surveys.

a. At the baseline, 724 adolescents were interviewed, but 3 respondents had to be excluded from the analysis because of missing household data.

frequently identified in the literature as critically important for reproductive health, especially for young people: prenatal care, institutional delivery, and knowledge about HIV/AIDS. The variables for prenatal care and institutional delivery refer to the first pregnancy of young married women because no pregnancies were reported among young unmarried women.[3] The prenatal care variable is a dichotomous measure of whether or not the pregnant woman visited a trained provider (doctor, nurse, or trained clinician) for prenatal care at least once. The institutional delivery variable is a dichotomous measure of whether or not the delivery (or miscarriage or abortion) for the first pregnancy was at a medical facility (hospital, clinic, or nursing home). Since general awareness of HIV/AIDS at baseline was already very high (over 90 percent), we use for this study a more sophisticated dichotomous measure—whether or not the respondent could correctly list at least two modes of HIV transmission. Response options considered correct were unsafe sexual contact, needle sharing, mother-to-child transmission, and blood transfusion.

Independent Variables

DEFINING DISADVANTAGE. The term *disadvantaged* refers here to adolescent girls and boys and their families who are worse off than others in the same population on several dimensions.[4] We examine disadvantage by the respondent's household economic status and the respondent's own education, rural-urban residence, and gender. The inclusion of these criteria is based on qualitative data showing that they are at least as important as wealth in defining disadvantage in our project areas. Gender and rural-urban residence are defined as dichotomous variables. Education is defined by years of schooling completed. Economic status is defined and measured in terms of household wealth, as elaborated below.

MEASURING HOUSEHOLD WEALTH. The Nepal Adolescent Project did not collect data on household income or consumption. Consequently, we measure household wealth in terms of household assets (for details, see annex 11.2). Other studies have shown that household assets are a reasonable proxy for household income or consumption (Montgomery and others 2000; Filmer and Pritchett 2001). We obtained the asset information from the NAP household questionnaire, which includes questions about each household's ownership of consumer items ranging from a radio to a television and car and about land ownership, home ownership, source of drinking water, toilet facilities, and other characteristics related to household wealth status.

From these data, following the approach used by Gwatkin and others (2000), we created an asset index that provides a single measure of household wealth. Each individual is then assigned the value or score of the asset index for his or her household.

Data Analysis

We compare the relationship between various measures of disadvantage and the three dependent variables at baseline and endline for the study and control sites using multivariate analysis. If our intervention design had targeted specific individuals, such analysis would be done on a pooled sample of individuals at baseline and endline, with dichotomous variables for study-control and for baseline-endline. Because, however, the interventions were at the community level, the NAP data provide, essentially, two cross-sectional samples at baseline and endline. Thus, we present analyses separately by the samples for study-baseline, study-endline, control-baseline, and control-endline and use significance tests to test the differences in coefficients between baseline and endline in study versus control sites.[5]

The three dependent variables also apply to different subsamples of adolescents. The two pregnancy-related variables (prenatal care and institutional delivery) are applicable only to young married women. Because the interventions targeted the age 14–21 group for these service delivery–related outcomes, we track this cohort and compare the outcomes for the age 18–25 group at endline. The dependent variable on knowledge regarding modes of HIV transmission applies to the full sample of adolescents—males and females, married and unmarried. Here, we compare the age 14–21 group at baseline and endline. The age 14–17 group at endline is included in the comparison because information-related interventions were aimed at the entire community, including younger adolescents. The age 22–25 group is excluded only because knowledge levels among youths in the older age groups are so high that there is no variation to explain. Lack of variation is also an issue for the entire urban sample, and so we limit the analysis of this third variable to the rural sites.

For the multivariate analyses, a continuous wealth variable is used in every case, although the particular continuous variable used depends on the outcome being considered. For the prenatal care and institutional delivery outcomes, we pooled the urban and rural samples and used a continuous wealth variable with the household asset scores for the combined urban and rural areas. For the HIV/AIDS knowledge outcome, the rural continuous wealth variable is used because the analysis is limited to the rural sample.

To visually highlight our findings, we also occasionally use bivariate graphs to show the association between an outcome and household wealth. For the bivariate analysis, households were ranked by asset score and divided into poor and nonpoor (for institutional delivery) or into quartiles (for HIV knowledge), with a different grouping used depending on the sample size for the health outcome analyzed. All sample individuals were assigned the wealth group of the household in which they resided.

Means and Distributions for Variables in the Analysis

Table 11.2 presents the descriptive frequencies with means and the range of values, where relevant, for outcome variables and key independent variables. The first set of frequencies is for the subsample of young women who have ever been pregnant. The sample size here is fairly small, posing limitations for the multivariate analysis. Because the cohort aged during the intervention period, the mean age at endline is higher than at baseline for both study and control sites. Also, in both sites the proportional representation of rural women increases from baseline to endline, indicating that urban women were less likely to have had a pregnancy by endline. In part because of the greater representation of rural women in this subsample, the wealth score shows only minimal change from baseline to endline in both sites. This group of women is somewhat better educated by the endline in both sites.

Interestingly, the overall change in the two maternal health outcome variables does not indicate an improved scenario in the study sites as opposed to the control sites. For prenatal care, the mean declined in the study site while increasing minimally in the control site. For institutional delivery, the change was positive for both sites but substantially more so in the control site than in the study site. To some degree, these numbers reflect small sample sizes and also the worsening of a selection bias in the type of women who are likely to experience first pregnancy at a young age. They also indicate that the overall impact of the participatory interventions was not universally positive. Our evaluation of a wide range of results (Mathur, Mehta, and Malhotra 2004) indicates that for direct measures of reproductive health outcomes, the impact of the participatory approach was mixed, with some negative, some neutral, and some positive results. The balance, however, favored more positive results than did the standard approach. The participatory approach was significantly more successful in showing positive change in more fundamental and indirect determinants of reproductive health such as youths' and young women's empowerment, age at marriage, and social norms (Mathur, Mehta, and Malhotra 2004).

Table 11.2. *Sample Means and Distributions for Variables in the Analysis, Nepal*

Variable	Study baseline	Study endline	Control baseline	Control endline
Subsample for prenatal care and institutional delivery: married young women with pregnancy experience				
Independent variables				
Mean age in years	19.5	22.1	19.1	21.6
(range in parentheses)	(14–21)	(18–25)	(14–21)	(18–25)
Percentage living in rural areas	41.1	57.5	60.7	69.5
Mean wealth score	−0.47	−0.51	−1.33	−1.13
(range in parentheses)	(−2.9, 3.7)	(−3.4, 3.8)	(−2.9, 2.2)	(−3.4, 3.3)
Mean years of schooling	4.1	4.8	2.9	3.3
Dependent variables				
Percentage receiving prenatal care	71.4	58.8	53.6	56.8
Percentage using institutional delivery	48.2	51.9	32.1	47.4
N	56	80	56	95
Subsample for knowledge of modes of HIV/AIDS transmission: rural male and female youths				
Independent variables				
Mean age in years	17.2	17.1	17.0	17.2
(range in parentheses)	(14–21)	(14–21)	(14–21)	(14–21)
Mean wealth score	0.56	0.65	0.07	−0.15
(range in parentheses)	(−2.3, 4.2)	(−2.5, 10.1)	(−2.3, 3.8)	(−2.5, 13.2)
Percentage female	53.7	49.7	57.6	50.5
Mean years of schooling	4.6	5.6	4.2	5.2
Dependent variable				
Percentage who know at least two modes of HIV transmission	45.1	82.4	45.6	80.5
N	175	157	198	202

Source: Nepal Adolescent Project, 1999 baseline adolescent and household surveys and 2003 endline adolescent and household surveys.

The second part of table 11.2 presents descriptive statistics for the rural sample of married and unmarried young men and women and the variable on knowledge regarding modes of HIV transmission. For the overall sample of rural young people, the improvements in education from baseline to endline are more substantial than for the selective sample of young women who have had pregnancies. The change in the outcome variable of interest is also more substantial from baseline to endline in both control and study sites. At baseline, less than 50 percent of respondents could accurately name at least two modes of transmission, but by the endline the proportion was closer to 80 percent.

Findings

Our results from various vantage points indicate that the participatory approach was more successful than the nonparticipatory intervention in reducing advantage-based differentials in youth reproductive health outcomes. This is generally true for the three indicators presented here—prenatal care, institutional delivery, and knowledge of HIV/AIDS transmission.

Overlap in Disadvantages

As a first analysis step, we examine disadvantage in the study and control communities and find a notable overlap in the incidence of the different types of disadvantage we measure in this population. The overlap between household wealth status and urban-rural status is especially striking. Our data show that the difference in wealth across the two settings is so large as to be almost synonymous with rural-urban residence itself. Figure 11.1, which shows the cutoff points for wealth quintiles for all four sites at baseline and endline, clearly illustrates the wide gap in rural-urban wealth. In the urban areas, not only is the curve for distribution of wealth much higher than in the rural areas; the cutoff for the poorest 20th percentile in the urban areas is also at a higher asset index score than the cutoff for the least poor 20th percentile in the rural area. This gap in the distribution of wealth across the two areas is apparent at both baseline and endline.

Two other measures of disadvantage—education and ethnicity—also overlap substantially with both wealth and rural-urban residence. Because of the high collinearity across these measures of disadvantage and the small sizes of the subsamples for some of our dependent variables, the effects of individual disadvantage-defining variables cannot always be disentangled in a multivariate setting. We therefore limit our multivariate analyses to basic models with minimal controls.[6] Where needed, we present bivariate graphs showing the relation of household wealth to the outcome in question.

Figure 11.1. Wealth Quintile Cutoff Points, Nepal

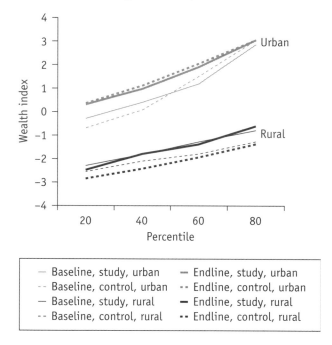

Source: Nepal Adolescent Project, 1999 baseline adolescent and household surveys and 2003 endline adolescent and household surveys.

Prenatal Care

Table 11.3 shows the effect of disadvantage, measured separately by rural-urban residence as well as by wealth, on the use of prenatal care by young married women for their first pregnancy. In all cases, the regression coefficients shown are from two models. Model 1a controls for age and shows the impact of residing in an urban as opposed to a rural area, and model 1b controls for age and shows the impact of wealth as a continuous variable.

Comparison of the coefficients for baseline with those at endline (model 1a) shows that the rural-urban differential is practically eliminated in the study sites but is essentially unchanged in the control sites. The coefficient for urban residence in the study site is 2.8 at baseline and is significant at the 0.001 level, whereas at the endline it is reduced to 0.22 and is no longer significant. The odds ratios indicate a dramatic turnaround: at baseline an urban young woman in the study site was 16 times more likely to get prenatal care than a rural young woman, but by the endline the ratio drops to 1.2.

Table 11.3. Prenatal Care: Regression Results, Study and Control Sites, Nepal

	Study		Control	
	Baseline *(age 14–21)*	*Endline* *(age 18–25)*	*Baseline* *(age 14–21)*	*Endline* *(age 18–25)*
Model 1a: urban vs. rural residence (controlling for age)				
Coefficient	2.80	0.22	1.32	1.16
Odds ratio	16.4	1.2	3.7	3.2
p-value	0.001	0.644	0.028	0.021
N	56	80	56	95
One-tailed *t*-test (*p*)	2.9 (0.00)		0.2 (0.42)	
Model 1b: wealth (controlling for age)				
Coefficient	1.01	0.20	0.66	0.36
p-value	0.005	0.189	0.017	0.010
N	56	80	56	95
One-tailed *t*-test (*p*)	2.3 (0.01)		1.1 (0.13)	

Source: Nepal Adolescent Project, 1999 baseline adolescent and household surveys and 2003 endline adolescent and household surveys.
Note: The *t*-tests are one-tailed to test the hypothesis that differentials by disadvantage are reduced from baseline to endline.

In the control site the initial contrast was less extreme: urban women were only 3.7 times more likely to get prenatal care than rural women. The differential shrinks to only 3.2 times more likely for the urban women and remains significant at the endline. Tests of significance between baseline and endline coefficients in each study and control site confirm a statistically significant decline in residence-based advantage in the study sites between the baseline and the endline; no significant change occurs in the control sites.

Model 1b shows similar results, using wealth as the key independent variable and again controlling for age. The beneficial impact of belonging to a wealthier family is substantial and significant in both study and control sites at baseline (more so in the study than in the control site). In the study site the coefficient for wealth is much smaller by the endline than at baseline and is no longer significant. By contrast, at the control site at endline, wealth remains an important differentiating factor in young women's access to prenatal care. Again, significance tests confirm that the baseline-endline change is significant in the study sites but not in the control sites.[7]

Institutional Delivery

Table 11.4 shows the regression results for the relationship between disadvantage and young women's delivery of their first pregnancies in a medical facility. Model 2a shows the extent to which rural-urban differentials shifted from baseline to endline. Again, the results are much more encouraging in the study sites than in the control sites. At baseline, and in both study and control sites, institutional delivery is a rare occurrence in rural compared with urban areas: in the study site urban young women are over 15 times more likely to have an institutional delivery than rural women, and in the control site they are over 13 times more likely to do so. Although differences remain in the study site by the endline, they are substantially reduced: the

Table 11.4. Institutional Delivery: Regression Results, Study and Control Sites, Nepal

	Study		Control	
	Baseline (age 14–21)	*Endline (age 18–25)*	*Baseline (age 14–21)*	*Endline (age 18–25)*
Model 2a: urban vs. rural residence (controlling for age)				
Coefficient	2.75	1.52	2.61	3.05
Odds ratio	15.6	4.6	13.5	21.3
p-value	0.000	0.002	0.000	0.000
N	56	79	56	95
One-tailed *t*-test (*p*)	1.4 (0.08)		−0.4 (0.66)	
Model 2b: wealth (controlling for age)				
Coefficient	0.62	0.68	1.42	0.85
p-value	0.019	0.001	0.000	0.000
N	56	79	56	95
One-tailed *t*-test (*p*)	−0.2 (0.57)		1.5 (0.07)	

Source: Nepal Adolescent Project, 1999 baseline adolescent and household surveys and 2003 endline adolescent and household surveys.

Note: The *t*-tests are one-tailed to test the hypothesis that differentials by disadvantage are reduced from baseline to endline.

odds ratio is down to 4.6, and the urban-rural coefficient decreases from 2.75 to 1.52, a statistically significant difference between baseline and endline. By contrast, the differentials actually increase in the control sites, where at endline young women in the urban area are 21 times more likely to have institutional deliveries than their rural counterparts.

At a bivariate level, wealth differentials (poor-nonpoor ratios) show a similar, although less dramatic, pattern. At baseline both study and control sites show substantial differentials between the better off and the poor: the poor-nonpoor ratio in institutional deliveries is 0.32 in the study sites and 0.24 in the control sites (figure 11.2).[8] As a result of the intervention, differentials are reduced more in the study sites than in the control sites, largely because of improved access by the poor in the study sites. By the endline, the improvement in access to institutional delivery affects only the poorer 50 percent of the population in the study site, whereas in the control sites both the better off and the poor gain from the interventions. As a result, at the endline the poor-nonpoor ratio in institutional deliveries improves to 0.54 in the study sites but only to 0.35 in the control sites.

The multivariate analysis for the relationship between wealth and institutional delivery, however, is not consistent with this interpretation. As model 2b in table 11.4 shows, when the measure for wealth is used as a continuous variable and the age of the respondent is controlled for, there is little change between baseline and endline in the study sites, but there is a more dramatic reduction in the control sites. Our diagnostics show that the relationship between wealth and institutional delivery for the study and control sites is highly sensitive to how the wealth variable is defined. When wealth is defined as a continuous variable and in a linear relationship, the control sites show a stronger improvement, but when it is defined as a dichotomous variable, or with a squared term, and in a curvilinear relationship, the study sites show a stronger improvement. This is because in the control sites much of the increase in institutional deliveries is at the extreme ends of the wealth continuum, while in the study sites much of the improvement is among those in the middle.

Knowledge of HIV Transmission

The factors generating disadvantage in knowledge of HIV transmission modes are somewhat different from and broader than those applying to prenatal care and institutional delivery. A major reason for this is the broader sample base to which this indicator applies: married and unmarried young men and women. As many studies on youths and adults have noted,

Figure 11.2. *Delivery in a Medical Facility: First Pregnancy, Poor and Nonpoor Young Married Women, Nepal*

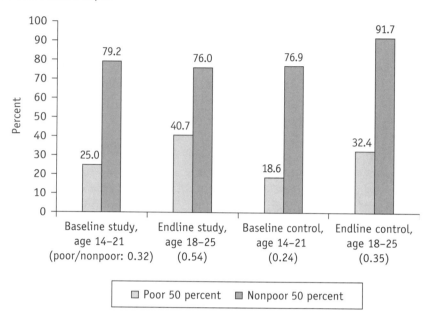

Source: Nepal Adolescent Project, 1999 baseline adolescent and household surveys and 2003 end-line adolescent and household surveys.

women are at a relative disadvantage in comparison with men in access to information and knowledge on sexual and reproductive issues in general and HIV/AIDS in particular (Weiss, Whelan, and Gupta 1996; World Bank 2004). Thus, gender, along with poverty and rural-urban residence, is an important basis for disadvantage.

Figure 11.3 presents a bivariate graph of wealth-based inequalities in knowledge of at least two modes of HIV transmission for the study and control sites at baseline and endline. A larger sample size than was available for maternal care allows us to use wealth quartiles in the bivariate analysis rather than just poor-nonpoor ratios, thus capturing a more nuanced picture of the relationship between disadvantage and HIV knowledge. As the figure shows, the overall proportion of those who can correctly identify at least two modes of HIV transmission is fairly similar for both the study and control sites, with a substantial improvement from baseline to endline for both. The degree of improvement, however, varies by wealth score: by the endline, the differentials by wealth in knowledge of HIV transmission are less

Figure 11.3. *Knowledge of At Least Two Modes of HIV Transmission, by Wealth Quartile, Young Men and Women Age 14–21, Nepal*

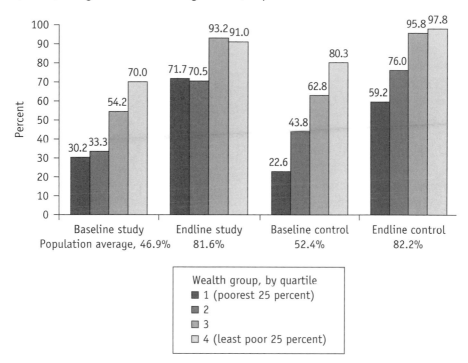

Source: Nepal Adolescent Project, 1999 baseline adolescent and household surveys and 2003 endline adolescent and household surveys.

marked in the study site than in the control site. In particular, at endline, young people from the poorest quartile are closer in knowledge to the remainder of the population in the study sites than in the control sites.

To further explore these differentials, we present three multivariate models in table 11.5. Model 3a shows the effect of being male rather than female, controlling only for age; model 3b shows the effect of gender and schooling; and model 3c further includes a continuous variable for household wealth. The multivariate models present data only for the rural areas, since in the urban areas knowledge levels for everyone were high at endline.

Model 3a shows that in the rural study site at baseline, differentials in knowledge of HIV transmission by gender, although not statistically significant, favored males: young men were 1.5 times more likely than young women to identify at least two modes of transmission. By the endline, this

Table 11.5. *Knowledge of HIV/AIDS Transmission: Rural Study and Control Sites, Nepal*

	Study		Control	
	Baseline	*Endline*	*Baseline*	*Endline*
Model 3a: gender (controlling for age)				
Coefficient male vs. female (0 = female)	0.41	−0.28	−0.21	1.23
Odds ratio	1.5	0.8	0.8	3.4
p-value	0.211	0.430	0.531	0.000
One-tailed t-test (p)	1.4 (0.07)		−3.1 (0.99)	
Model 3b: gender and education (controlling for age)				
Coefficient male vs. female (0 = female)	0.18	−0.71	−1.23	0.74
Odds ratio	1.2	0.5	0.3	2.1
p-value	0.612	0.086	0.003	0.034
One-tailed t-test (p)	1.6 (0.05)		−3.7 (0.99)	
Coefficient education	0.21	0.46	0.39	0.35
Odds ratio	1.2	1.6	1.5	1.4
p-value	0.001	0.000	0.000	0.000
One-tailed t-test (p)	−2.2 (0.98)		0.5 (0.32)	
Model 3c: gender, education, and wealth (controlling for age)				
Coefficient male vs. female (0 = female)	0.17	−0.73	−1.22	0.74
Odds ratio	1.2	0.5	0.3	2.1
p-value	0.634	0.079	0.003	0.034
One-tailed t-test (p)	1.7 (0.05)		−3.6 (0.99)	
Coefficient education	0.22	0.46	0.40	0.35
Odds ratio	1.2	1.6	1.5	1.4
p-value	0.002	0.000	0.000	0.000
One-tailed t-test (p)	−2.1 (0.98)		0.1 (0.48)	
Coefficient wealth	−0.05	−0.09	−0.08	−0.05
p-value	0.619	0.510	0.586	0.625
One-tailed t-test (p)	0.2 (0.41)		−0.2 (0.55)	
N	175	157	198	202

Source: Nepal Adolescent Project, 1999 baseline adolescent and household surveys and 2003 endline adolescent and household surveys.

Note: The t-tests are one-tailed to test the hypothesis that differentials by disadvantage are reduced from baseline to endline.

small male advantage disappears, and the odds of males' knowing more are less than 1 (but not statistically significant). The disappearance of the male advantage from baseline to endline in the study site is statistically significant, however. By contrast, no significant gender differences are apparent at the baseline in the control site, but by the endline, young men in the control site are more than three times more likely than young women to know how HIV is transmitted.

Model 3b sheds further light on this pattern. In both sites, at both baseline and endline, education is positively and significantly associated with knowledge of HIV transmission. In fact, there is little change between baseline and endline in the effect of education. In the study site by the endline, a baseline advantage for men seems to have disappeared, and women are significantly more likely to have correct knowledge of HIV transmission than men: men are only half as likely as women to correctly list two modes of transmission (odds ratio, 0.5). Significance tests between baseline and endline coefficients show that this shift is significant. This suggests that because men are more likely than women to be educated and the educated are much more likely to know about HIV transmission, only by controlling for the confounding effects of education can we see the true effect of the intervention in reducing gender disparities in HIV knowledge. In the control site, on the contrary, even after controlling for education, and thus for men's advantage on the schooling front, young men are still more likely than young women to be aware of HIV transmission modes. In fact, there is no significant change in the gender differentials between baseline and endline in the control site.

Adding in a variable for household wealth (model 3c) makes no difference to the gender or education coefficients. The wealth variable itself has a very minor coefficient and is insignificant, suggesting that for knowledge of HIV transmission, education and gender, not wealth, are defining aspects of disadvantage.

Summary of Findings

Our analysis shows that for the population in this study, change in the relationship between disadvantage and health knowledge or behavior depends on both the measure used to define disadvantage and the specific health outcome in question. For access to prenatal care services and institutional delivery, the key aspect of disadvantage is urban-rural residence. Household wealth is significant for prenatal care only. For knowledge of HIV transmission, gender and educational differences are key. On balance, our analysis shows that for most of the measures used to define disadvantage, the participatory approaches in the study sites were more successful in increasing access or knowledge for the disadvantaged than the more standard approaches used in the control sites.

Why Did the Participatory Approach Work?
The Processes behind the Results

Our broader results indicate that the participatory approach, although generally more positive in its outcomes, is by no means a panacea. The overall evaluation of the study concluded that the participatory approach required significant investment of time and resources by both implementers and community. Moreover, a number of immediate outcomes of interest were not significantly more positive in the study sites than in the control sites, although they were in the end (Mathur, Mehta, and Malhotra 2004). The broader conclusions are also reflected in our analysis, where we find that the participatory approach is usually, but not universally, more effective in reducing differentials due to disadvantage by rural-urban residence, wealth, and gender.

The qualitative and participatory data collected for the Nepal Adolescent Project make it possible to elaborate on some of the reasons for the greater success of the participatory approach in reducing disadvantage-based differentials in the use of reproductive health services by young people and in health outcomes among them. According to our analysis of these data, at least three important aspects of the greater effectiveness of the participatory approach were at work: (1) facilitating coproduction of services, (2) empowering youths and adults and increasing the accountability of service providers and policy makers to the community, and (3) increasing community demand for information and services.

1. COPRODUCTION. The nature of adolescent reproductive health makes it especially amenable to coproduction and self-service by clients, and the participatory intervention design substantially facilitated such coproduction. Qualitative data from the study sites underscore the emergence of well-informed and trained peers and more reliable social networks as critical sources of service provision for young people. Based on findings from the needs assessment, the study site interventions tapped and strengthened social networks for information exchange and counseling, while the control site interventions did not. Moreover, young people's understanding of what services actually mean and how to best use the options available to them

showed more substantial improvement in the study sites. As one of the young men who participated in the study site interventions said in the end-line survey, in response to a question about where youths seek advice on love and marriage (a taboo subject in the community):

> We don't go to the subhealth post, hospitals, FCHVs [family and child health volunteers] because they cannot solve our problem. We can talk with friends and peer educators, they can help in case of severe problem. (*male urban youth, study site, endline)*

2. EMPOWERMENT AND ACCOUNTABILITY. As a result of the active effort to impart information and build decision-making structures and coalitions, the participatory intervention was substantially more successful in empowering youths and adult community members and increasing the accountability of providers and policy makers to the communities. One factor was that the participatory structures (committees, task forces, and youth clubs) set up in the study sites fostered community skills in consensus building, decision making, planning, organizing, consulting, and demanding resources and accountability from various actors. For example, adults and youth learned to negotiate with the village development committee and felt that jointly, they could demand government funds to continue project activities. Empowerment and demand for accountability are also apparent from the data documenting the change in the client-provider relationship in the study sites. Not only were the providers trained by the program to be more youth-friendly, courteous, and responsive; young people in the community were also made aware that they can enforce these expectations. Both male and female respondents noted this:

> Earlier, the service provider used to give a very bad response if anyone went for counseling hence feared and felt embarrassed to go . . . but now with the help of the program, the service providers show cordial behavior and maintain confidentiality. Due to this the adolescents as well as the adults have started to go for health and counseling services. *(rural male and female youths, study site)*

3. COMMUNITY DEMAND. Finally, in the study sites the greater focus not just on altering reproductive health outcomes but also on changing fundamental social norms and institutions was a major factor in increasing demand for information and services among the disadvantaged. The evaluation data for the full study demonstrate that the participatory approach had a significant impact on a number of the broader contextual factors that

have long-term consequences for reproductive health outcomes, including entry into marriage and childbearing, secondary schooling, mobility, and social spaces for young women (Mathur, Mehta, and Malhotra 2004). The results also indicate that the enabling environment for good reproductive health has improved in the study sites because the participatory approach has generated a new mindset in the communities marked by a deeper, more sophisticated understanding of youth reproductive health and its implications. Community members are better able to understand and articulate the basic connections between youth reproductive health and a range of critical life outcomes. They are also clearer about how family, gender, and social structures and norms constrain healthier sexual and reproductive behaviors. This richer, enhanced understanding is a sign of sustainability of the demand for youth reproductive health services in the long run.

Limitations and Implications for Future Studies

Our study has limitations that need to be considered in designing future studies and analyses of this kind. One such limitation—or choice to be considered—is associated with conducting a micro household and community-based study versus a large, macro survey. Although the micro household study design provides a unique perspective that is more in-depth than macro studies can be, it has analytical limitations that arise mainly from small sample size. One of our main constraints has been the small sample sizes for some outcomes of interest that prevented us from considering certain key reproductive health outcomes such as contraceptive use. For the outcomes we were able to analyze, small sample sizes restricted our ability to use sophisticated regression models. But the community-based nature of the data did allow more in-depth, qualitative analyses. These were a huge asset in defining disadvantage and poverty in a manner that was contextually appropriate to our study and control communities in rural and urban Nepal and in analyzing causes of the observed patterns of disadvantage and change.

As highlighted in this chapter, wealth, residence, education, caste, and gender are all important measures of disadvantage in the Nepali context. No single variable, however, captures disadvantage completely. Using an index based solely on household wealth or a measure of urban-rural residence captures most but not all levels of disadvantage in this population. Other measures such as gender or education capture different dimensions of disadvantage than do wealth or urban-rural residence. Thus, no measure of disadvantage that was used succeeded in fully capturing the extent to which groups with multiple disadvantages suffer. An alternative for future consideration in this and other work is to develop a broader measure of disadvantage by creating an index that not only includes wealth or asset ownership but also accounts for the other relevant factors contributing to disadvantage. Whether a combined index or separate measures of disadvantage should be used will depend on the question to be answered.

Another important point is that because the availability of health services in or near the rural and urban communities was a factor in site selection, it could not be used as a factor in the analysis. Finally, as noted earlier, the study employed a longitudinal study design in that we studied a cohort of young people over time, but we could not duplicate a true panel design by following the same individuals. Unfortunately, most recent studies of youth reproductive health issues in the developing world have found it difficult and practically impossible to overcome the challenges involved in setting up a true panel design (Magnani and others 2001).

Conclusions

The study results suggest that empowerment and accountability issues, which are considered essential for improving health for the poor, can be operationalized at multiple levels. Our work shows that in addition to macrolevel initiatives, smaller scale community-level efforts can be targeted to achieve these outcomes. In fact, macro policy efforts have much to learn from the participatory processes implemented at the grassroots. Such community-based participatory projects are usually not well documented or evaluated. This study presents a rare rigorous evaluation of the benefits and pitfalls of using participatory approaches to improve reproductive health outcomes and expand access to services by disadvantaged clients. As such, it adds significantly to the literature on the role of participation in diminishing the disadvantages faced by those who are worst off: poor, rural, uneducated, female clients.

Our results show that the participatory approach can provide clients, especially those who are disadvantaged, with choices and mechanisms for engaging with health and social systems. These approaches and mechanisms have strengthened the power of young people in our study communities in negotiating for appropriate, accessible, and accurate information and services from providers and policymakers. This, in turn, has increased the accountability of providers to these clients.

Perhaps most critically, our study reinforces the literature on the need for broader definitions of disadvantage. Poverty is irrefutably a key and powerful measure of disadvantage. Nonetheless, in many rural communities in the developing world the most disadvantaged owe their condition to complex and interwoven interactions between various contextual factors. To arrive at a full measure of disadvantage in any one community, these context-specific factors need to be fully considered. Beyond this, even at a broader, generalizable level, our study and others that examine inequalities in health show that analyses of poverty as a measure of disadvantage need to be accompanied by analyses of rural-urban residence, gender, and educational access as important markers of social, cultural, and economic differentials.

Annex 11.1. Data and Methodology

See annex table 11.1.

Annex 11.2. Measurement of Household Wealth

Household wealth in our analysis is measured in terms of household assets. From the data in our study on household asset ownership, and following the approach used by Gwatkin and others (2000), we created an asset index that ranked households by their asset score. We calculated asset indexes separately for baseline and endline. In addition to one overall baseline and one endline index, we created separate urban and rural indexes at baseline and endline, following the approach taken by Pande and Yazbeck (2003). Our creation of separate rural and urban indexes is based on the likelihood that the same asset has different possible valuations in different contexts. For instance, owning a bicycle might score high (and thus indicate a wealthy household) in a rural area, whereas the same asset may be common enough in an urban area that it does not indicate a particularly wealthy household. More specifically, based on our understanding of the study and control sites, it was clear to us that the rural sample is much poorer than the urban sample, and thus we expected the entire rural wealth distribution to be very different from that for urban areas. To retain comparability across urban and rural areas, and across baseline and endline samples, assets are defined identically for the most part.[9]

Specifically, the overall and urban asset indexes take into account whether a household has a flush toilet, a pit toilet, a water source in the residence or yard, electricity, radio, black-and-white television, color television, telephone, bicycle, motorcycle, refrigerator, or car; whether a household owns its house; and whether a household owns any land, owns land in rural

Annex Table 11.1. Data Sources, Samples, and Research Tools, Nepal Adolescent Project

Methodology	Baseline and formative research (January 1999–March 2000)	Endline (April to November 2003)	Monitoring and process documentation (November 2000–March 2003)
Quantitative (study and control sites)	• Household survey, N = (965) • Adolescent survey, age 14–21, N = (724) • Adult survey, age 30+, N = (752) • Service provider survey, N = (59)	• Household survey, N = (1,003) • Adolescent survey, age 14–25, N = (979) • Adult survey, age 30+, N = (654) • Service provider survey, N = (62)	• Facilitator reports on participation in intervention activities (231) • Mystery client survey at midpoint and endpoint (48)
Qualitative (study and control sites)	• Key informant interviews (3) • In-depth interviews (14) • Focus group discussions (10)	Focus group discussions (16)	Facilitator reports on intervention activities (same as above)
Participatory (study sites only)	9 participatory activities with 4 to 5 groups each: • Community mapping • Mobility mapping • Free listing and ranking • Lifelines • Body mapping • Reproductive health problem trees • Reproductive health service matrix	5 participatory activities with 20 groups each: • Mobility mapping • Lifelines • Reproductive health problem trees • Reproductive health service matrix • Trend analysis	67 community group assessments at midpoint and endpoint

235

areas (and if so, how much), or owns land in urban areas. The only asset excluded from the rural index was ownership of urban land, since only two rural respondents at baseline, and only three at endline, owned any urban land.

Each asset was assigned a weight or factor score generated through principal component analysis, using programs generated by Stata (StataCorp 1997). The resulting raw asset scores were standardized in relation to a standard normal distribution with a mean of zero and a standard deviation of one. For each household, the scores reflecting the distribution of assets for that household were summed to generate a household asset score as follows:

$$\text{Household asset score} = \left(\frac{\text{value of asset variable} - \text{unweighted mean of asset variable}}{\text{unweighted standard deviation of asset variable}}\right)$$
$$\times \text{"raw" asset factor score}$$

Notes

We would like to thank our U.S. and Nepal-based partners, the Andrew W. Mellon Foundation, EngenderHealth, New Era, and the BP Memorial Foundation, whose efforts and contributions made this work possible.

1. The two rural sites, located in the Terai, in Nawalparasi and Kawasoti Districts near the border with India, are about 80 kilometers apart and have about 200 households each. They were selected because they each have a secondary school, a range of health service providers, access to a main road, access to electricity, and at least one working NGO. They thus represent the more developed Nepali village. Communities in the urban area were defined as extended neighborhoods in a specific geographic area with shared facilities for schooling, commercial, and social services and a governance structure as one ward within the larger municipality. The two urban communities selected, located about 20 kilometers apart and with about 300 households each, were drawn from middle-class suburbs on the outskirts of Kathmandu. They met the basic criteria described above and also had a more developed infrastructure and wider range of options for transportation, schooling, employment, health services, and leisure activities.

2. Because of the community-based nature of this project, the baseline and endline are two independent samples rather than a longitudinal sample of the same cohort. In reality, however, for the lagged cohort samples (ages 14–21 and 18–25), there is substantial overlap in the individuals in the sample from baseline to endline.

3. Because the respondents are young women with a recent first pregnancy, recall bias is expected to be negligible.

4. There is considerable debate on defining inequality in health (Alleyne, Casas, and Castillo-Salgado 2000; Gakidou, Murray, and Frenk 2000; Gwatkin 2000).

Although pure inequality—that is, health inequality between any two individuals—is important in its own right, in this chapter we focus on inequalities in access to health information or services systematically associated with economic status, gender, rural-urban residence, or educational attainment at the time of the study. Other research has examined the extent of unjustness or inequity related to various inequalities (Le Grand 1987) and the potential ethical dilemmas posed by focusing on reducing inequalities in health relative to improving health for all (Wagstaff 2001). We acknowledge the importance of these debates, but they are outside the scope of this study.

5. Although we were tracking a cohort of adolescents, the samples are likely to contain repeat observations of the same individual. These repeat observations, however, cannot be identified, and so we would not be able to correct for them as would be necessary for a pooled time-series analysis.

6. For all outcomes, models were run with combinations of the following variables: age, education, gender, rural-urban residence, and household wealth. Due to sample size limitations, interaction models were not possible. Only final regression models are shown here.

7. To see how wealth interacted with rural-urban residence, we also ran regressions separately by urban and rural areas, but these did not yield meaningful results, largely because of the small sample sizes. The issue of sample selection was also problematic in the urban areas. Between baseline and endline, urban areas showed a large decline in pregnancies, and the pregnancies that did occur were heavily skewed toward the poorest.

8. As noted, because of the small sample size for institutional delivery, we use poor-nonpoor ratios rather than tertiles, quartiles, or quintiles.

9. In some cases, because of small sample sizes for certain categories of assets for either rural or urban areas, definitions may differ between rural and urban areas. Asset definitions, scores, and household quintile cutoffs for urban and rural samples are available from the authors on request.

References

Alleyne, George A. O., Juan Antonio Casas, and Carlos Castillo-Salgado. 2000. Equality, equity: why bother? *Bulletin of the World Health Organization* 78(1): 76–77.

Cornwall, A., and J. Gaventa. 2001. Bridging the gap: Citizenship, participation, and accountability. *PLA Notes* 40: 32–36.

Filmer, Deon, and Lant H. Pritchett. 2001. Estimating wealth effects without expenditure data—or tears: An application to educational enrollments in states of India. *Demography* 38(1): 115–32.

Gakidou, E. E., C. L. J. Murray, and J. Frenk. 2000. Defining and measuring health inequality: An approach based on the distribution of health expectancy. *Bulletin of the World Health Organization* 78(1): 42–54.

Gwatkin, Davidson. 2000. Health inequalities and the health of the poor. *Bulletin of the World Health Organization* 78(1): 3–17.

Gwatkin, Davidson, Shea Rutstein, Kiersten Johnson, Rohini Pande, and Adam Wagstaff. 2000. Socio-economic differences in health, nutrition and population— 45 countries. Health, Nutrition and Population Department, World Bank, Washington, DC. http://web.worldbank.org/WBSITE/EXTERNAL/TOPICS/ EXTHEALTHNUTRITIONANDPOPULATION/EXTPAH/0,,contentMDK: 20216957~menuPK:400482~pagePK:148956~piPK:216618~theSitePK:400476,00 .html.

Le Grand, J. 1987. Equity, health and health care. *Social Justice Research* 1: 257–74.

Magnani, Robert J., Lynne Gaffikin, Estella Maria Leão de Aquino, Eric E. Seiber, Maria de Conceição Chagas Almeida, and Varja Lipovsek. 2001. Impact of an integrated adolescent reproductive health program in Brazil. *Studies in Family Planning* 32(3): 230–43.

Mathur, S., A. Malhotra, and M. Mehta. 2001. Adolescent girls' life aspirations and reproductive health in Nepal. *Reproductive Health Matters* 9(17): 91–100.

Mathur, S., M. Mehta, and A. Malhotra. 2004. Youth reproductive health in Nepal: Is participation the answer? International Center for Research on Women and EngenderHealth, Washington, DC, and New York.

McCauley, A. P., and C. Salter. 1995. Meeting the needs of young adults. *Population Reports,* Series J, 43. Baltimore: Johns Hopkins School of Public Health, Population Information Program.

Mensch, B., J. Bruce, and M. Greene. 1998. The uncharted passage: Girls' adolescence in the developing world. Population Council, New York.

Montgomery, Mark R., Michele Gragnolati, Kathleen A. Burke, and Edmundo Paredes. 2000. Measuring living standards with proxy variables. *Demography* 37(2): 155–74.

Nepal, Ministry of Health; New ERA; and others. 2002. *Nepal Demographic and Health Survey 2001.* Calverton, MD: Family Health Division, Ministry of Health, Nepal; New ERA; and ORC Macro.

Norman, Jane. 2001. Building effective youth-adult partnerships. *Transitions* 14(1): 10–14.

Pande, Rohini P., and Abdo S. Yazbeck. 2003. What's in a country average? Income, gender, and regional inequalities in immunization in India. *Social Science and Medicine* 57(11): 2075–88.

Senderowitz, J. 1998. Involving youth in reproductive health projects. Research, Program and Policy Series, FOCUS on Young Adults/Pathfinder International, Washington, DC.

———. 1999. Making reproductive health services youth friendly. Research, Program and Policy Series, FOCUS on Young Adults/Pathfinder International, Washington, DC.

StataCorp. 1997. *Stata Statistical Software: Release 5*. College Station, TX: Stata Corporation.

UNFPA (United Nations Population Fund). 2004. Population issues. Supporting adolescents and youth: Fast facts. New York. http:www.unfpa.org/adolescents/facts.htm.

Wagstaff, A. 2001. Economics, health and development: Some ethical dilemmas facing the World Bank and the international community. *Journal of Medical Ethics* 27(4): 262–7.

Weiss, Ellen, Daniel Whelan, and Geeta Rao Gupta. 1996. Vulnerability and opportunity: Adolescents and HIV/AIDS in the developing world. International Center for Research on Women, Washington, DC.

World Bank. 2004. *World development report 2004: Making services work for poor people*. New York: Oxford University Press.

Part IV

Latin America Studies

12

Argentina: Assessment of Changes in the Distribution of Benefits from Health and Nutrition Policies

Leonardo C. Gasparini and Mónica Panadeiros

Argentina has been in a deep recession since 1998. Public spending has fallen dramatically, and borrowing abroad has been impossible since the country's default. Targeting scarce public resources to the needy has become more than ordinarily important and difficult. Not an easy job at any time in a country like Argentina, where universal programs were the rule for decades, targeting now has to contend with falling incomes. Many people—not just the poor—feel entitled to public assistance.

This study addresses the distributional incidence of social policies in Argentina. Analysis is focused on health and nutrition policies for pregnant women and for children under five years of age. Individual and household information from two Living Standards Measurement Surveys (1997 and 2001) is used to identify beneficiaries of public programs.

The study is intended to help answer two sets of questions:

- Who are the beneficiaries of the publicly financed programs for pregnant women and children? Are these programs pro-poor? Which programs are more pro-poor? Did the structure of beneficiaries change between 1997 and 2001? Did the programs become less (or more) pro-poor?
- Why did public programs become less (or more) pro-poor between 1997 and 2001?

The first set of questions is tackled through benefit-incidence analysis. Public health and nutrition programs, although open to everyone, are intended mainly to benefit the poor, who usually have nutritional problems and lack private health insurance. Some nonpoor people, however, also benefit from public provision, attracted by the low cost (most publicly provided health services are free) and reasonable quality.

To shed light on the second question, we decompose changes in the benefit-incidence results for a particular service into three components: changes in individual and household characteristics linked to the decision to consume a service; changes in the way decisions on whether to consume the service are made; and changes in the public versus private decision on where to consume the service. Both aggregate and microeconometric decompositions are applied to obtain estimates of these three components.

Health, Nutrition, and Distribution in Argentina

Health and nutrition have generally been good in Argentina compared with other Latin American countries.

Health

Argentina's health system is organized around a strong public sector that, besides regulating health services, owns and operates an extensive network of public hospitals and primary health care centers. Expenditures on health by the three levels of government, federal, provincial, and municipal, account for 25 percent of the welfare system in Argentina (DGSC 2001). The public health system is universal in the sense that everyone is entitled to use most services at public health facilities. In practice, public expenditures are targeted mainly to low- and middle-income families because more affluent households usually opt for private treatment.

Most public health policies are channeled through the network of public hospitals and primary health care centers, where people have access to all sorts of health services, mostly free of charge. Our analysis is concentrated on the following services for pregnant women and children under five: antenatal care, attended delivery, visits to a physician, medicines, hospitalizations, and immunization.[1]

Nutrition

Although nutrition problems have been infrequent in Argentina—a country abundant in food—press coverage of child deaths caused by malnutrition has led to public debate about nutrition issues.

Public nutrition programs targeted to needy children have been small in size and coverage. Babies are provided with milk while under medical supervision at public hospitals or primary health care centers. Children benefit from nutrition programs delivered through selected kindergartens and schools and local feeding centers (*comedores*) and sometimes delivered directly to the home. Some nutrition programs are targeted to extremely poor localities; examples are Programa Alimentario Nutricional Infantil (PRANI) and Pro-Huerta. The economic crisis and the increase in malnutrition forced the government to institute some emergency nutrition programs in 2002.

In this chapter we study three publicly provided nutrition services: milk for babies at public health facilities, meals in kindergartens, and meals at local feeding centers.

Mean Income and Distribution

Argentina's economic performance over the past three decades has been disappointing. Figure 12.1 shows large cyclical fluctuations in disposable mean income, with no signs of a rising trend. During the period covered by this analysis, income fell substantially: per capita disposable income in real terms dropped 13 percent between 1997 and 2001 according to National Accounts estimates.

Figure 12.1. Mean Disposable Income, Argentina, 1980–2002

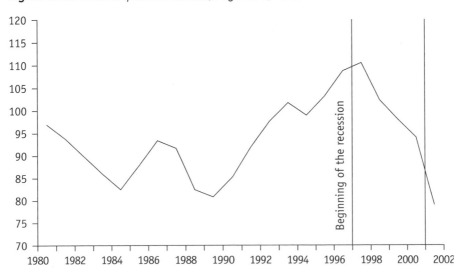

Source: National Accounts data.

Along with a stagnant economy, Argentina has suffered dramatic transformations in income distribution (Gasparini 2003). Inequality and poverty have substantially increased over the past three decades (figures 12.2 and 12.3). The Gini coefficient for household per capita income distribution in Greater Buenos Aires, an urban region with a third of the Argentinean population, increased from 0.345 in 1974 to 0.538 in 2002 (CEDLAS 2003). The poverty headcount ratio, using the official poverty line, was about 5 percent in Greater Buenos Aires in 1980, 28.9 percent in 2000, and a dramatic 54.3 percent by 2002, reflecting the economic crisis. In few countries has poverty increased so much so fast in the absence of a war or a natural disaster.[2]

Who Benefits from Health and Nutrition Policies?

Using a traditional benefit-incidence analysis of public spending on health and nutrition programs for pregnant women and children under five, we assess the targeting precision of average public spending. Benefits from a specific program are assigned to individuals according to their answers to a household survey on their use of that program.[3]

Figure 12.2. *Gini Coefficients for Household Per Capita Income, Greater Buenos Aires, 1980–2002*

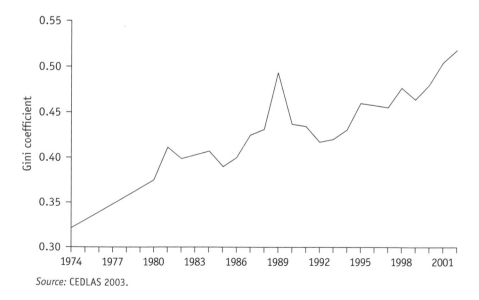

Source: CEDLAS 2003.

Figure 12.3. Poverty Headcount Ratio, Greater Buenos Aires, 1980–2002

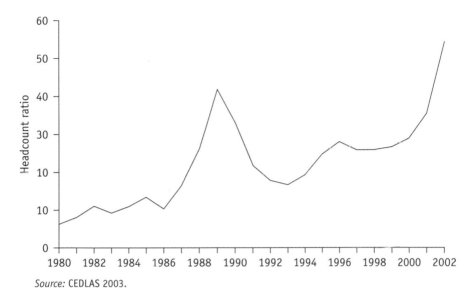

Source: CEDLAS 2003.

The Data

Benefit-incidence analyses require household surveys with data on a welfare indicator and information on the use of social programs. Argentina has conducted two recent Living Standards Measurement Survey questions on the use of various health and nutrition services. The first survey, Encuesta de Desarrollo Social (EDS), was carried out in 1996–7. It includes about 75,000 individuals (representing 83 percent of the total population) living in urban areas. The second survey, Encuesta de Condiciones de Vida (ECV), with similar coverage and questionnaires, was conducted in 2001.[4]

Welfare Indicators

A crucial stage in a benefit-incidence analysis is sorting households by a welfare indicator. Among the variables usually included in a household survey, household consumption adjusted for demographics is the best proxy for individual welfare (Deaton and Zaidi 2002). Unfortunately, most household surveys in Argentina, including those in the EDS and the ECV, do not have household-expenditure questions. Here we mostly use household income adjusted for demographics—equivalized household income—as the individual welfare indicator.[5]

In annex table 12.2, individuals with consistent answers and positive reported household incomes are grouped in income deciles. The table shows distribution of per capita household income and equivalized household income by decile for 1997 and 2001, and annex table 12.3 shows various inequality indexes for both distributions for those years.[6] Inequality increased significantly between 1997 and 2001. This result is robust to changes in the inequality index and the distribution considered. As annex table 12.4 shows, poverty also increased significantly over the period.

Use of Health Services and Nutrition Programs

This study focuses on health and nutrition programs targeted to pregnant women and children under five. Annex table 12.5 shows total population and number of children by quintile of the distribution of equivalized household income. By construction, quintiles have 20 percent of total population, but since the number of children per household decreases as income rises, the share of children is not uniform along the income distribution. For instance, the share of children under five was 30.1 in the bottom quintile in 1997, and it was 12.1 in the top quintile. This fact has fundamental consequences for the distributional incidence of public programs directed to children. Even a universal program for all children will be pro-poor, given the inverse correlation between the number of children and household income. This relationship became less strong between 1997 and 2001 as a consequence of a decline in the fertility of low-income families relative to other income groups, implying a potential reduction in the targeting of social policies.[7]

From the surveys, we are able to identify households that use public health services and nutrition programs for children and pregnant women. The rest of this section is devoted to analyzing the use of these services and computing benefit-incidence results.

Antenatal Care

Mothers of children under age two are asked whether they used antenatal care while pregnant.[8] The surveys also ask about the month of the first antenatal care visit, the frequency of tests, and the site of most visits. Annex table 12.6 and figure 12.4 show the results by equivalized household income quintile for 1997 and 2001. Antenatal care is widespread in Argentina, even for poor mothers; mothers of 97.1 percent of the children in 1997 and 97.7 percent in 2001 made at least one visit. In the bottom income distribution quintile, that share rose from 94.8 to 97.6 percent during the same period.

Figure 12.4. *Use of Antenatal Care, Argentina*

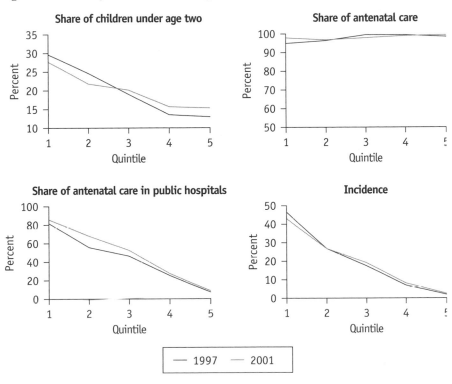

Source: Authors' calculations based on SIEMPRO (1997, 2000).

Differences across quintiles are more evident with respect to the number of visits, the month of the first visit, and the visit site. On average, poor mothers make the first visit after the third month of pregnancy, while mothers from nonpoor households make it after a month and a half of pregnancy. The share of pregnant women with more than four visits increases significantly with household income, from about 70 percent in the first quintile to 95 percent in the top quintile. Most poor mothers go to public hospitals or primary health care centers for antenatal care, whereas nonpoor mothers frequent private institutions. The differences are significant: in 2001, 85.6 percent of mothers in the bottom quintile, but only 9 percent in the top quintile, reported receiving antenatal care in public facilities. During the economically depressed period studied, the share of visits to public facilities increased along income distribution lines. The average rose from 51.6 to 54.9 percent between 1997 and 2001.

The government finances public health facilities. With the help of government resources (for example, doctors' and nurses' salaries, supplies, and a portion of capital costs), public hospitals and centers are able to provide most antenatal care free of charge. A usual assumption is that the beneficiaries of the public program are the users of the subsidized service and their families. By using a free public service, a family saves the cost of buying that service, which is assumed to be equal to the average cost of public provision.[9]

To find the beneficiaries of each public program, we identify the potential users of the service (mothers with children under age two, in the case of antenatal care), the effective use of the service, and the choice of public or private facilities. Annex table 12.6 shows two incidence results for antenatal care according to whether the number of visits is taken into account (H2) or is not considered (H1) in the calculations.[10] In both cases, subsidies for antenatal care in public facilities are highly pro-poor, but the bias weakens when the number of visits (H2) is considered. In 1997 more than 40 percent of all beneficiaries of the program belonged to the first income distribution quintile. The share of beneficiaries in the top quintile was around 2 percent. This pro-poor pattern is basically the consequence of a greater concentration of children under age two at the bottom of the income distribution and a sharp decrease in the choice to use public facilities at higher incomes.

The targeting precision of the public subsidy for antenatal care decreased between 1997 and 2001 (figure 12.4). This change seems to be a consequence mainly of a reduction in the share of children under age two in the bottom quintile and an increase in the use of public facilities by middle- and high-income households. In the next section, we analyze this point in greater detail.

Attended Delivery

Most deliveries in urban Argentina are assisted by a medically trained person. Even in the bottom quintile, the proportion of attended deliveries is close to 100 percent (annex table 12.7). The share of normal births has decreased over time, especially in the bottom quintiles. The share of cesarean sections is still increasing significantly at higher household incomes. More than half of all deliveries are attended at public facilities. This share has increased slightly in recent years. Deliveries in public facilities are much more frequent for poor than for nonpoor mothers. In 2001, 83.4 percent of deliveries by mothers in the bottom quintile were in public facilities, but the figure was only 11.3 percent for mothers from the least poor quintile. Because fertility is higher and the use of public facilities is more widespread among poor households, the subsidy for attended deliveries in public facilities is decidedly pro-poor.

We have also computed incidence results assuming that cesarean deliveries cost twice as much as vaginal deliveries. Because the share of cesarean deliveries increases with income, incidence results under this assumption are much less pro-poor.

Visits to a Doctor

Both the 1997 and 2001 surveys ask parents about visits to a doctor for their children age 0 to 4, but there are differences in the questionnaires. The 1997 survey first asks about the child's health status (Has the child felt sick or had an accident in the last 30 days?) and then reports consultations with a physician only for "sick" children. This two-stage procedure misses information about visits to a doctor for routine checkups of well children. The 2001 survey asks about any consultations with a physician, irrespective of the subjective assessment of a child's health status. The large differences in the share of children seen by a doctor shown in annex table 12.8 (32.7 percent in 1997 and 53.8 percent in 2001) is very likely attributable to this difference in the questionnaires. If in 2001 we restrict the analysis to children reported sick, the shares are similar (32.7 percent in 1997 and 29.3 percent in 2001). Patterns also differ with income distribution. The share of children under five who visited a doctor the month before the survey is more sensitive to household income in the 2001 survey than in the 1997 survey. This is a sign that taking a well child to a doctor is more common in wealthier households than in poorer ones.

Two other differences undermine the comparison: only the 1997 survey records the number of visits during the month, and only the 1997 survey has information on visits to public facilities that are not completely free of charge and are partially financed with user charges. Despite the methodological differences, results for both 1997 and 2001 clearly indicate a pro-poor profile of public subsidies for services offered by doctors in public facilities. Around 70 percent of the beneficiaries of these subsidies are individuals in the two poorest quintiles of the population. Leakages to nonpoor households are small.

Comparisons can also be made by ignoring in 2001 individuals not reported as sick (even when it is known that they went to see a doctor) and ignoring in 1997 the available information on the number of visits and partial financing of visits. This alternative (labeled H2 in annex table 12.8) suggests a reduction in the precision of public subsidy targeting for visits to doctors in public facilities.

The 1997 survey includes a question on waiting time. A person in the lowest quintile waits an average of 79 minutes for a doctor to see a child. The average waiting times for the other quintiles are 75, 56, 55, and 45 minutes, respectively. This significant difference in waiting time is probably one factor accounting for the lower probability that a child from a poor household will visit a doctor, even when the service is free of charge.

Medicines

At public health facilities some medicines are free or are sold at subsidized prices. The targeting precision of these subsidies can be studied with the help of household surveys. Again, the two-stage questionnaire of 1997 and the lack of detail in the 2001 questions on the financing of medicines blur the comparative results. Nevertheless, annex table 12.9 unambiguously suggests a pro-poor profile of public subsidies for medicines prescribed for children in public facilities. Around 50 percent of these drugs go to children from households in the bottom quintile of the equivalent household income distribution. The targeting precision of this public program was clearly reduced between 1997 and 2001.

Hospitalizations

According to the household survey responses, on average 8.4 percent of children under five are hospitalized each year (annex table 12.10). The number did not change between 1997 and 2001. During that period, the use of public facilities slowly increased along the lines of income distribution.

Vaccination

Immunization of children under five is widespread in Argentina; in 2001, 99 percent of children received at least one dose of the bacille Calmette-Guérin (BCG) vaccine against tuberculosis (see annex table 12.11).[11] The corresponding shares for the Sabin and measles vaccines were 95.4 and 72.8 percent, respectively. Most children get their shots at public facilities. Even children from wealthier households participate in public immunization programs, but since poor households have more children and some children from nonpoor families use private facilities, the incidence of public immunization programs is still clearly pro-poor. For instance, in the case of BCG, 30.6 percent of the vaccines go to children in the poorest quintile, and 10.5 percent benefit children in the top quintile. (The 2001 survey does not record information on the use of public facilities for vaccination, so all incidence results refer to 1997.)

Nutrition Programs

The three levels of government in Argentina run a variety of nutrition programs. The survey captures those that make available milk for babies in hospitals, food in some public kindergartens, and meals in local feeding centers. Annex tables 12.12 through 12.14 show significant differences in targeting across these programs. The share of total benefits accruing to the poorest 20 percent of the population in 2001 ranges from 77.3 percent for meals in local feeding centers to 41.7 percent in public kindergartens. Local feeding centers are usually situated in public schools in poor neighborhoods.

The coverage of these nutrition programs increased dramatically between 1997 and 2001. For instance, only 2.6 percent of poor children attended local centers to get free meals in 1997, but by 2001, 20.2 percent of them did.

Like health services in public hospitals, the hospital milk delivery program seems to have become less targeted over time. In the case of food in kindergartens, changes seem to have been pro-poor, and they were somewhat neutral for local feeding centers.

Summarizing Incidence Results

The literature has developed a range of graphic and analytical instruments for summarizing information on the incidence of public programs. In figures 12.5 through 12.10 we show concentration curves for various health and nutrition programs. Individuals are sorted according to their equivalized household income. The concentration (Lorenz) curve shows the cumulative share of total benefits (income) from a given program accruing to the poorest nth of the population. Concentration curves above the Lorenz curve characterize progressive programs; curves above the diagonal (the "perfect equality line") are associated with pro-poor programs (Lambert 1993).[12]

Concentration curves do not differ significantly among health programs, with the exceptions of immunization programs, which are less pro-poor, especially the quadruple (DPT plus *Haemophilus influenzae* type B) vaccine and the measles, mumps, and rubella (MMR) vaccines (figures 12.5 and 12.6). Figure 12.7 shows substantial differences between typical concentration curves for a health service and for a vaccination program. Curves for nutrition programs are estimated with less precision, considering the scope of these programs (figure 12.8). Curves for meals in local feeding centers are above the curves for the other nutrition programs.

Targeting precision seems to have decreased since 1997 for all health services considered, according to the concentration curves shown in figure 12.9. The same comment applies to milk in public hospitals and primary

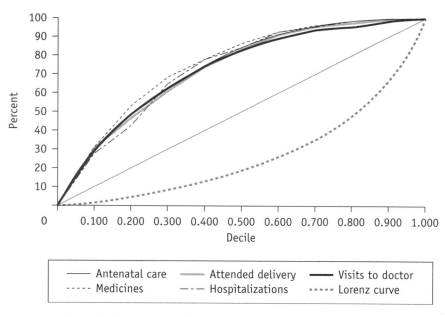

Figure 12.5. *Concentration Curves, Health Services, Argentina, 1997*

Legend:
— Antenatal care — Attended delivery — Visits to doctor
---- Medicines —— Hospitalizations ···· Lorenz curve

Source: Authors' calculations based on SIEMPRO (1997).

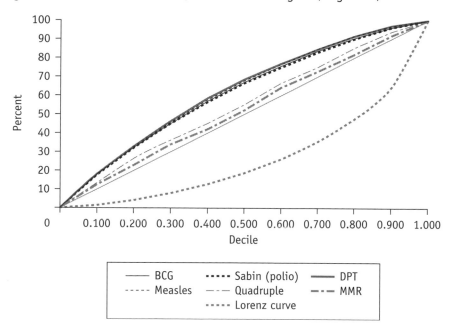

Figure 12.6. *Concentration Curves, Immunization Programs, Argentina, 1997*

Legend:
— BCG ····· Sabin (polio) — DPT
---- Measles —— Quadruple —·— MMR
···· Lorenz curve

Source: Authors' calculations based on SIEMPRO (1997).
Note: BCG, bacille Calmette-Guérin (tuberculosis) vaccine; DPT, diphtheria, pertussis, and tetanus vaccine; MMR, measles, mumps, and rubella vaccine; quadruple, MMR plus Haemophilus influenzae type B vaccine.

Figure 12.7. Concentration Curves, Visits to a Doctor and BCG Vaccination, *Argentina, 1997*

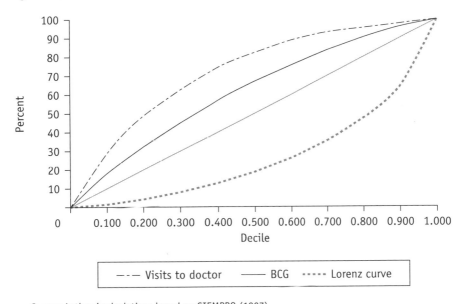

Source: Authors' calculations based on SIEMPRO (1997).
Note: BCG, bacille Calmette-Guérin (tuberculosis) vaccine.

Figure 12.8. Concentration Curves, Nutrition Programs, *Argentina, 1997*

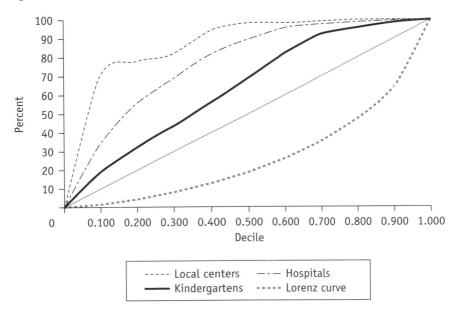

Source: Authors' calculations based on SIEMPRO (1997).

Figure 12.9. Concentration Curves, Antenatal Care, Attended Delivery, Medicines, and Hospitalizations, 1997 and 2001

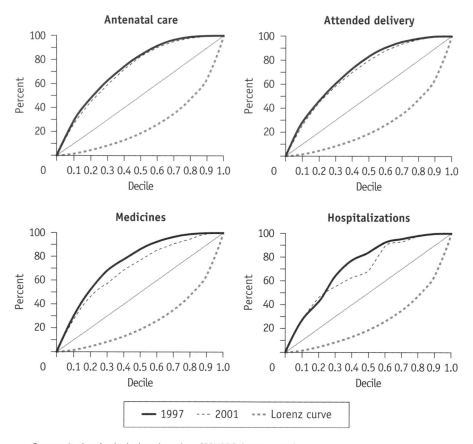

Source: Authors' calculations based on SIEMPRO (1997, 2000).

health care centers (figure 12.10). There is no clear pattern for changes in meals in kindergartens and local feeding centers.

Annex table 12.15 shows the concentration index (CI) for each service, a measure of the extent to which a particular variable is distributed unequally across income strata (Lambert 1993). Negative numbers reflect pro-poor programs. The higher the CI in absolute value, the more pro-poor is the program.

All health and nutrition programs considered are pro-poor. The most pro-poor is the program of meals in the local feeding center, followed by milk in hospitals, all health services, and immunization programs. Between

Figure 12.10. *Concentration Curves, Nutrition Programs, 1997 and 2001*

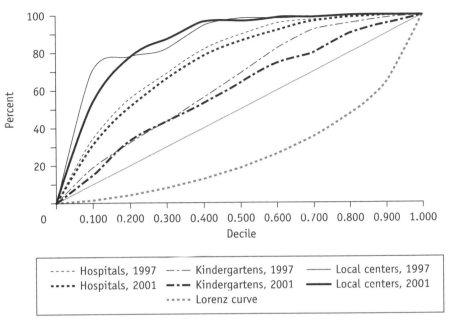

Source: Authors' calculations based on SIEMPRO (1997, 2000).

1997 and 2001, targeting precision decreased in the health services for which comparable data are available. The same is true of the milk delivery programs. For other nutrition programs, changes were insignificant.

Characterizing Changes in Targeting

Benefit-incidence results are derived by aggregating individual decisions on the consumption of publicly provided services. A household will consume a service if at least one of its members is eligible for it, if the person (or his or her parents) decides to consume the service, and if the person decides to do it in the public sector. Accordingly, differences in a program's targeting over time or across regions are the result of differences in the three stages described above. It is relevant to identify to what extent the change in a program's targeting accuracy results from changes in the sociodemographic structure of the population or from changes in household decisions on the consumption of the service (whether to use it or not, and where to use it). In this section, we tackle this issue using aggregate and microeconometric decompositions.

Aggregate Decompositions

Suppose we group total population into quintiles $h = 1, \ldots, 5$ according to their equivalized household income. The proportion of total users of a health service j in a public facility who belong to quintile h in time t is denoted b_{hjt}. These proportions are the inputs of any benefit-incidence measure. If b_{hjt} is decreasing in income, the public program j is said to be pro-poor. The value b_{hjt} can be written:

$$b_{hjt} = q_{hjt} \bullet a_{hjt} \bullet p_{hjt},$$

where $q_{hj}t$ is the proportion of people who qualify for service j who belong to quintile h, a_{hjt} is the rate of use of service j in quintile h relative to the population mean, and p_{hjt} is the share of users in the public sector in h relative to the population mean. Differences among quintiles in the value of b are driven by differences in q, a, and p.

Let us illustrate this decomposition with the case of antenatal care by medically trained persons. By definition, only pregnant women qualify for this service. If pregnant women are not uniformly distributed along the income distribution, the value of q will differ across quintiles. In most countries, fertility rates decrease with income, which implies that the value of q decreases with income for health services related to pregnant women and children. All other things constant, this pattern will imply a pro-poor bias for any health service directed to that population.

The relative use of a service (summarized by a) is the second determinant of the incidence results. Keeping all else constant, if, in contrast to pregnant women from nonpoor households, most women from poor households decide not to see a medically trained person, the value of a will increase with income.

Finally, the choice between public or private care is the third crucial determinant of the incidence results. If poor pregnant women choose a public facility more often than nonpoor women, the value of p will decrease with income.

Differences in the pattern of the bs, and then in the incidence results over time and across regions, depend on differences in factors on the right-hand side of the equation. We use this simple decomposition to obtain a preliminary characterization of differences in incidence results over time and across regions in Argentina.

Annex table 12.16 shows the results of the decomposition of incidence results by quintile for different health programs. The first three sets of rows in each panel of the table reproduce results from annex tables 12.6, 12.7, 12.9, and 12.10. The distribution of potential users, the participation decision, and the choice between public or private care determine the incidence results in row set 4. The differences in incidence by quintile are reported in row 5.

There is a clear reduction in the degree of targeting of the public antenatal care program. In 1997, 46.5 percent of total beneficiaries of that program belonged to the bottom quintile of the equivalized income distribution; in 2001 the share fell to 43.3 percent. This drop of 3.2 percentage points has its complement in the gains of 1.6 for quintile 3, 1.0 for quintile 4, and 0.6 for the top quintile. Row set 6 helps us characterize the incidence changes by showing decomposition results. The Potential users line shows incidence results if we change the distribution of pregnant women (row set 1) between 1997 and 2001 but keep fixed the participation rates and the public or private decisions at the values of a given year. Since the values of a and p can be fixed at two alternative years, in the table we report the average over the four possible simulations.[13]

The distribution of pregnant women became less pro-poor between 1997 and 2001, implying a 1.4 drop in the incidence on the bottom quintile. This means that with everything constant, the demographic changes would explain a sizeable part of the decrease in the precision of subsidy targeting to antenatal care in public hospitals and primary health care centers. Poor women are now more likely to be seen by medically trained personnel. This increase in participation (combined with the changes in the rest of the distribution) implies an increase (0.9 points) in incidence on the bottom quintile. The last effect, labeled Public provision, seems the most relevant. Although the use of public hospitals increased for poor people, it increased proportionally more for the rest of the population. This effect implies a sizeable drop in the precision of targeting in the bottom quintile.

For attended deliveries, participation rates are assumed to be unchanged because no information is available for 2001. The reduction in targeting precision on the bottom quintile between 1997 and 2001 is again a consequence of the reduction in the relative fertility rate of poor women and the relative increase in the use of public facilities by nonpoor women. In contrast with the case of antenatal care, the first effect seems to be the dominant one. Similar results are obtained for public subsidies to medicines. The incidence of public hospital admissions increased somewhat for the bottom quintile and decreased considerably for the second one, leading to a decline in the overall precision of targeting as measured by the concentration index. The decrease for the second quintile is explained by a relative reduction in fertility, a large drop in the share of hospitalized children, and a less pronounced increase in the use of public facilities than in other quintiles of the distribution.

The reduction in the precision of targeting of the nutrition programs for milk in hospitals and primary health centers and for meals in local feeding centers is attributable to a decline in the fertility rates of poor people and to a large increase in the participation of people from other quintiles of the distribution in nutrition programs (annex table 12.17).

Microsimulations

The aggregate decompositions, although informative, are only rough approximations of the effect on the benefit-incidence results of changes in the structure of the population, the decision to consume a given health service, and the public or private choice. A more sophisticated analysis can be performed with the help of microeconometric (or microsimulation) decomposition techniques.[14] Suppose we want to analyze changes between t and t' in the concentration index for the program of visits to doctors in public facilities. The idea behind this methodology is to simulate for each individual the counterfactual decision of whether to visit a doctor in a public facility in time t if certain factors were those of time t' instead of those observed in time t.[15] We consider three sets of factors that can be alternatively changed between t and t': the characteristics of each individual (and the individual's family), the way these characteristics are linked to the decision to visit a doctor, and the way these characteristics are linked to the choice to attend a public facility instead of a private one.

To implement this methodology, we estimate econometric models of the decision to visit a doctor, and the conditional decision to attend a public facility, as functions of various individual and household characteristics.[16] Changes in the concentration index are decomposed into three effects. The *population effect* is obtained by simulating the health decisions in time t if the individual and household characteristics were those of time t'; the *participation effect* comes from simulating each individual's health decisions in time t if the parameters governing the decision to visit a doctor were those of time t'; and the *public provision effect* is computed by assuming that the parameters governing the public versus private decision were those of time t'.

Annex table 12.18 reports the decomposition results. The first row reports the change in the absolute value of the concentration index between 1997 and 2001 for each health service, and the last three rows show the values of each effect.[17] The concentration index for the antenatal care program in public facilities declined 4.8 points between 1997 and 2001, implying less precise targeting. If the only change between 1997 and 2001 had been in the way individual decisions are made, the CI would have increased 0.4 points—a negligible change. The effect of changes in public versus private decisions between 1997 and 2001 contributed 1.7 points to the overall fall of the CI. The most significant factor in this decline was the change in population characteristics. Even keeping all other parameters constant, the change in characteristics would have contributed 3.5 points to the reduction in the CI. The reduction in the number of children in poor families is likely the main factor behind this result.

The population effect is also highly relevant for targeting attended deliveries, medicines, and hospitalizations. The public provision effect is negative except for attended deliveries, probably because an increasing number of middle- and high-income groups sought care at public hospitals as a result of the economic crisis. The participation effect is negligible in all cases except hospitalizations, a sign of the increase in hospitalizations of children from the poorest quintile.

Conclusions

This study analyzes targeting precision of health and nutrition policies for pregnant women and children under five in Argentina, using information from two Living Standards Measurement Surveys in 1997 and 2001. A benefit-incidence analysis tells us that public health and nutrition programs are pro-poor. The results of aggregate and microeconometric decompositions, however, suggest that incidence changes in the past five years have favored the nonpoor because of two factors: a substantial reduction in the fertility rate of poor couples, and an increase in the use of public facilities by wealthier households, probably triggered by the continuing economic crisis that began in 1998.

Annex Table 12.1. *Living Standards Measurement Surveys, Observations and Population Represented by the Sample. Argentina, 1997 and 2001*

	1997	*2001*
Observations		
Total	75,407	71,574
Men	36,439	34,556
Women	38,968	37,018
Population		
Total	29,991,693	31,959,425
Men	14,448,953	15,389,584
Women	15,542,740	16,569,841

Source: Authors' calculations based on SIEMPRO (1997, 2000).

Annex Table 12.2. *Mean Income by Decile, Argentina, 1997 and 2001*

	Per capita income		Equivalized income	
Decile	*1997*	*2001*	*1997*	*2001*
1	35.7	24.2	50.6	34.0
2	73.6	52.1	100.2	71.4
3	104.6	78.9	140.3	104.2
4	137.3	107.1	178.8	139.5
5	173.6	137.1	221.5	175.8
6	220.3	176.8	276.1	221.1
7	278.3	227.5	343.9	280.7
8	363.9	300.4	443.2	363.6
9	517.7	428.0	617.5	511.4
10	1,190.0	981.1	1,382.7	1,136.5
Mean	309.5	251.3	375.6	303.8

Source: Authors' calculations based on SIEMPRO (1997, 2000).

Annex table 12.3. *Income Distribution by Decile and Inequality Indexes, Argentina, 1997 and 2001*

	Per capita income		Equivalized income	
	1997	*2001*	*1997*	*2001*
Share of deciles (percent)				
1	1.2	1.0	1.3	1.1
2	2.4	2.1	2.7	2.3
3	3.4	3.1	3.7	3.4
4	4.4	4.3	4.8	4.6
5	5.6	5.5	5.9	5.8
6	7.1	7.0	7.4	7.3
7	9.0	9.1	9.2	9.2
8	11.8	11.9	11.8	12.0
9	16.7	17.0	16.4	16.8
10	38.5	39.0	36.9	37.4
Income ratio				
10:1	33.3	40.6	27.3	33.4
90:10	11.3	13.7	9.7	11.7
95:80	2.3	2.3	2.2	2.2
Inequality indexes				
Gini	0.507	0.522	0.484	0.499
Theil	0.491	0.521	0.443	0.471
CV	1.410	1.481	1.291	1.350
A(0.5)	0.213	0.227	0.194	0.207
A(1)	0.380	0.406	0.348	0.374
A(2)	0.645	0.678	0.603	0.641
E(0)	0.477	0.520	0.427	0.468
E(2)	0.994	1.097	0.833	0.912

Source: Authors´ calculations based on SIEMPRO (1997, 2000).

Annex table 12.4. *Poverty Measures, Argentina, 1997 and 2001 Official Poverty Line*

	1997	*2001*
Headcount ratio	0.326	0.429
Poverty gap	0.143	0.226
FGT (2)	0.088	0.160

Note: FGT, Foster, Greer, and Thornbecke index.

Annex table 12.5. *Population and Child Population by Quintiles of Equivalized Household Income, Argentina, 1997 and 2001*

	Quintile					
	1	2	3	4	5	Total
1997						
Individuals						
All individuals						
Sample	17,084	15,362	14,820	13,620	12,524	73,410
Population	5,859,871	5,858,144	5,858,311	5,850,874	5,810,177	29,237,377
Children under 2						
Sample	1,456	972	799	605	472	4,304
Population	470,802	388,856	302,447	214,781	206,541	1,583,427
Children under 5						
Sample	2,446	1,645	1,326	1,074	792	7,283
Population	801,369	651,945	488,135	394,471	322,350	2,658,270
Share (percent)						
All						
Sample	23.3	20.9	20.2	18.6	17.1	100.0
Population	20.0	20.0	20.0	20.0	20.0	100.0
Children under 2						
Sample	33.8	22.6	18.6	14.1	11.0	100.0
Population	29.7	24.6	19.1	13.6	13.0	100.0
Children under 5						
Sample	33.6	22.6	18.2	14.7	10.9	100.0
Population	30.1	24.5	18.4	14.8	12.1	100.0

			Quintile			
	1	*2*	*3*	*4*	*5*	*Total*
2001						
Individuals						
All						
Sample	12,387	12,017	11,538	10,814	10,544	57,300
Population	4,832,178	4,832,686	4,831,489	4,829,508	4,815,221	24,141,082
Children under 2						
Sample	938	718	599	455	409	3,119
Population	353,412	278,273	257,517	199,744	193,819	1,282,765
Children under 5						
Sample	1,626	1,207	1,041	774	688	5,336
Population	608,055	472,205	445,167	340,094	318,925	2,184,446
Shares (percent)						
All						
Sample	21.6	21.0	20.1	18.9	18.4	100.0
Population	20.0	20.0	20.0	20.0	20.0	100.0
Children under 2						
Sample	30.1	23.0	19.2	14.6	13.1	100.0
Population	27.6	21.7	20.1	15.6	15.1	100.0
Children under 5						
Sample	30.5	22.6	19.5	14.5	12.9	100.0
Population	27.8	21.6	20.4	15.6	14.6	100.0

Source: Authors´ calculations based on SIEMPRO (1997, 2000).

Annex Table 12.6. *Antenatal Care by Quintiles of Equivalized Household Income, Argentina, 1997 and 2001*

	Quintile					
	1	2	3	4	5	Total
1997						
Children under 2 (percent)	29.7	24.6	19.1	13.6	13.0	100.0
ANC visits (percent)	94.8	96.3	99.5	99.4	98.4	97.1
Month of first visit	3.1	2.8	2.6	1.8	1.6	2.6
More than 4 visits (percent)	73.0	82.3	91.7	94.5	95.6	84.5
Visits in public hospital	81.6	56.0	46.0	25.7	7.6	51.6
Incidence (H1)	46.5	26.8	17.7	7.0	2.0	100.0
Incidence (H2)	42.1	27.3	20.1	8.2	2.3	100.0
2001						
Children under 2 (percent)	27.6	21.7	20.1	15.6	15.1	100.0
ANC visits (percent)	97.6	96.5	97.6	98.5	99.2	97.7
Month of first visit	3.6	2.4	2.1	2.0	1.7	2.5
More than 4 visits (percent)	69.6	83.0	87.8	91.0	94.8	83.1
ANC visits in public hospital	85.6	68.1	52.4	27.7	9.0	54.9
Incidence (H1)	43.3	26.8	19.3	8.0	2.5	100.0
Incidence (H2)	38.2	28.2	21.4	9.2	3.0	100.0

Source: Authors´ calculations based on SIEMPRO (1997, 2000).
   Note: H1, calculated without taking number of visits into account; H2, calculated taking number of visits into account.

Annex Table 12.7. *Attended Deliveries by Quintiles of Equivalized Household Income, Argentina, 1997 and 2001*
(percent)

	Quintile					
	1	2	3	4	5	Total
1997						
Children under 2	29.7	24.6	19.1	13.6	13.0	100.0
Attended delivery	98.3	99.4	99.9	100.0	100.0	99.3
Caesarean section	21.4	27.4	37.4	38.3	45.6	31.1
Delivery in public hospital	79.5	59.4	49.1	27.3	10.9	53.4
Incidence (H1)	44.5	27.7	17.9	7.1	2.7	100.0
Incidence (H2)	34.6	27.4	23.9	9.7	4.4	100.0
2001						
Children under 2	27.6	21.7	20.1	15.6	15.1	100.0
Attended delivery	98.3	99.4	99.9	100.0	100.0	99.3
Caesarean section	28.2	33.3	38.4	39.8	47.9	36.0
Delivery in public hospital	83.4	67.5	49.5	33.0	11.3	55.0
Incidence (H1)	41.9	27.0	18.4	9.5	3.2	100.0
Incidence (H2)	35.8	27.1	21.3	11.4	4.5	100.0

Source: Authors′ calculations based on SIEMPRO (1997, 2000).

Note: The 2001 survey does not record the share of attended deliveries. In computing incidence results, we assume no changes between 1997 and 2001. H1, calculated without taking into account differential costs of vaginal delivery and caesarean sections; H2, assumes that the cost of caesarean sections is twice the cost of normal births.

Annex Table 12.8. *Visits to a Doctor by Quintiles of Equivalized Household Income, Argentina, 1997 and 2001*
(Percent, except as otherwise indicated)

	Quintile					
	1	2	3	4	5	Total
1997						
Children under 5	30.1	24.5	18.4	14.8	12.1	100.0
Reported sick	33.6	36.6	34.5	37.3	37.1	35.5
Saw a doctor if reported sick	90.7	90.8	92.4	94.4	95.4	92.2
Saw a doctor	30.5	33.3	31.9	35.2	35.4	32.7
Number of visits	2.5	2.4	2.2	2.4	2.5	2.4
Publicly financed (1)[a]	77.4	56.5	42.5	20.5	10.3	48.0
Publicly financed (2)[b]	83.0	61.5	45.0	22.3	11.1	51.7
Incidence (H1)	47.0	29.2	14.4	6.6	2.9	100.0
Incidence (H2)	45.1	29.6	15.6	6.9	2.8	100.0
2001						
Children under 5	27.8	21.6	20.4	15.6	14.6	100.0
Reported sick	31.3	34.7	35.9	31.8	44.3	35.0
Saw a doctor if reported sick	81.3	79.0	84.7	85.0	90.7	83.8
Saw a doctor (calculated as product of two preceding rows)	25.4	27.4	30.4	27.1	40.2	29.3
Saw a doctor (actual answers)	46.7	51.2	54.9	57.3	65.9	53.8
Publicly financed	89.7	68.1	45.4	23.5	8.6	50.6
Incidence (H3)	42.8	27.7	18.7	7.7	3.1	100.0
Incidence (H2)	43.2	27.5	19.1	6.7	3.4	100.0

Source: Authors´ calculations based on SIEMPRO (1997, 2000).

Note: The "Reported sick" row and the "Saw a doctor" rows refer to the 30 days preceding the survey. For 1997, H1 refers to publicly financed, taking into account the differences between partial and total financing and including differences in the number of visits; H2 refers to publicly financed, ignoring the difference between partial and total financing and differences in number of visits. For 2001, no breakdown between partial and public financing is available. H3 is computed using the row "Saw a doctor (actual answers)"; H2 is computed using the row "Saw a doctor (calculated)."

a. Takes into account the difference between partial and total financing.

b. Does not take into account the difference between partial and total financing.

Annex Table 12.9. *Medicines by Quintiles of Equivalized Household Income,*
Argentina, 1997 and 2001
(percent)

| | Quintile | | | | | |
	1	2	3	4	5	Total
1997						
Children under 5	30.1	24.5	18.4	14.8	12.1	100.0
Prescribed medicines	25.1	27.0	27.2	29.5	26.9	26.8
Received medicines	96.7	94.9	97.7	96.4	97.3	96.5
Publicly financed	49.7	29.2	21.4	10.1	3.1	27.2
Incidence (H1)	51.6	26.1	14.8	6.1	1.4	100.0
2001						
Children under 5	27.8	21.6	20.4	15.6	14.6	100.0
Prescribed medicines	54.6	55.0	59.6	56.8	63.5	57.6
Received medicines	94.5	94.5	97.0	96.4	99.4	96.3
Publicly financed	64.8	36.4	25.9	19.1	8.0	32.3
Incidence (H2)	49.4	21.7	16.3	8.7	3.9	100.0
Incidence (H1)	47.3	24.4	16.5	8.2	3.7	100.0

Source: Authors' calculations based on SIEMPRO (1997, 2000).
Note: H1, ignores population that does not self-report being sick; H2, includes population that
does not self-report being sick.

Annex Table 12.10. *Hospitalizations by Quintiles of Equivalized Household Income,*
Argentina, 1997 and 2001
(percent)

| | Quintile | | | | | |
	1	2	3	4	5	Total
1997						
Children under 5	30.1	24.5	18.4	14.8	12.1	100.0
In hospital last year	8.8	10.6	6.9	7.1	7.0	8.4
Publicly financed	84.3	70.5	62.1	29.1	9.2	63.1
Incidence	42.5	35.0	15.1	5.9	1.5	100.0
2001						
Children under 5	27.8	21.6	20.4	15.6	14.6	100.0
In hospital last year	9.6	6.8	10.9	9.1	4.5	8.4
Publicly financed	91.9	66.0	67.3	35.1	15.0	65.4
Incidence	44.5	17.5	27.1	9.1	1.8	100.0

Source: Authors' calculations based on SIEMPRO (1997, 2000).

Annex Table 12.11. Vaccines by Quintiles of Equivalized Household Income,
Argentina, 1997
(Percent, except as otherwise indicated)

	Quintile					
	1	*2*	*3*	*4*	*5*	*Total*
BCG						
Children under 5	30.1	24.5	18.4	14.8	12.1	100.0
Received vaccine (1997)	97.5	98.0	99.2	99.2	95.7	98.0
Received vaccine (2001)	99.1	98.4	99.2	97.4	99.6	98.8
Doses (number)	1.0	1.1	1.1	1.1	1.0	1.1
Publicly financed	98.4	98.4	96.3	91.7	85.3	95.5
Incidence	30.6	25.5	18.9	14.5	10.5	100.0
Sabin						
Children under 5	30.1	24.5	18.4	14.8	12.1	100.0
Received vaccine (1997)	93.9	94.6	94.9	97.1	96.4	95.0
Received vaccine (2001)	93.9	96.1	95.1	95.6	97.7	95.4
Doses (number) (1997)	3.3	3.3	3.4	3.4	3.3	3.3
Doses (number) (2001)	3.4	3.4	3.4	3.4	3.4	3.4
Publicly financed	98.6	98.2	96.0	91.3	82.7	95.0
Incidence	30.6	24.9	18.8	15.0	10.8	100.0
DPT						
Children under 5	30.1	24.5	18.4	14.8	12.1	100.0
Received vaccine (1997)	87.1	90.0	86.2	86.4	72.8	85.8
Received vaccine (2001)	80.8	82.0	77.9	79.6	82.9	80.6
Doses (number) (1997)	3.2	3.2	3.3	3.3	3.3	3.3
Doses (number) (2001)	3.5	3.5	3.5	3.6	3.5	3.5
Publicly financed	66.7	46.1	33.3	17.6	10.4	36.3
Incidence	48.4	27.9	14.7	6.4	2.6	100.0
Measles						
Children under 5	30.1	24.5	18.4	14.8	12.1	100.0
Received vaccine (1997)	71.8	73.2	74.1	78.6	65.4	72.8
Doses (number) (1997)	1.1	1.1	1.1	1.1	1.1	1.1
Publicly financed	98.2	98.2	95.7	91.1	80.5	94.7
Incidence	31.6	25.7	18.7	15.0	9.0	100.0

			Quintile			
	1	*2*	*3*	*4*	*5*	*Total*
Quadruple						
Children under 5	30.1	24.5	18.4	14.8	12.1	100.0
Received vaccine (1997)	28.5	30.4	40.5	51.1	60.2	38.4
Received vaccine (2001)	67.0	72.2	79.4	76.9	86.4	75.0
Doses (number)	3.0	2.9	3.2	2.9	3.1	3.0
Publicly financed	97.4	93.4	89.8	79.5	74.2	87.4
Incidence	25.2	19.7	20.9	17.5	16.8	100.0
MMR						
Children under 5	30.1	24.5	18.4	14.8	12.1	100.0
Received vaccine (1997)	15.0	19.2	26.2	29.4	43.4	23.6
Received vaccine (2001)	72.3	68.9	71.3	72.0	79.0	72.3
Doses (number)	1.2	1.3	1.2	1.3	1.2	1.2
Publicly financed	95.1	92.6	89.9	74.3	73.5	84.8
Incidence	21.0	22.3	21.2	16.9	18.6	100.0

Source: Authors' calculations based on SIEMPRO (1997, 2000).
Note: BCG, bacille Calmette-Guérin (tuberculosis) vaccine; DPT, diphtheria, tetanus, and pertussis vaccine; MMR, measles, mumps, and rubella vaccine; quadruple, DPT plus the *Haemophilus influenzae* type B vaccine.

Annex Table 12.12. *Milk for Babies in Hospitals by Quintiles of Equivalized Household Income, Argentina, 1997 and 2001*
(percent)

			Quintile			
	1	*2*	*3*	*4*	*5*	*Total*
1997						
Children under 5	30.1	24.5	18.4	14.8	12.1	100.0
Received milk	24.1	16.6	12.8	8.8	11.6	16.4
Publicly financed	91.8	80.4	74.7	28.2	4.7	74.2
Incidence	55.0	26.9	14.5	3.0	0.5	100.0
2001						
Children under 5	27.8	21.6	20.4	15.6	14.6	100.0
Received milk	35.8	29.4	23.8	24.6	21.6	28.2
Publicly financed	92.0	82.4	54.2	31.6	6.2	65.5
Incidence	49.7	28.4	14.2	6.6	1.1	100.0

Source: Authors' calculations based on SIEMPRO (1997, 2000).

Annex Table 12.13. *Food in Kindergartens by Quintiles of Equivalized Household Income, Argentina, 1997 and 2001*
(Percent, except as otherwise indicated)

	Quintile					
	1	2	3	4	5	Total
1997						
Children under 5	30.1	24.5	18.4	14.8	12.1	100.0
Attend kindergarten	10.3	13.1	21.1	27.0	38.9	18.9
Attend public kindergarten	70.8	55.2	56.5	33.5	20.6	44.8
Number of meals	1.6	1.3	1.2	1.3	1.0	1.1
Incidence	31.4	20.0	24.2	16.0	8.3	100.0
2001						
Children under 5	27.8	21.6	20.4	15.6	14.6	100.0
Attend kindergarten	33.3	36.9	41.3	45.4	49.2	41.4
Attend public kindergarten	86.2	69.5	61.0	52.3	24.5	54.7
Number of meals	1.7	1.3	1.2	1.1	1.0	1.3
Incidence	41.7	21.0	19.2	12.6	5.5	100.0

Source: Authors´ calculations based on SIEMPRO (1997, 2000).

Annex Table 12.14. *Meals in Local Feeding Centers by Quintiles of Equivalized Household Income, Argentina, 1997 and 2001*
(Percent, except as otherwise indicated)

	Quintile					
	1	2	3	4	5	Total
1997						
Children under 5	30.1	24.5	18.4	14.8	12.1	100.0
Receive food in local centers	2.6	1.9	0.6	0.1	0.3	1.4
Receive food in public local centers	35.3	8.9	14.5	50.3	0.0	24.2
Number of meals	1.1	1.6	1.0	1.0	0.0	1.1
Incidence	78.1	16.2	4.1	1.7	0.0	100.0
2001						
Children under 5	27.8	21.6	20.4	15.6	14.6	100.0
Receive food in local centers	20.2	12.2	10.4	9.0	1.5	12.0
Receive food in public local centers	25.9	14.9	2.5	1.6	—	16.0
Number of meals	1.3	1.2	1.0	1.0	—	1.2
Incidence	77.3	19.4	2.3	1.0	0.0	100.0

Source: Authors´ calculations based on SIEMPRO (1997, 2000).

Annex Table 12.15. *Concentration Indexes, Health and Nutrition Programs, Argentina, 1997 and 2001*

	1997	2001
Health		
Antenatal care	−0.469 (−0.484, −0.458)	−0.429 (−0.445, −0.411)
Attended delivery	−0.453 (−0.464, −0.438)	−0.414 (−0.430, −0.391)
Visits to a doctor	−0.440 (−0.449, −0.431)	
Medicines	−0.510 (−0.535, −0.484)	−0.387 (−0.417, −0.366)
Hospitalizations	−0.466 (−0.499, −0.443)	−0.372 (−0.433, −0.331)
Immunization		
BCG	−0.223 (−0.235, −0.214)	
Sabin	−0.216 (−0.228, −0.202)	
DP	−0.241 (−0.253, −0.230)	
Measles	−0.234 (−0.245, −0.219)	
Quadruple	−0.085 (−0.108, −0.052)	
MMR	−0.040 (−0.075, −0.012)	
Nutrition		
Milk in hospitals	−0.544 (−0.557, −0.528)	−0.496 (−0.515, −0.479)
Meals in kindergartens	−0.279 (−0.330, −0.199)	−0.195 (−0.233, −0.151)
Meals in local centers	−0.754 (−0.793, −0.708)	−0.724 (−0.745, −0.695)

Source: Authors´ calculations based on SIEMPRO (1997, 2000).

Note: BCG, bacille Calmette-Guérin (tuberculosis) vaccine; DPT, diphtheria, tetanus, and pertussis vaccine; MMR, measles, mumps, and rubella vaccine; quadruple, DPT plus *Haemophilus influenzae* type B vaccine. Numbers in parentheses are the limits of the 95 percent confidence intervals for the concentration index estimates. Intervals are computed by bootstrapping techniques, with 200 replications. For details, see Gasparini and Panadeiros (2004).

Annex Table 12.16. *Aggregate Decomposition of Incidence Results, Health Services, Argentina, 1997 and 2001*
(percent)

	Quintile					
	1	2	3	4	5	Total
Antenatal care						
1. *Potential users*						
1997	29.7	24.6	19.1	13.6	13.0	100.0
2001	27.6	21.7	20.1	15.6	15.1	100.0
2. *Participation*						
1997	94.8	96.3	99.5	99.4	98.4	97.1
2001	97.6	96.5	97.6	98.5	99.2	97.7
3. *Public provision*						
1997	81.6	56.0	46.0	25.7	7.6	51.6
2001	85.6	68.1	52.4	27.7	9.0	54.9
4. *Incidence*						
1997	46.5	26.8	17.7	7.0	2.0	100.0
2001	43.3	26.8	19.3	8.0	2.5	100.0
5. *Difference*	−3.2	0.0	1.6	1.0	0.6	
6. *Effects*						
Potential users	−1.4	−2.1	1.7	1.4	0.4	
Participation	0.9	−0.2	−0.5	−0.1	0.0	
Public provision	−2.7	2.4	0.4	−0.2	0.1	
Attended deliveries						
1. *Potential users*						
1997	29.7	24.6	19.1	13.6	13.0	100.0
2001	27.6	21.7	20.1	15.6	15.1	100.0
2. *Participation*						
1997	98.3	99.4	99.9	100.0	100.0	99.3
2001	98.3	99.4	99.9	100.0	100.0	99.3
3. *Public provision*						
1997	79.5	59.4	49.1	27.3	10.9	53.4
2001	83.4	67.5	49.5	33.0	11.3	55.0
4. *Incidence*						
1997	44.5	27.7	17.9	7.1	2.7	100.0
2001	41.9	27.0	18.4	9.5	3.2	100.0
5. *Difference*	−2.6	−0.8	0.5	2.4	0.4	
6. *Effects*						
Potential users	−1.5	−2.2	1.7	1.5	0.6	
Participation	0.0	0.0	0.0	0.0	0.0	
Public provision	−1.1	1.5	−1.2	1.0	−0.1	

| | Quintile | | | | | |
	1	2	3	4	5	Total
Medicines						
1. *Potential users*						
1997	30.1	24.5	18.4	14.8	12.1	100.0
2001	27.8	21.6	20.4	15.6	14.6	100.0
2. *Participation*						
1997	24.2	25.6	26.6	28.5	26.2	25.9
2001	51.6	52.0	57.8	54.8	63.1	55.5
3. *Public provision*						
1997	49.7	29.2	21.4	10.1	3.1	27.2
2001	64.8	36.4	25.9	19.1	8.0	32.3
4. *Incidence*						
1997	51.6	26.1	14.8	6.1	1.4	100.0
2001	49.4	21.7	16.3	8.7	3.9	100.0
5. *Difference*	−2.2	−4.4	1.4	2.6	2.5	
6. *Effects*						
Potential users	−1.7	−1.9	2.3	0.7	0.6	
Participation	0.6	−0.9	0.6	−0.6	0.3	
Public provision	−1.1	−1.6	−1.5	2.6	1.6	
Hospitalizations						
1. *Potential users*						
1997	30.1	24.5	18.4	14.8	12.1	100.0
2001	27.8	21.6	20.4	15.6	14.6	100.0
2. *Participation*						
1997	8.8	10.6	6.9	7.1	7.0	8.4
2001	9.6	6.8	10.9	9.1	4.5	8.4
3. *Public provision*						
1997	84.3	70.5	62.1	29.1	9.2	63.1
2001	91.9	66.0	67.3	35.1	15.0	65.4
4. *Incidence*						
1997	42.5	35.0	15.1	5.9	1.5	100.0
2001	44.5	17.5	27.1	9.1	1.8	100.0
5. *Difference*	2.0	−17.5	12.0	3.2	0.3	
6. *Effects*						
Potential users	−1.8	−2.2	3.0	0.6	0.4	
Participation	2.7	−12.2	8.7	1.6	−0.8	
Public provision	1.1	−3.2	0.4	0.9	0.7	

Source: Annex tables 12.6–12.10; authors' calculations based on SIEMPRO (1997, 2000).

Annex Table 12.17. *Aggregate Decomposition of Incidence Results, Nutrition Programs, Argentina, 1997 and 2001*
(percent)

	Quintile					
	1	2	3	4	5	Total
Milk in hospitals						
1. *Potential users*						
1997	30.1	24.5	18.4	14.8	12.1	100.0
2001	27.8	21.6	20.4	15.6	14.6	100.0
2. *Participation*						
1997	24.1	16.6	12.8	8.8	11.6	16.4
2001	35.8	29.4	23.8	24.6	21.6	28.2
3. *Public provision*						
1997	91.8	80.4	74.7	28.2	4.7	74.2
2001	92.0	82.4	54.2	31.6	6.2	65.5
4. *Incidence*						
1997	55.0	26.9	14.5	3.0	0.5	100.0
2001	49.7	28.4	14.2	6.6	1.1	100.0
5. *Difference*	−5.3	1.5	−0.2	3.5	0.5	
6. *Effects*						
Potential users	−1.1	−1.9	2.3	0.5	0.2	
Participation	−5.9	1.8	1.6	2.4	0.1	
Public provision	1.7	1.6	−4.2	0.7	0.2	
Meals in local centers						
1. *Potential users*						
1997	30.1	24.5	18.4	14.8	12.1	100.0
2001	27.8	21.6	20.4	15.6	14.6	100.0
2. *Participation*						
1997	2.6	1.9	0.6	0.1	0.3	1.4
2001	20.2	12.2	10.4	9.0	1.5	12.0
3. *Public provision*						
1997	35.3	8.9	14.5	50.3	0.0	24.2
2001	25.9	14.9	2.5	1.6	0.0	16.0
4. *Incidence*						
1997	81.1	12.1	4.8	2.0	0.0	100.0
2001	75.6	20.4	2.8	1.2	0.0	100.0
5. *Difference*	−5.5	8.3	−2.0	−0.8	0.0	
6. *Effects*						
Potential users	−0.5	−0.8	0.7	0.6	0.0	
Participation	−8.6	−3.9	2.5	9.9	0.0	
Public provision	3.2	13.0	−5.2	−10.9	0.0	

Source: Annex tables 12.12 and 12.14; authors' calculations based on SIEMPRO (1997, 2000).

Annex Table 12.18. *Microeconometric Decompositions (Microsimulations): Change in the Absolute Value of Concentration Index, Argentina, 1997–2001*

	Antenatal care	Attended deliveries	Medicines	Hospitalizations
Difference	−0.048	−0.052	−0.116	−0.072
Participation	0.004	0.000	−0.008	0.021
Public provision	−0.017	0.006	−0.036	−0.057
Population	−0.035	−0.058	−0.072	−0.036

Source: Authors' calculations based on SIEMPRO (1997, 2000).

Notes

We are grateful for the outstanding research assistance of Julieta Trías of the Universidad Nacional de La Plata and Eugenia Orlicki of the Fundación de Investigaciones Económicas Latinoamericanas. We also thank Daniel Bergna and seminar participants at a workshop of the World Bank's Reaching the Poor Program for useful comments and suggestions. This chapter is a condensed version of part of a study entitled "Targeting Health and Nutrition Policies: The Case of Argentina" prepared for the World Bank's Reaching the Poor Program. The full study is available from the authors on request.

1. The extended version of this paper (Gasparini and Panadeiros 2004) also contains information on postnatal care, medical studies and analysis, treatment of chronic diseases, and HIV/AIDS testing of pregnant women.

2. Trends in inequality and poverty for the rest of urban Argentina in the 1990s are similar to those depicted in figures 12.2 and 12.3 for Greater Buenos Aires. The levels vary significantly, however, across regions. For instance, whereas in the city of Jujuy in the northwest of the country the poverty headcount ratio is 57.3 percent, in Río Gallegos in the Patagonia region it is 11 percent, and in the city of Buenos Aires it is 10 percent.

3. See van de Walle and Nead (1995) and van de Walle (1998). More recent assessments of these techniques and their problems are found in Bourguignon, Pereira da Silva, and Stern (2002) and Carneiro, Hansen, and Heckman (2002). For benefit-incidence analysis in Argentina, see Flood, Gasparini, and Harriague (1993); Harriague and Gasparini (1999); Gasparini and others (2000); and DGSC (2002).

4. The sample frame for both surveys is the same. Migration was not relevant in the period under analysis.

5. Equivalized household income is computed here as total household income divided by the number of adult equivalents in the household raised to a power of 0.9 in order to consider moderate consumption economies of scale within the household. We use the official adult equivalent scale for Argentina. See Gasparini and Panadeiros (2004) for details.

6. Weighted statistics are used throughout this chapter. Weights to expand the sample to the population were provided by the Instituto Nacional de Estadística y Censos (INDEC).

7. Marchionni and Gasparini (2003) report a similar trend for Greater Buenos Aires, using information from the Encuesta Permanente de Hogares.

8. There is a selection bias because mothers are not asked about miscarriages or children who died, but since infant mortality is low in Argentina, this bias is probably small.

9. The factors used in producing the service are not considered beneficiaries of public provision. It is assumed that doctors and nurses could find similar jobs in the private sector if the public sector decided not to provide health services.

10. Theoretically, the number of visits is relevant for an incidence analysis. The surveys, however, record neither the exact number of visits (they only ask whether the mother made more than four visits) nor the type of facility visited (the surveys ask only where mothers made *most* of their visits).

11. Information on vaccinations was recounted by the mother and confirmed by inspection of a vaccination card.

12. For technical notes on quantitative techniques for health equity analysis, see the World Bank Website, http://www.worldbank.org/poverty/health/wbact/health_eq.htm.

13. Results are quite robust to changes in the base year.

14. For the application of microsimulation techniques to distributional problems, see Bourguignon, Ferreira, and Lustig (2004).

15. A more detailed explanation of the methodology is included in Gasparini and Panadeiros (2004) and can be obtained from the authors on request.

16. Details of the estimated models are given in Gasparini and Panadeiros (2004).

17. Changes do not exactly coincide with those in annex table 12.15 because observations with missing information for variables included in the models were dropped.

References

Bourguignon, François, Francisco H. G. Ferreira, and Nora Lustig, eds. 2004. *The microeconomics of income distribution dynamics in East Asia and Latin America*. New York: Oxford University Press.

Bourguignon, François, Luis Pereira da Silva, and Nicholas Stern. 2002. Evaluating the poverty impact of economic policies: Some analytical challenges. Presented at the International Monetary Fund Conference on Macroeconomic Policies and Poverty Reduction, Washington, DC, March 14–15.

Carneiro, P., K. Hansen, and J. Heckman. 2002. Removing the veil of ignorance in assessing the distributional impacts of social policies. Working paper, University of Chicago.

CEDLAS (Centro de Estudios Distributivos, Laborales y Sociales). 2003. Estadísticas distributivas en la Argentina. CEDLAS, Departamento de Economía, Universidad Nacional de La Plata.

Deaton, Angus, and Salman Zaidi. 2002. *Guidelines for constructing consumption aggregates for welfare analysis.* Living Standards Measurement Study Working Paper 135. Washington, DC: World Bank.

DGSC (Dirección de Gastos Sociales Consolidados). 2001. Caracterización y evolución del gasto público social. DGSC, Secretaría de Política Económica, Ministerio de Economía, Buenos Aires.

——. 2002. El impacto distributivo de la política social en la Argentina. DGSC, Secretaría de Política Económica, Ministerio de Economía, Buenos Aires.

Flood, M., L. Gasparini, and M. Harriague. 1993. Impacto distributivo del gasto público social: Argentina, 1991. *Anales de la XXVIII reunión de la Asociación Argentina de Economía Política.* Tucumán.

Gasparini, Leonardo. 2003. Argentina´s distributional failure. Inter-American Development Bank, Washington, DC.

Gasparini, Leonardo, and Mónica Panadeiros. 2004. Targeting health and nutrition policies: The case of Argentina. Fundación de Investigaciones Económicas Latinoamericanas, Buenos Aires.

Gasparini, Leonardo, Verónica Alaimo, Fernando Cuenin, Mariano Rabassa, and Guillermo Vúletin. 2000. El impacto distributivo del gasto público en sectores sociales en la Provincia de Buenos Aires: Un análisis en base a la Encuesta de Desarrollo Social. *Cuadernos de economía* 50. La Plata

Harriague, M., and L. Gasparini. 1999. El impacto redistributivo del gasto público en los sectores sociales. *Anales de la XXXIV reunión de la Asociación Argentina de Economía Política.* Rosario.

Lambert, P. 1993. The distribution and redistribution of income. Manchester University Press.

Marchionni, M., and L. Gasparini. 2003. Tracing out the effects of demographic changes on the income distribution: The case of Greater Buenos Aires, 1980–2000. Working paper, Universidad Nacional de La Plata.

SIEMPRO (Subsecretaría de Proyectos Sociales). 1997. Encuesta de desarrollo social (EDS). SIEMPRO, Secretaría de Desarrollo Social, Buenos Aires.

——. 2001. Encuesta de condiciones de vida (ECV). SIEMPRO, Secretaría de Desarrollo Social, Buenos Aires.

van de Walle, Dominique. 1998. Assessing the welfare impacts of public spending. *World Development* 26(3): 365–79.

van de Walle, Dominique, and Kimberly Nead. 1995. *Public spending and the poor: Theory and evidence.* Baltimore: Johns Hopkins University Press.

13

Brazil: Are Health and Nutrition Programs Reaching the Neediest?

Aluísio J. D. Barros, Cesar G. Victora, Juraci A. Cesar,
Nelson Arns Neumann, and Andréa D. Bertoldi

Social inequalities represent a major problem in Latin America. As pointed out in *Human Development Report 2003* (UNDP 2003), of the 12 countries that rank highest in income concentration, 6 are in Latin America. (The other 6 are in Africa.) The Latin American countries with the greatest income inequality are Brazil, Nicaragua, Honduras, Paraguay, Chile, and Colombia, in descending order of their Gini coefficients, which range from 60.7 to 57.1.

Health inequalities are recognized by the Pan American Health Organization as "the leading health problem" in the Americas (PAHO 1998). Reducing such inequalities is not a simple task, however. Knowledge about the impact of health interventions on the inequalities is imperfect, and some interventions may actually increase inequalities instead of reducing them (Victora and others 2000).

A common strategy is to target health programs at the poorest people. Nutrition supplementation projects—milk supplements, family ration distribution, school meals in poor neighborhoods, and so on—are classic examples. In Brazil such projects were popular until about 10 years ago, but, beset by difficulties in the management and distribution of food, they have given way to programs that offer money allowances to the poorest families on condition that the families keep their children in school and bring them to health facilities regularly.

Meanwhile, health service strategy has been heading away from targeting specific groups and toward universal coverage since the creation of the Sistema Único de Saúde (SUS—Unified Health System) by Brazil's 1988 constitution. The SUS offers free and comprehensive health care to anyone, regardless of contribution or affiliation. In a country with huge social disparities, the SUS has been an important mechanism for equalizing access to services, as can be seen, for example, by comparing health services with dental services (Barros and Bertoldi 2002), which are not widely offered within the SUS.

Programs Studied

In this study we evaluate to what extent four current Brazilian health programs, some universal and some targeted, cover the neediest. These programs, selected for their importance, national coverage, and availability of data, are the national immunization program, the national antenatal care program, the Family Health Program (Programa Saúde da Família, PSF), and the Pastorate of the Child. The first two are universal, intended for the whole population. The third is also universal, but it was designed to start with the poorest people and expand gradually. Unlike the first three programs, which are operated by the government, the Pastorate of the Child is run by a nongovernmental organization (NGO) linked to the Catholic Church. The Pastorate of the Child is the only strictly targeted initiative of the four; it is directed at very poor families or at families with malnourished children.

National Immunization Program

The National Immunization Program was created in 1973 with the objective of eradicating vaccine-preventable diseases. By 1988 vaccine coverage for illnesses included in the official list was slightly above 60 percent. Efforts were made to improve the program, and by 1991 coverage was officially reported to be 90 percent or more for measles, for diphtheria, pertussis, and tetanus (DPT), and for tuberculosis (bacille Calmette-Guérin vaccine, BCG), with polio lagging, at about 76 percent (de Miranda and others 1995). From 1994 to 2002, the total number of doses administered rose from nearly 31 million to more than 162 million, and coverage of individual vaccines was high—more than 95 percent for all vaccines in the official calendar.[1]

Since 2000, in addition to polio, measles, BCG, and DPT, vaccines against *Haemophilus influenzae* type B, hepatitis B, mumps, and rubella have been made available through the public health service. The vaccines are freely available in public health centers and polyclinics for routine vaccination of children and the elderly. National immunization campaigns are organized regularly, with vaccination stations scattered in health facilities, supermarkets, shopping malls, and community centers.

Despite this effort, full immunization coverage has not yet been achieved. Using data from the Brazil Demographic and Health Survey (DHS) of 1996, we have shown that only 75 percent of children between 12 and 23 months old had received all doses of the vaccines prescribed by the basic immunization calendar—that is, one BCG, three DPT, and three polio (authors' unpublished data). Very similar results were found in a study carried out in the city of Porto Alegre (de Miranda and others 1995). In Ceará, a state where strong efforts were directed toward child health, coverage for all the vaccines prescribed for the first year was 89 percent in 1994 (Victora and others 2000).

National Antenatal Care Program

In 1984 Brazil's Ministry of Health launched the Program of Integral Assistance to Women's Health (PAISM). Antenatal care was already provided through the primary health care system, but it was felt that it had to be strengthened. With the creation of the Sistema Único de Saúde, the conditions were laid for the antenatal care program to be offered widely. Local health authorities are responsible for the program, and services are delivered at primary health care facilities. The basic guidelines for the local programs recommend a first antenatal visit in the first three months of pregnancy and additional visits every four weeks thereafter for uncomplicated pregnancies. The visits should include, at minimum, a check for edema and measurement of blood pressure, uterine height, and fetal heart frequency. A few laboratory tests are also routine, plus immunization against tetanus, if necessary. Antenatal care coverage is high: more than 90 percent of women have at least one checkup, and the average is more than six consultations (Monteiro, França Júnior, and Conde 2000; Coutinho and others 2002; Trevisan and others 2002). The same studies, however, also show variation in the prevalence of adequate care, defined as a first consultation in the first 20 weeks of pregnancy and at least six consultations overall. In Juiz de Fora (Minas Gerais State), 26.7 percent of the women had adequate antenatal care (Coutinho and others 2002); in Caxias do Sul (Rio Grande do Sul State), 35.2 percent (Trevisan and others 2002); and in Pelotas (Rio Grande do Sul State), 37 percent (Silveira, Santos, and Costa 2001). In São Paulo City, by contrast, the figure was 69 percent (Monteiro, França Júnior, and Conde 2000).

Family Health Program (PSF)

Since the creation of the Family Health Program by the Ministry of Health in 1994, Brazil's primary health system has been undergoing a reform designed to bring it closer to households. To this end, there has been a shift from the traditional static health center—a primary health facility typically staffed by a pediatrician, an obstetrician, and an adult clinician, plus nurses and secretarial personnel—to family health teams responsible for outreach as well as passive service. This shift has been gaining momentum in recent years.

The PSF was created to reorganize primary health care by instituting teams made up of a general practitioner, a registered nurse, a nurse assistant, and four community health workers. Each team is in charge of up to 1,000 families, or about 4,500 individuals. The rationale behind the PSF is to offer health care that assigns priority to preventing disease and promoting health, in addition to providing curative care. Services are delivered at health facilities or, whenever necessary, through home visits. The composition of the PSF team was designed to encourage bonding with the people covered in order to foster a sense of mutual responsibility toward health.[2]

In most municipalities the plan for implementation of the program is to start in the poorest areas and areas not yet covered by primary health care. The Ministry of Health offers incentives to municipalities that attain coverage of more than 70 percent of the population, paying approximately $20,000 per team per year, compared with $10,000 for municipalities with coverage below 5 percent. If this policy is maintained, the PSF should replace the traditional health centers in a few years. As of October 2003, according to data from the national program office, the Northeast Region had the highest coverage, 49.8 percent. Coverage for the Central-West, South, North, and Southeast Regions was 38.9, 33.7, 31.0, and 26.0 percent, respectively.

Pastorate of the Child

The Pastorate of the Child (Pastoral da Criança) was launched in 1983 as an initiative of the Catholic Church. The Pastorate's purpose is to work directly with families in their homes to promote such cultural values as fraternity, social coresponsibility, and ecumenism; to reduce malnutrition, infant mortality, and social marginalization; and to foster integrated child development.

At the core of the program are the volunteer leaders, mainly women, who visit the enrolled families to provide information on suitable infant-feeding strategies, especially breastfeeding, and to monitor growth by measuring and weighing all children monthly. The leaders also teach families about immunization and use of oral rehydration therapy. As they gain experience, the volunteers also help with respiratory infections and the prevention of domestic accidents. The work done is always voluntary, and most leaders devote one day a month to it.

Pastorate leaders are recruited from the local community to work with up to 15 neighborhood children. The leaders are trained for their main duties, described in the Pastorate Leader's Guide. Because an information system was developed to monitor and evaluate the activities promoted by the Pastorate, not only can the tasks performed be quantified, but a health profile of the communities assisted can also be drawn.

According to data from the Pastorate management (www.pastoraldacrianca.org.br), in 2000, 100 percent of Brazil's 27 states and 61 percent of all parishes were served by the Pastorate. In all, 3,555 municipalities are covered by 133,134 leaders, and, on average, 1.6 million children under age six are seen by the program each month (roughly equivalent to 10 percent of the Brazilian population). The Pastorate also runs literacy projects and income generation programs for adults and broadcasts a weekly radio program over 1,343 stations.

Available data on the program are limited, but they suggest a less optimistic situation. In Criciúma (Santa Catarina State), less than 5 percent of the children were covered by the Pastorate, and dropouts were frequent (Neumann and others 1999).

Research Questions

Our main hypothesis is that coverage of universal programs such as immunization and antenatal care is high overall but is lower among the poorest, especially when the quality of service is taken into account. We also hypothesize that although targeted programs assist mostly the poorest, a fair degree of leakage (that is, coverage of nonpoor persons) occurs and that coverage among the extremely poor is limited.

Using existing information from surveys, as well as new data collected from PSF-covered areas in Porto Alegre (Rio Grande do Sul State), we assess the performance of the four health programs described above with respect to their coverage of the poor and their focus (targeting). Where suitable data (mainly from the Porto Alegre PSF study) are available, the reasons for the observed results on coverage and focus are explored.

Methods

The analyses are intended to describe how the benefits of the programs assessed were distributed across the population, classified in terms of wealth. One indicator used was focus—that is, the percentage of the benefit going to the poor, with benefit in this case represented by program coverage (Habicht, Mason, and Tabatabai 1984). To give a more complete picture of program performance, the full distribution of economic status for the population served by the programs studied is presented in the results.

Coverage, defined as the proportion of the population assisted by the program, was also calculated, both for the whole population and by economic stratum. The coverage indicators can be directly estimated from the data sets based on cross-sectional surveys that are representative of the whole population.

Inequalities in coverage can be assessed by ratios of differences between the poorest and the richest, typically comparing the 20 percent poorest with the 20 percent richest. Inequalities were also evaluated by measures of coverage concentration derived for each program. These concentration measures have the advantage of including the whole distribution under study instead of only the extreme groups, as in ratio and difference measures (Kakwani, Wagstaff, and van Doorslaer 1997). The concentration index, a Gini-like measure, is defined as twice the area of a Lorenz-type concentration curve. This curve is obtained by plotting the cumulative distribution of an outcome against the respective percentile of the population ordered by income (or other socioeconomic indicator).[3]

Economic classification is a critical issue in equality analysis. The approach used here was based on information for household assets, which was available from each study. Using this information, asset index scores were developed for each household. The technique used in constructing the index scores was principal component analysis, as proposed by Filmer and Pritchett (2001) and applied in several other studies (for example, Gwatkin and others 2000). After the asset score was created, the households were divided into quintiles. The whole process took into account the sampling strategy of each study and thus included weighting, stratification, and correction for clustering, as necessary. The results are expressed as quintiles of households. Because there are more people per household in some quintiles (especially the poorer ones) than in others, the number of individuals can vary from quintile to quintile of households. Our focus population, the poor, was defined as the households in the study population in the first (poorest) quintile or the individuals living in such households.

A criterion for assessing adequacy of the antenatal program was needed, and the Kessner criterion (modified by Takeda) for adequate antenatal care was used. Care was classified as adequate if the mother attended at least six consultations, starting in the first 20 weeks of pregnancy (Silveira, Santos, and Costa 2001). This criterion has been tested against other approaches and performed better (Delgado-Rodriguez and others 1997).

For immunization, a simple criterion already used in other studies (de Miranda and others 1995) was applied. Children age one year or more were considered fully immunized if they had received at least one dose of BCG and three doses of the polio and DPT vaccines.

All the analyses were performed with Stata Release 8.0 (StataCorp. 2003).

Data Sources

Data from four cross-sectional studies were used. Of these, the Demographic and Health Survey (DHS) was a large national survey; the other three, which were carried out by the authors, dealt with specific population groups in selected Brazilian cities and states.

Demographic and Health Survey, 1996

DHS surveys, undertaken in many countries using a common approach, are designed to collect information on fertility and family planning, maternal and child health, child survival, and other reproductive health topics. The DHS program includes modules on the household, on women of reproductive age, and on the children born to these women. Health status outcomes and use of health services for specific conditions include occurrence of some diseases of infancy and childhood, mortality under age five (including neonatal, postneonatal, and infant mortality), nutritional status of children and mothers, access to antenatal and delivery care, breastfeeding, family planning, and fertility. These surveys do not include modules on household consumption and income.

The DHS survey conducted in Brazil in 1996 (Pesquisa Nacional sobre Demografia e Saúde, PNDS) included 13,283 households, a sample designed to be representative of the whole country except the rural area of the North Region. The results can be disaggregated by state and for some metropolitan areas such as São Paulo, Rio de Janeiro, and Porto Alegre. The survey was carried out by the Sociedade Civil Bem-Estar Familiar no Brasil (BEMFAM) and was supported by the United Nations Population Fund

(UNFPA), the United Nations Children's Fund (UNICEF), Brazil's Ministry of Health, the Brazilian Institute of Geography and Statistics (Instituto Brasileiro de Geografia e Estatística, IBGE), and the U.S. Agency for International Development (USAID).[4] Our study uses DHS data in assessing the antenatal and immunization programs.

Criciúma Study, 1996

The study of Criciúma, Santa Catarina State, southern Brazil, was carried out by N. A. Neumann and colleagues in 1996 and was funded by the Pastorate of the Child. The sample included 2,208 children under age three who were selected using a stratified two-stage sampling scheme. Extensive information on family characteristics, including family income and ownership of a variety of goods, and on utilization of health services were collected from the mothers. In particular, coverage by the Pastorate and characteristics of the assistance being provided were carefully recorded (Neumann and others 1999). This data set was used to assess the Pastorate of the Child, as well as the government antenatal care program.

Sergipe Study, 2000

The study carried out in 2000 in the state of Sergipe, northeastern Brazil, by J. A. Cesar and colleagues was funded by the World Health Organization's Department of Child and Adolescent Health. It was based on a two-stage sample designed to be representative of households in the state with at least one child under five and included 1,785 children from urban and rural areas. Extensive information on family characteristics, including family income and ownership of a variety of assets, and on utilization of health services was collected from the mothers. In addition, qualitative data on the PSF and other health-related initiatives were gathered from mothers, health workers, nurses, and doctors through focus group discussions, in-depth interviews, and interviews with experts. The study provided data for assessing the PSF and the immunization and antenatal care programs.

Porto Alegre PSF Study, 2003

A cross-sectional study funded by the World Bank under the Reaching the Poor Program was carried out in Porto Alegre, the capital of Rio Grande do Sul State, by A. J. D. Barros between July and September 2003. Porto Alegre, with approximately 1.3 million people according to the 2000 census, is one of the richest cities in Brazil, yet it is encircled by poor neighborhoods where part of the population is deeply deprived.

At the time of the study, 56 PSF units had been operating in the city for more than six months. The population covered by these units (that is, living in their catchment areas) was estimated at 143,000. A sample of 900 households was selected through two-stage cluster sampling. The primary units were 45 areas covered by PSF units, and the secondary units were the households, 20 of which were selected in each primary sampling unit. Through standardized interviews, data concerning household assets and infrastructure were collected, together with information on access to and utilization of health services, health expenditure and financing, and satisfaction with health services. All individuals living in the selected households were included in the study. The economic classification of the sample was done using the wealth index (*indicador econômico nacional*, IEN) proposed by Barros and Victora (2005), in which an asset score was developed through principal component analysis using a set of 13 variables from the 2000 Brazilian Census. The proposed asset score was calculated for each household in our sample. Instead of dividing the households into quintiles based on the study sample, they were classified according to the distribution of the wealth index for the whole city of Porto Alegre (referred to as IEN/POA), using the cutoff points presented in the Barros and Victora paper. This strategy allowed the sample, which included only households in areas covered by the PSF, to be classified into wealth quintiles relative to the population of the whole city. Thus, households belonging to the first reference quintile are among the 20 percent poorest in the entire city, not in the sample alone.

Findings about Distribution

This section describes how benefits from the four programs assessed are distributed in the population, with an emphasis on population coverage and focus on the poor. All the results presented are original, the product of analyses performed on the data sets described above.

National Immunization Program

Both the DHS and the Sergipe study indicated that about 20 percent of children age one to four years had not received all doses of the basic immunization scheme (one BCG, three DPT, and three polio). Table 13.1 shows a significant difference across wealth quintiles only for the DHS, where incomplete immunization is more than twice as frequent among the poorest

Table 13.1. *Prevalence and Inequality of Incomplete Immunization among Children Age 12 Months and Older, by Wealth Quintile, Brazil DHS (1996) and Sergipe Study (2000)*
(Percent except as indicated)

Wealth quintile	DHS (N = 3,827)	Sergipe (N = 1,436)
1 (poorest)	33.4	28.0
2	16.4	20.4
3	14.2	20.6
4	11.9	15.5
5 (least poor)	15.3	17.8
Entire sample	19.3	20.5
p	<0.001	0.176
Concentration index	–0.218	–0.108

Source: Brazil DHS 1996; data for Sergipe from study by Cesar and others.
Note: DHS, Demographic and Health Survey.

than among the least poor. The concentration index is –0.218, indicating the concentration of incomplete immunization in the poor population. Data from Sergipe also point to a higher prevalence of incomplete immunization among the poorest, although the disparity is not significant, and yield a concentration index of –0.108. The lower inequality in the Sergipe study than in the DHS is linked to the much wider national coverage of the DHS, which includes both the richest and the poorest regions of the country.

Turning to the focus of the program, in the DHS 21 percent of the fully immunized children were from the poorest quintile of households, which included 26 percent of all children. In Sergipe 17.8 percent of fully immunized children were from the poorest group, which accounted for 19.7 percent of all children. Given that the immunization program is universal, high focus was not expected. Nevertheless, coverage is clearly lower among the poorest, contrary to the idea of program universality.

Antenatal Care

The availability of data about antenatal care in three of the studies we drew on is an indication of the program's importance in Brazil. It is certainly one of the most traditional programs delivered through the primary care network. The quality criterion used, proposed by Kessner, is widely accepted

Table 13.2. *Proportion of Mothers Receiving Inadequate Antenatal Care (Kessner Criterion) by Wealth Quintile, Three Studies, Brazil*
(Percent except as indicated)

Wealth quintile	DHS (1996)	Sergipe (2000)	Criciúma (1996) Total sample	Criciúma (1996) SUS users	Percentage of children in Criciúma sample using SUS
1 (poorest)	70.0	49.1	37.8	38.7	93.8
2	43.5	48.3	27.9	29.2	89.4
3	27.4	35.3	24.6	29.3	77.4
4	19.1	30.2	21.0	26.5	65.1
5 (least poor)	13.6	18.7	15.9	24.6	37.1
Entire sample	38.4	35.7	25.9	30.7	74.3
P	<0.001	<0.001	0.003	0.166	<0.001
Concentration index	−0.317	−0.183	−0.162	−0.009	

Source: Brazil DHS 1996; data for Sergipe from study by Cesar and others; data for Criciúma from Neumann and others (1999).
Note: DHS, Demographic and Health Survey; SUS, Sistema Único de Saúde.

and, as mentioned, performs better than other criteria (Delgado-Rodriguez and others 1997).

In the three studies, the overall proportion of mothers receiving inadequate antenatal care ranged from 25.9 percent in Criciúma to 38.4 percent in the whole country (table 13.2). In Criciúma it was possible to isolate the children who used the SUS as their primary source of health care, and in this group the prevalence of inadequate antenatal care was 30.7 percent.

Inequality across wealth quintiles was again evident from the data. As expected, the DHS, with its much wider area, showed the highest concentration index for inadequate care, −0.317. Inadequate coverage was about five times higher in the poorest quintile than in the least poor. The Sergipe study yielded the second-highest concentration index, −0.183, close to the −0.162 for Criciúma. The latter, located in a wealthy part of the country, presented the lowest prevalence of inadequate care, but the degree of inequality was comparable to that in Sergipe, as measured by the concentration index and the ratio of poor to least poor. When, however, only SUS users from Criciúma were considered, the concentration index was −0.009, and no significant difference across wealth quintiles was found. The lower degree of inequality was attributable to higher prevalence of noncoverage in the better-off quintiles. Wealthy SUS users had antenatal care coverage similar to that of the middle quintile of the whole sample. SUS users are a minority in the least poor quintile (37.1 percent), while in the poorest they are the absolute majority (93.8 percent).

On the focus issue, the proportions of poor children among those receiving adequate antenatal care were 13.1, 13.6, and 17 percent, respectively, for

Figure 13.1. *Distribution of the Population Covered by the Pastorate of the Child by Wealth Quintile and Weight-for-Age Z-Score, Indicating Program Focus (Incidence), Criciúma, 1996*

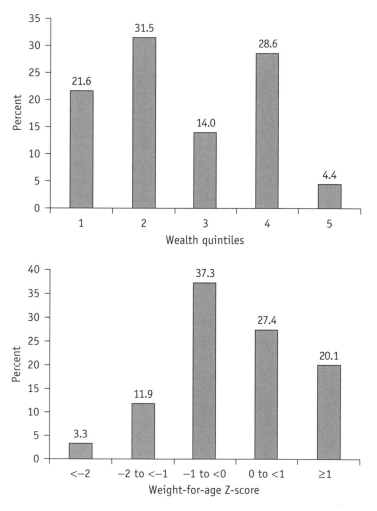

Source: Neumann and others 1999.

the DHS, Sergipe, and Criciúma, while proportions of poor children in the whole sample were 26.9, 20.4, and 20 percent, respectively. Focus in this universal program is low.

Pastorate of the Child

The Pastorate of the Child is the only fully targeted program analyzed in this chapter. As explained earlier, the Pastorate is meant to concentrate on undernourished children and on children from the poorest families. Measuring program focus is, therefore, more relevant than for the programs discussed above. As shown in figure 13.1, among the children covered by the Pastorate, 21.6 percent were from the poorest quintile of households, and almost 32 percent were from the second quintile. The distribution of nutritional status among covered children (figure 13.1) follows closely the distribution of the total population presented in table 13.3, suggesting that the program fails to concentrate on malnourished children.

Table 13.3. *Coverage of the Pastorate of the Child by Wealth Quintile and by Children's Weight-for-Age Z-Score, Criciúma, 2003*

	Percentage of children surveyed	Coverage (percent)
By wealth quintile		
1 (poorest)	20.0	4.8
2	26.6	5.3
3	16.0	3.9
4	20.1	6.4
5 (least poor)	17.3	1.1
Entire sample	100	4.5
P		0.049
By children's weight-for-age Z-score		
<−2	5.4	2.7
−2 to <−1	16.4	3.3
−1 to <0	32.4	5.2
0 to <1	29.4	4.2
≥1	16.4	5.5
Entire sample	100	4.5
P		0.169

Source: Neumann and others 1999.

Coverage of the program was low, at 4.5 percent of all children (table 13.3). Only the richest quintile had distinctly lower coverage, but the significance was borderline. The highest coverage was achieved in the fourth quintile. No significant difference was found for coverage by nutritional status. In absolute terms, the severely malnourished children had the lowest coverage, and the best nourished had the highest coverage.

Family Health Program (PSF)

The PSF is in different phases of implementation in various places in Brazil. We studied it in the city of Porto Alegre, where it is relatively new, and in the state of Sergipe, where it has been much more widely implemented. Although the PSF is not targeted explicitly toward the poor, the plan is for its implementation to start in the poorest areas and in those not yet covered by a primary health unit. The potential program beneficiaries are all residents of the units' catchment areas (who are referred to here as PSF residents). Because a number of these individuals will never use the public service, we also conducted some analyses with service users in Porto Alegre—that is, those who reported having used the PSF at least once in the previous six months (referred to as PSF users).

In Porto Alegre the program focus was estimated at 36 percent—the proportion of the population living in the catchment area of PSF facilities that belonged to the poorest 20 percent of the city's residents. Considering only actual PSF users, focus was 41 percent. An additional 28 percent of PSF users came from the second-poorest 20 percent of the population. Thus, in all, nearly 70 percent of those using PSF services belonged to the poorest 40 percent of the population. (The full distributions are shown in figure 13.2.) Total PSF coverage in the city was estimated at 10.8 percent, and the coverage of the poorest 20 percent was 19.3 percent (table 13.4).

In Sergipe 27 percent of the residents of areas served by the PSF were in the poorest 20 percent of the population, compared with 36 percent in Porto Alegre (see figure 13.2). Focus was thus lower in Sergipe than in Porto Alegre. Coverage, however, was higher: more than 55 percent of the poorest 20 percent of Sergipe residents were in areas where the PSF was active, compared with only 19 percent in Porto Alegre. The same was true at the middle and higher economic levels. In Sergipe 25 percent of all people in the highest 20 percent of the population lived in PSF-served areas, a figure 10 times higher than in Porto Alegre (table 13.4).

The differences observed are probably attributable to the different stages of implementation of the program in the two sites. At the beginning, cover-

Figure 13.2. *Distribution of Wealth Status for Residents of Areas Covered by the Family Health Program (PSF), Porto Alegre and Sergipe, and for PSF Users, Porto Alegre*

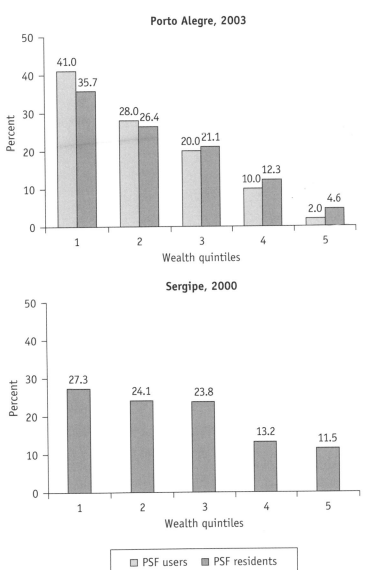

Source: Neumann and others 1999.

Table 13.4. *Family Health Program (PSF) Coverage by Wealth Quintile, Porto Alegre (2003) and Sergipe (2000)*
(percent)

Wealth quintile	Porto Alegre N = 3,827	Sergipe N = 1,436
1	19.3	55.1
2	14.3	49.2
3	11.4	42.6
4	6.7	31.1
5	2.5	24.9
Entire sample	10.8	41.1

Source: For Porto Alegre, data from study by Barros; for Sergipe, data from study by Cesar and others.

age is low and focus is high, as observed in Porto Alegre. Later, with increased overall coverage, focus decreases, but coverage is still higher among the poor.

Findings about Reasons for the Distribution

The programs studied had markedly different profiles of distribution in the population served. Further data on the programs are explored to establish, to the extent possible, why that is so.

Immunization and Antenatal Care Programs

The universal preventive programs—immunization and antenatal care—that are studied here showed similar patterns: reasonably high coverage of the whole population and low focus on the poor. That is what is expected from universal programs. But when coverage is stratified according to decreasing wealth, the result is a consistent reduction in coverage.

Barriers to the utilization of these services by the poor may be present at one or more levels in the path leading to the actual use of preventive health services (figure 13.3). Poorer people may be less aware of the benefits of the programs because they are less likely than the better off to be reached by educational messages. Furthermore, given their harsh living conditions, they may assign less importance than the better off to preventive care. Even if the poor perceive a need for preventive care, they may fail to seek it because of personal barriers such as lack of money or transportation or a

Figure 13.3. *Simple Model of Health Service Utilization*

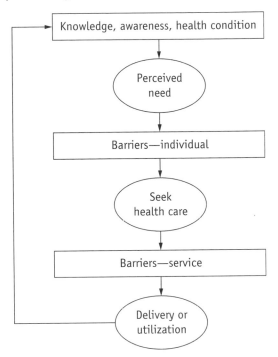

negative perception of health services (resulting from frequent rescheduling, expectations of long waiting times, and similar considerations). Finally, obtaining access to the desired program or service may be limited by service-related deficiencies such as already fully booked service rosters, long waits, and difficulties in obtaining laboratory exams. We discuss below the evidence concerning each group of possible obstacles to service utilization.

Starting with the barriers closest to utilization—those related to the service itself—our data suggest that access to health services is not an important problem. Among those who sought health care, either curative or preventive, only 6 percent failed to get medical attention, although this was more common among the poor ($p = 0.02$) than among the better off (figure 13.4). About a third of those who failed to get care gave as the reason that the service was fully booked. Other common reasons were that the doctor was unavailable, that the waiting time was too long, and that the specialized service or doctor needed was not available at the facility visited. The high access to health services is confirmed by other studies based on the 1998 National Household Sample Survey (PNAD) carried out by the IBGE.

Figure 13.4. *Percentage of the Population That Failed to Seek or to Receive Medical Attention on the First Attempt, by Wealth Quintile, Porto Alegre, 2003*

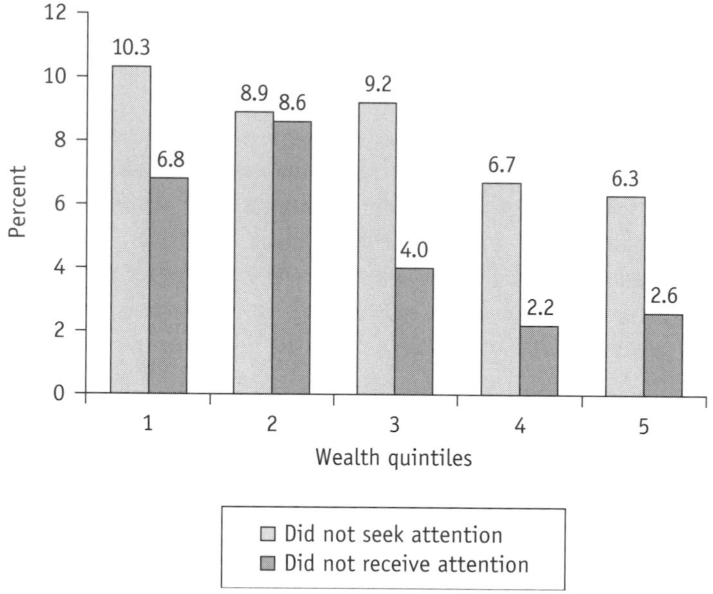

Source: Data from study by Barros.

These found access to health services in general to be about 97 percent (IBGE 2000; Barros and Bertoldi 2002).

Access to referral services was lower. In the Porto Alegre study 12 percent of the individuals reported that they failed to get the laboratory exams requested, and 23 percent did not obtain access to a specialist doctor when referred by the generalist.

Another indication of service availability is that 27 percent of the Porto Alegre sample received medical care in the 15 days before the interview, with no significant difference by wealth quintile. Despite similar utilization, there was a clear difference in motives for the consultation across economic groups. Among the worse off, an illness was more commonly (65 percent) cited as a motive than among the better off (16 percent). Conversely, prevention was more common among the richest quintile (51 percent) than among the poorest (23 percent).

As for personal barriers to use of health services, among those reporting a need for medical attention in Porto Alegre, 9 percent did not seek care. There was no significant difference among wealth quintiles (figure 13.4).

More than a third of the respondents blamed lack of time. Other reasons included reported negligence about the person's own health, the time required to book an appointment (including getting in line early in the morning), and other difficulties with scheduling appointments.

We do not have data on barriers related to knowledge, awareness, or motivation (see the first box in figure 13.3), but a 2000 study of antenatal care in Caxias do Sul, near Porto Alegre (Trevisan and others 2002), showed that the main reported motive for not attending antenatal care was lack of information about its importance. Nevertheless, only 5 percent of mothers failed to attend.

Negative perceptions of the quality of public health services could potentially reduce utilization, but studies consistently show high levels of user satisfaction with both public and private health services. In a study to assess user satisfaction with antenatal care within the Brazilian public health system (Ribeiro and others 2004), 86 percent of users rated the service as either good (22 percent) or excellent (64 percent). Satisfaction with health services in general was also high (86 percent good and very good) in the 1998 national household survey (IBGE 2000). In the Porto Alegre PSF study a similar proportion (84 percent) of users rated the service as good or very good.

Contrasting with this picture of high access to and high satisfaction with public health services, we found in the Porto Alegre study a strong association between economic level and type of service used. Figure 13.5 shows a steep decrease in the use of public sector primary health care with increasing economic well-being. Conversely, use of private services (private health insurance or direct payment) increased with economic level ($p < 0.001$). Higher utilization of public hospital outpatient and emergency services was also observed among the better off.

Important differences in the use of public sector primary health care according to health insurance coverage were found (figure 13.6). In all wealth quintiles, insured individuals were less than half as likely as the uninsured to use government services.

Using a Poisson regression model with utilization of primary health care as the outcome, we assessed the effect of health insurance coverage after adjustment for the effect of wealth (Barros and Hirakata 2003). Having private health insurance reduced the use of primary health care by 63 percent (adjusted relative risk = 0.37; 95 percent confidence interval = 0.26–0.52). There was no interaction between health insurance and wealth. Coverage by private health insurance was 6.5 percent in the poorest quintile, increasing to nearly 70 percent among the richest ($p < 0.001$).

Figure 13.5. *Where Respondents Sought Health Care for the First Time during Previous 15 Days, by Wealth Quintile, Porto Alegre, 2003*

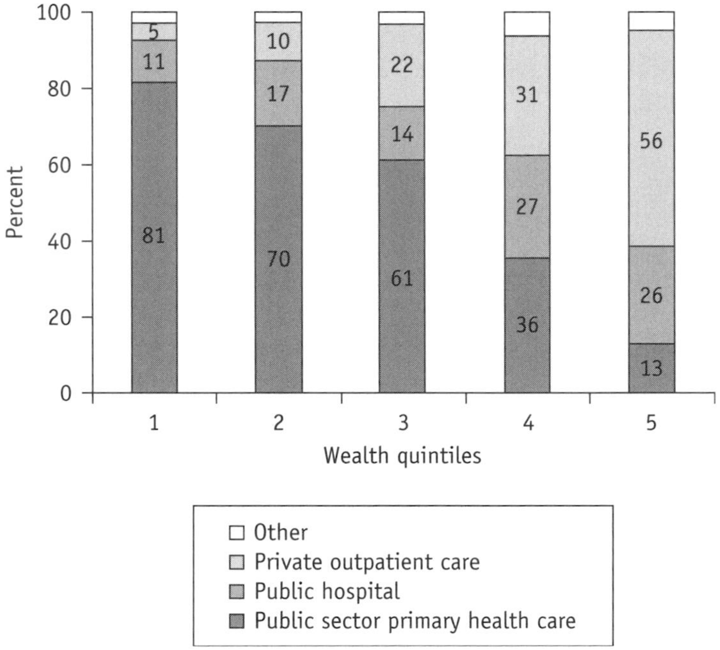

Source: Data from study by Barros.
Note: χ^2 test, $p < 0.001$.

Putting the evidence together, the low coverage of preventive programs among the poorest does not seem to be caused by difficulties in delivering services, given the general high access to and utilization of services. The high rates of self-exclusion from public services observed among the wealthy and among privately insured individuals indicate that important problems are being perceived by users but are not clearly captured by the available studies. These problems are probably related to waiting times, hours of operation, and limitations in access to specialized services and complementary exams (laboratory and imaging).

User awareness may also pose problems at the distal end of our model. As reported in the Caxias do Sul study (Trevisan et al. 2002), poor patients may not be aware of or convinced of the importance of immunization and antenatal programs. Perhaps they do not even know about the recommended immunization schedule or the recommended number and frequency of ante-

Figure 13.6. *Use of Primary Health Care among Users of a Health Service in the Previous 15 Days, by Wealth Quintile and Health Insurance Coverage, Porto Alegre, 2003*

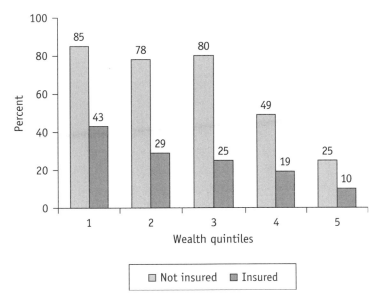

Source: Data from study by Barros.
Note: For both variables, $p < 0.001$.

natal consultations. This possibility is supported by a study showing that low maternal schooling was the main factor associated with incomplete immunization in the Northeast Region among public health service users, even after controlling for family income (da Silva and others 1999).

Family Health Program (PSF)

Unlike the first two programs, the PSF showed higher coverage among the poor. The reason is likely related to the factors discussed above. Better-off individuals and the privately insured migrate to private services for both primary care with a general physician and specialist care. Our study was not designed to investigate in detail why this happens. Still, despite a general preference for private services, the PSF and public services play an essential role in providing health care to the poorest and manage to offset the advantage of the better off, resulting in similar access rates for nonpoor and poor.

The same program may exhibit different behavior with respect to focus and coverage over its life span. In its initial stages the PSF in Porto Alegre had high focus and low coverage. In Sergipe coverage was much higher, and focus was lower. The results are very much in accordance with the proposed targeted implementation of the PSF.

Pastorate of the Child

Finally, the Pastorate of the Child, a program whose importance is recognized worldwide, and the only targeted program studied here, failed to give priority to the neediest as defined by economic or nutritional criteria. Neumann and others (1999) identified an important problem of dropout. Among mothers who had participated in the Pastorate at some point, 70 percent had left the program, mainly because of migration, lack of time, or interruption of the Pastorate leader's visits. But it is unlikely that these motives can explain the low focus.

An alternative explanation is program efficacy. If children covered by the program experience improved growth, they shift to higher Z-score groups, giving the impression that covered children are better nourished than the rest. It is unlikely, though, that this could fully explain the results.

The dependence of the program on the leader's volunteer activities can be a limiting factor for focus and coverage of the poorest because the most deprived communities may be those where recruiting leaders is more difficult or where leaders' work is less intensive or less regular. Improved targeting and better incentives to keep children under surveillance are needed.

Limitations

National data and data from several locations were used. Even so, only a fraction of current health programs and services was studied, and the investigation does not reflect Brazil's wide regional diversity. The consistency of the results, however, suggests that despite temporal and regional variations, the picture presented is credible.

The search for solutions to social, economic, and health inequalities involves the documentation of such inequalities, but the reasons behind them also have to be uncovered. Long-term, complex social processes are at work, as well as real or perceived health service deficiencies. We have explored this issue within the limits of the available information. For a better understanding, specific quantitative and qualitative studies will be needed. For example, a qualitative study carried out in Pelotas in southern Brazil showed that the public saw public health facilities in the city's periurban slums as poor substitutes for the good-quality private health care used by the wealthy (Behague, Goncalves, and Dias da Costa 2002). In-depth assessment of quality of care is important to ensure that equality is measured not only by use of services but also by how well people are being served.

Implications

We have shown that health care coverage is lower among the poor than among the wealthy for the two universal programs studied: immunization and antenatal care. The Pastorate of the Child, the only targeted program studied, also showed low coverage, as well as low focus and a high dropout rate. Coverage of the poor by the PSF was higher than coverage of the wealthy because of its targeted implementation. But this higher coverage was also attributable to self-exclusion by the better off: the wealthier the individuals, the less they used the service. We also showed that coverage by private health insurance reduced the use of the PSF by more than 60 percent. Asked why people would choose to use the PSF, most mentioned the proximity of the facility, and very few brought up quality of care.

Interpretation of the results requires some caution because the programs studied are directed at different populations and involve very different approaches. The immunization program, for instance, requires the presence of the child for a very short time on a limited number of occasions. Antenatal care involves medical consultations, laboratory exams, and so on. PSF utilization encompasses preventive activities but is most frequently related to treatment of illness.

The differences can be revealing. The Brazilian experience with successful immunization is globally recognized. The last case of polio in Brazil was in 1989, and the disease was officially declared eradicated in 1994. For the past two years no autochthonous measles cases have been reported. The immunization program is widely seen as of good quality and the vaccines as reliable. Although we did not have data on where children received their vaccines, private immunization clinics are known to be few and seldom used. Most children, nonpoor and poor, get their vaccines at the health centers. But even though the program was perceived as being of good quality and highly accessible, as well as free, coverage among the poor was much lower than among the better-off.

The record of the immunization program contrasts with the case of general PSF utilization, where constraints related to quality or to ease of access put the wealthier off. The results we presented are in agreement with the conclusions of the qualitative primary health care study of Pelotas by Behague, Goncalves, and Dias da Costa (2002), in which people voiced their distaste for the units. Paradoxically, several quantitative studies among users have shown high reported satisfaction, but one may wonder whether subjects provide valid answers when interviewed at a service site by someone who looks like a government official (IBGE 2000; Trad and others 2002).

All told, action on several fronts seems necessary if public health services for the poor are to be improved:

- Empower users, especially the poorest, by informing them about the importance of each program, what is expected from the user, and what the user should expect from the service—and create channels for complaints to be heard.
- Instead of simply expanding primary health care by increasing the number of service units, improve accessibility to the service by reducing waiting times, the need to line up very early in the morning, and other inconveniences.
- Improve access to referral services such as laboratory exams and specialists.
- Continue to monitor and evaluate programs with an equity lens by repeating exercises such as the present study and expanding them to cover other health programs.
- Feed back results of equity studies to decision makers and to the general population.

Notes

1. The data are from Datasus, http://tabnet.datasus.gov.br/cgi/pni/dpnimap.htm.

2. For further information on the PSF, see its Website, http://portal.saude .gov.br/saude/visao.cfm?id_area=149.

3. A clear and practical approach to concentration curves and indexes is available at the World Bank Website "Quantitative techniques for health equity analysis: Technical notes," http://www.worldbank.org/poverty/health/wbact/health_eq.htm.

4. Details about the Brazilian and other DHS surveys can be found at the DHS Website, www.measuredhs.com.

References

Barros, Aluísio J. D., and Andréa D. Bertoldi. 2002. Desigualdades na utilização e no acesso a serviços odontológicos: Uma avaliação em nível nacional. *Ciência e Saúde Coletiva* 7(4): 709–17.

Barros, Aluísio, and Vânia N. Hirakata. 2003. Alternatives for logistic regression in cross-sectional estimates: An empirical comparison of models that directly estimate the prevalence ratio. *BMC Medical Research Methodology* 3: 21. http://www.biomedcentral.com/1471-2288/3/21.

Barros, A. J., and C. G. Victora. 2005. A nationwide wealth score based on the 2000 Brazilian Demographic Census. *Revista de Saúde Pública* 39(4).

Behague, D. P., H. Goncalves, and J. Dias da Costa. 2002. Making medicine for the poor: Primary health care interpretations in Pelotas, Brazil. *Health Policy and Planning* 17(2): 131–43.

Coutinho. T., M. T. B. Teixeira, S. Dain, J. D. Sayd, and L. M. Coutinho. 2002. Adequação do processo de assistência pré-natal entre as usuárias do Sistema Único de Saúde em Juiz de Fora-MG. *Revista Brasileira de Ginecologia e Obstetrícia* 25(10): 717–24.

da Silva, A. A., U. A. Gomes, S. R. Tonial, and R. A. da Silva. 1999. Cobertura vacinal e fatores de risco associados à não-vacinação em localidade urbana do Nordeste brasileiro 1994. *Revista de Saúde Pública* 33(2): 147–56.

Delgado-Rodriguez, M., M. Gomez Olmedo, A. Bueno Cavanillas, and R. Galvez Vargas. 1997. Comparison of 2 indexes of prenatal care and risk of preterm delivery [in Spanish]. *Gaceta Sanitaria* 11(3): 136–42.

de Miranda, A. S., I. M. Scheibel, M. R. Tavares, and S. M. Takeda. 1995. Avaliação da cobertura vacinal do esquema básico para o primeiro ano de vida. *Revista de Saúde Pública* 29(3): 208–14.

Filmer, Deon, and Lant H. Pritchett. 2001. Estimating wealth effects without expenditure data—or tears: An application to educational enrollments in states of India. *Demography* 38(1): 115–32.

Gwatkin. Davidson R., Shea Rutstein, Kiersten Johnson, Rohini Pande, and Adam Wagstaff. 2000. Socio-economic differences in health, nutrition, and population in Brazil. HNP/Poverty Thematic Group, World Bank, Washington, DC. http://poverty.worldbank.org/library/view/4135/.

Habicht, J. P., John B. Mason, and H. Tabatabai. 1984. Basic concepts for the design of evaluation during programme implementation. In *Methods for the evaluation of the impact of food and nutrition programmes*, ed. David E. Sahn, Richard Lockwood, and Nevin S. Scrimshaw, 1–25. Tokyo: United Nations University.

IBGE (Instituto Brasileiro de Geografia e Estatística). 2000. *Acesso e utilização de serviços de saúde: PNAD 1998*. Rio de Janeiro: IBGE.

Kakwani, Nanak, Adam Wagstaff, and Eddy van Doorslaer. 1997. Socioeconomic inequalities in health: Measurement, computation, and statistical inference. *Journal of Econometrics* 77(1): 87–104.

Monteiro, Carlos Augusto, Ivan França Júnior, and Wolney Lisboa Conde. 2000. Evolução da assistência materno-infantil na cidade de São Paulo (1984–1996). *Revista de Saúde Pública* 34(6 suppl.): 19–25.

Neumann, N. A., C. G. Victora, R. Halpern, P. R. Guimaraes, and J. A. Cesar. 1999. A Pastoral da Criança em Criciúma, Santa Catarina, Brasil: Cobertura e características sócio-demográficas das famílias participantes. *Cadernos de Saúde Pública* 15(3): 543–52.

PAHO (Pan American Health Organization). 1998. *Leading Pan-American Health.* Report 287. Washington, DC.

Ribeiro, J. M., R. Costa Ndo, L. F. Pinto, and P. L. Silva. 2004. Atenção ao pré-natal na percepção das usuárias do Sistema Único de Saúde: Um estudo comparativo. *Cadernos de Saúde Pública* 20(2): 534–45.

Silveira, D. S., I. S. Santos, and J. S. Costa. 2001. Atenção pré-natal na rede básica: Uma avaliação da estrutura e do processo. *Cadernos de Saúde Pública* 17(1): 131–39.

StataCorp. 2003. *Stata Statistical Software: Release 8.0.* College Station, TX: Stata Corporation.

Trad. L. A. B., A. C. Bastos, E. Santana, and M. O. Nunes. 2002. Estudo etnográfico da satisfação do usuário do Programa de Saúde da Família (PSF) na Bahia. *Ciência e Saúde Coletiva* 7(3): 581–89.

Trevisan. Maria do Rosario, Dino Roberto Soares de Lorenzi, Natacha Machado de Araújo, and K. Ésber. 2002. Perfil da assistência pré-natal entre usuárias do Sistema Único de Saúde em Caxias do Sul. *Revista Brasileira de Ginecologia e Obstetrícia* 24(5): 293–99.

UNDP (United Nations Development Programme). 2003. *Human development report 2003. Millennium Development Goals: A compact among nations to end human poverty.* New York: UNDP. http://www.undp.org/hdr2003/pdf/hdr03_complete.pdf.

Victora, C. G., J. P. Vaughan, F. C. Barros, A. C. Silva, and E. Tomasi. 2000. Explaining trends in inequities: Evidence from Brazilian child health studies. *Lancet* 356(9235): 1093–98.

14

Peru: Is Identifying the Poor the Main Problem in Reaching Them with Nutritional Programs?

Martín Valdivia

How well social programs reach the poor has been a long-standing social policy question in developing and developed countries. As J. S. Mill observed, the key issue in designing policies to alleviate poverty is "giving the greatest amount of needful help with the smallest amount of undue reliance on it" (Besley and Kanbur 1993, 67). The question is not only about who receives the benefits but also about their impact and cost. These concerns pertain both to the poor who urgently need cash or in-kind transfers and to the nonpoor who have to pay for these benefits and on whose support the political sustainability of social programs depends.

The answer to the question requires a definition of who the neediest are, what they need most, and what is the best way to provide them with it. But the complications do not end there. Next, the neediest have to be identified—not as simple a job as it may first appear. Being concerned about program costs, we cannot just ask the individuals who belong to the group defined as "the neediest"—say, the poor, who lack the income to purchase a basket of basic needs. If we did, many nonpoor would be tempted to say they are poor in order to receive the transfers. But the cost of finding out who is truly poor may be high, so program officers have to live with imperfect solutions. The consideration of incentives and administrative costs leads us to the notion of an optimal but imperfect level of targeting (Besley and Kanbur 1993). Tullock (1982) adds another rationale for less-than-perfect targeting: the nonpoor usually have more political power than the poor, so some leakage may be necessary to avoid eroding the political base that sustains a social program. This argument is controversial but is relevant to the current debate, especially with reference to established programs.

Several instruments have been developed for targeting the poor at a reasonable cost. Proxy means-tested programs are used to identify the poor on the basis of observable, easily collected information such as residential neighborhood, dwelling characteristics, family size, and age composition. This method is cheaper than the ideal of trying to collect unbiased income or expenditure information, but in practice, it still seems expensive. Sometimes, excluding certain individuals within a locality from program benefits is also complicated, especially when program officers do not agree with the results of the proxy means instrument. Poverty maps, used to identify neighborhoods where the neediest are concentrated, can further reduce costs while at the same time sparing program officers the dilemma involved in the exclusion of a group of individuals and families. Finally, programs can be designed in a way that discourages the nonpoor from participating. The possibilities range from altering the nature of the transfer itself, by offering low-wage jobs or low-income-elasticity goods such as food, to establishing certain procedures for receiving transfers, such as long waits in line (Alderman and Lindert 1998). The use of these instruments varies across programs, and targeting performance is a result of a combination of instruments.

This discussion of targeting is highly relevant in the current Peruvian context, where several important sectors within the public administration and civil society share the objective of reorganization of social policy. Many of the advances have concentrated on restructuring public food programs under the Program for the Integral Protection of Childhood, now administered by the National Food Assistance Program (PRONAA).[1] This institution was in charge of organizing the transfer of the food programs to local governments. Over the past two years, PRONAA itself and the Vaso de Leche (Glass of Milk) program have gone through a number of corruption-related media scandals and have experienced heavy leakage of benefits to the nonpoor. Several evaluations have been done on the various kinds of leakage affecting these programs. All this attention reflects the growing importance of the issue in Peru.[2]

Research Questions

In this chapter I analyze the targeting performance of a subset of targeted public food programs in Peru on the basis of information from the Living Standards Measurement Surveys (LSMSs). The programs are Vaso de Leche, the school breakfast program, and several small early childhood nutritional programs with similar objectives and procedures, aggregated under the category ECHINP. Unlike most previous studies, this one focuses on individual data on who benefits from programs, which allows checking not only the extent to which transfers reach poor families but also whether transfers are indeed received by the intended age groups. In addition, I follow two interesting methodological lines that provide important insights for the evaluation of the targeting performance of the programs. One explores the sensitivity of estimated targeting errors to changes in the poverty line; the second analyzes the extent to which the targeting performance of different programs changes with their size and timing. Unlike the case in previous studies, the marginal analysis presented here for the school breakfast and Vaso de Leche programs compares information for two years (1997 and 2000) so that individual data can be used instead of regional averages.

The Programs and the Data

Public food programs have come under close scrutiny in Peru following large increases in their number and budgets during the 1990s. Several new, uncoordinated programs, with confusing or overlapping objectives, were created under a number of government agencies.[3]

The programs analyzed in this study are the largest public programs targeting the health and nutrition of children in Peru. In 2000 the total combined budget for Vaso de Leche, the school breakfast program, and the ECHINP aggregate was equivalent to $195 million, representing more than 80 percent of all public resources allocated to food programs (table 14.1). Vaso de Leche,

Table 14.1. *Total Budget for Selected Public Food Programs, Peru, 1998–2000 (Thousands of U.S. dollars)*

Program	1998	1999	2000
Vaso de Leche	97,645	90,273	93,159
School breakfast	68,013	73,547	67,935
Early childhood nutritional programs (ECHINP)	38,324	55,471	34,673
Subtotal	203,982	219,291	195,767
Total budget, all food and nutritional programs	234,565	266,967	240,278

Sources: For 1998 and 1999, STPAN (1999); for 2000, Instituto Cuánto (2001).

with an annual budget of $93 million in 2000, is the largest food program, closely followed by the school breakfast program, with $68 million. The ECHINP aggregate is much smaller, with a budget of $35 million.

With household-level information from the 2000 LSMS, we can also compare program sizes by the number of individuals reporting themselves as program beneficiaries (figure 14.1). By this measure, the largest program was Vaso de Leche (3.1 million), followed by the school breakfast program (about 2.6 million). Unlike the case of Vaso de Leche, the number of beneficiaries of the school breakfast program closely matches the number reported by the program. The Secretaría Técnica de Política Alimentaria Nutricional (STPAN 1999) reports that Vaso de Leche is based on a total of 4.9 million beneficiaries but that according to some case studies, program beneficiaries may be overestimated by as much as 100 percent.

In addition to having the smallest budget, the ECHINP aggregate appears to have the smallest number of beneficiaries, and the difference is even larger than for the first two programs, suggesting that per capita transfers are also larger.

Figure 14.1. *Size of Selected Public Programs, Peru, 2000*

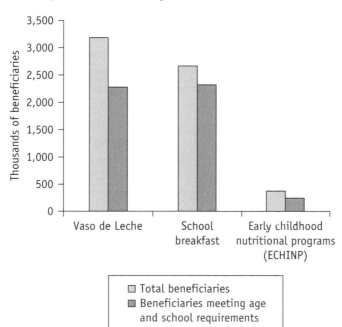

Source: LSMS 2000 (Instituto Cuánto 2000).

School Breakfast Program

The school breakfast program targets public primary school children. It was created in 1992 to improve nutrition for children age 4–13 to enable them to enhance their educational achievements and attendance. The program is funded by the central government through two public institutions: the National Food Assistance Program (PRONAA) and the Social Investment Fund (FONCODES). Coordination between the two agencies seemed loose, but FONCODES tended to concentrate on rural areas.

Breakfast, delivered to public schools during recreation periods, is organized by local mothers' committees.[4] It theoretically consists of a cup of a milklike beverage, fortified with cereals, and six small fortified biscuits and is the same for all children regardless of age. In practice, local committees make adjustments to incorporate local inputs, mainly milk and grains.[5]

In principle, PRONAA and FONCODES identify beneficiary schools on the basis of the poverty level of the district in which the schools are located, and the number of students registered in primary levels determines the number of breakfasts delivered. In practice, these criteria work for new areas, but transfer levels for older neighborhoods are maintained even when nutritional risk or poverty has manifestly been reduced.

Vaso de Leche

The Vaso de Leche program, started in 1984, was designed to target children under age six and pregnant or breastfeeding women. It has, however, heavy leakage toward older children (7 to 13 years old) and the elderly.[6] In that sense, it overlaps significantly with the school breakfast program. The treasury funds the program through the municipalities, which buy food and transfer it to the registered local mothers' committees. The committees then organize distribution to registered households. The process often implies a reduction in rations, as committees tend to increase the number of registered beneficiaries.

Distribution takes place in the municipal building, another community building, or the homes of elected local leaders. The ration varies by committee, but it usually includes 250 milliliters of milk, as well as cereals and other products, and it is often unprepared when delivered.[7] This is a key difference between Vaso de Leche and the school breakfast program, and one that facilitates allocation among household members according to the food preferences of the mothers or household head, regardless of program guidelines.

The size of the transfer to municipalities is based on the poverty level in the district, but the transfer received by the household is affected by the number of committees registered in the municipality and the number of families registered with the committees. Again, as with the school breakfast program, history affects practice. The committees are in charge of verifying poverty among families in their neighborhoods and the presence of children in the prescribed age range. There are no clear rules for updating information, and it is often claimed that many families remain beneficiaries although they are no longer poor or do not have children in the prescribed age group.

Early Childhood Nutritional Programs (ECHINP)

For the ECHINP category, I have selected and aggregated five relatively small programs with similar objectives and target populations. All of them focus on children under age three. Four have exclusively nutritional objectives: the Nutritional Assistance Program for High-Risk Families (PAN-FAR), operated by the Ministry of Health; the Infant Feeding Program (PAI), operated by the Ministerio de Promoción de la Mujer y Desarrollo Humano (PROMUDEH); and two other programs, Niños and Nutrición Infantil, run by nongovernmental organizations (NGOs).[8] The fifth program is the PRO-MUDEH integral child-care program, Wawa-Wasi, which targets poor children under age three. All these programs deliver precooked food rations (*papillas*) for children under three but use different locations for distribution.[9] PANFAR uses Ministry of Health facilities and personnel. Other programs' distribution mechanisms rely heavily on the participation of the beneficiaries' mothers and often use the community center or preschool buildings.

In the case of the Ministry of Health programs, public health facilities are responsible for identifying the family's socioeconomic status. Some health centers have developed means-testing instruments, but others rely more on the subjective impressions of social assistants. Beneficiaries are also recruited through the centers' extramural activities, in which they register information on the socioeconomic characteristics of the families and seek out newborns and pregnant women. Rules vary by center, but families classified as poor or indigent are offered the baskets of the applicable program. Still, the subjectivity of the process allows for significant leakage.

These programs are intended to help nutritionally vulnerable children, but each defines nutritional risk differently. PANFAR, for instance, looks for families with parents who have a primary education at most and with unstable employment status, more than three children under age five, pregnant and breastfeeding women at nutritional risk, or women who have recently given birth (Gilman 2003). A family is eligible if it has four of the above characteristics or if some of the children under five are undernourished. Eligibility is reviewed every six months, and the subsidy is withdrawn if no child under five is undernourished. This process generates a perverse incentive for which anecdotal evidence is often cited.

Table 14.2 summarizes the key characteristics of the food programs analyzed in this study. As indicated above, the empirical analysis uses the infor-

Table 14.2. Summary Analysis of Selected Public Food Programs, Peru

Item	School breakfast	Vaso de Leche	Early childhood nutritional programs (ECHINP)
Start of program	1992, PRONAA funding 1993, FONCODES funding	December 1984	PANFAR, 1988 Wawa-Wasi, 1994
Type of transfer	Food ration (prepared)	Food ration (precooked)	Food ration (precooked)
Delivery mechanism	Public schools	Mothers' clubs	Ministry of Health facilities
Primary target group	Children age 4–13 attending public primary schools	Children under age 6; pregnant and breastfeeding woman	Children under age 3 at nutritional risk
Secondary target groups	None	Children age 7–13; tuberculosis patients; elders	None
Geographic targeting	Yes	Yes	No
Household/ individual targeting	No	No	Yes
Target population size[a]	5,159,807	8,802,312	2,074,662
Target (poor) population size[b]	3,439,627	5,651,974	1,384,366

Sources: Author's compilation; for target population size, LSMS 2000 (Instituto Cuánto 2000).

Note: FONCODES, Social Investment Fund; PANFAR, Nutritional Assistance Program for High-Risk Families; PRONAA, National Food Assistance Program.

a. Target population within the age and school restriction of the program.

b. Target poor population within the age and school restriction of the program.

mation available in the Peruvian LSMS surveys. The LSMS is a multipurpose household survey with a representative sample at the national level and for seven regional domains. It collects information on many dimensions of household well-being such as consumption, income, savings, employment, health, education, fertility, nutrition, housing and migration, expenditures, and use of public social services.

The benefit-incidence information comes from social programs module 12 in the LSMS questionnaire. The first question asks the key informant whether any household member benefited from each program in the 12 months prior to the survey date. If the answer is positive, she is asked to identify those household members. For the most part, I use the 2000 LSMS, which includes a sample of 3,997 households and 19,957 individuals. For the marginal incidence analysis, I compare two rounds of the LSMS (1997 and 2000) that have different sample sizes but similar sampling procedures and questionnaires in the relevant modules.

Measurement Issues and Methodology

Lack of sufficient resources for social spending is the norm in developed and developing countries worldwide, although the size and nature of their needs differ substantially. Most public programs are forced to identify a target group on the basis of need or urgency. For nutritional programs, priorities are often defined in terms of vulnerability, which is related to income, age, and gender. Thus, in developing countries poor children and poor women of reproductive age are usually identified as the most vulnerable groups. In this context, it is always relevant to know to what extent public programs attend to individuals or families outside the target population (type 1 error, leakage) and to what extent part of the target population does not receive the transfers (type 2 error, undercoverage). To estimate the magnitude of these errors, the first task is to define the poor and identify the age group that is most vulnerable. Some of those decisions may have a significant impact on the evaluation of the targeting performance of public health programs.

The *poor* can be defined as any individual or household that cannot afford to purchase a consumption basket of basic needs designated by a group of local experts. In Peru, for instance, most poverty studies work with a basic consumption basket and a basic food basket. Inability to purchase a basic food basket identifies the *extremely poor*.

With a household survey, we can estimate all household members' expenditures or income and use this estimate to determine whether members are poor, assuming that resources are pooled within the household. A usual practice is to estimate per capita income or expenditures and compare it with the value of an individual consumption basket.[10] We can use the poverty indicator to define the measures of leakage and undercoverage, but for many programs poverty is not the only criterion for defining a target group. In fact, all the programs analyzed here specify children of various ages as the priority target population.[11] Enforcing that priority can be somewhat problematic if the program allows for food intake within the household because household heads can easily decide to distribute the food according to their preferences rather than the preference established by the program. In that sense, we report here two measures of leakage: (1) any case of a beneficiary who is nonpoor, is out of the age range, or does not attend a public school and (2) nonpoor beneficiaries.

We can use the two measures of targeting errors to evaluate the performance of a particular program over time or to compare two or more programs. If program A has a lower leakage rate and a lower undercoverage rate than program B, we can say that program A has a better targeting performance than program B. The evaluation is more complicated if program A has a lower leakage rate but a higher undercoverage rate. Some analysts, concerned only about leakage, would then rank program A first. Nevertheless, it can be argued that it is easier for smaller programs (with higher undercoverage) to have less leakage. That could be because operators are especially careful at the initial or pilot stages of a program but also because smaller programs are usually under less political pressure than larger ones to distort their allocation procedures.

Several issues need to be considered when analyzing absolute and relative targeting performance in search of policy implications. Here we discuss two of them: the arbitrariness of the poverty line, and the fact that the size of the leakage is not necessarily a measure of the way an expansion or contraction of a program affects the targeted population.

Targeting Errors and the Poverty Line

A key issue with the use of the targeting errors defined above is that they do not look at the entire distribution of beneficiaries across the expenditure distribution but only at whether they are above or below the poverty line. The poverty line approach has at least two limitations. The first concerns its arbitrariness and is particularly important if some individuals above the poverty line are not significantly different from some of those below the line in terms of, say, nutritional vulnerability. The second limitation is that a program may have many beneficiaries just above the poverty line while another program may have many beneficiaries farther above the poverty line.

With respect to the arbitrariness of the poverty line, it is important to keep in mind that program officers usually cannot observe beneficiaries' per capita expenditures and are limited to proxies based on the characteristics of the locality (geographic targeting) or of the dwelling and the family. In this sense, program leakage may come about because many beneficiaries just above the poverty line have dwelling and family characteristics similar to some who are below the poverty line. More important, they may face similar nutritional risk, so that the decision to identify such beneficiaries as a leakage is questionable.

These considerations lead us to explore the robustness of the measures of targeting errors defined above to changes in the poverty line to see if the program ranking changes significantly as we move the poverty line upward or downward. For these factors to be significant in aggregate terms, they have to imply a systematic bias in the sense that many individuals above (below) the poverty line should be considered appropriate (inappropriate) beneficiaries. An additional condition is a significant concentration of children, beneficiaries or not, around the standard poverty line.

One way to analyze the sensitivity of the presented measures of incidence focuses on the leakage rate, using concentration curves to compare the targeting performance of the programs under analysis. A concentration curve for the beneficiaries of a program lets us know the proportion of beneficiaries who belong to any first expenditure or income percentile of the population.[12] If we focus on one point of the expenditure distribution, say x, then we can use $1 - C(x)$ as a measure of the leakage rate. In addition, if the concentration curve for program A is above that for program B, it can be said that program A has a lower leakage rate for all levels of the poverty line.[13] We need to be careful with these comparisons, however, for they could be somewhat misleading when comparing programs that focus on populations with different poverty levels.

Marginal Incidence Analysis

The proportions of poor and nonpoor benefiting from a program at any time may not be a good indicator of how an expansion or contraction would affect the poor. There are arguments for both early and late capture by the nonpoor, based on the presence of positive participation costs that differ for the poor and nonpoor and change with the scale of the program (Lanjouw and Ravallion 1998). The higher cost of reaching remote areas is typically the argument advanced for early capture. Late capture could result because whereas small pilot projects are more carefully monitored and under less political pressure than larger projects, expansion would invariably transfer the program to public officials with less expertise and fewer compatible incentives. Political pressures or bribes that distort resource allocation are also more likely as a program expands.

Furthermore, political distortions can affect the dynamics of beneficiary selection. A good system for identifying beneficiaries can imply low leakage rates at the beginning. Later, leakage increases because households that escape poverty or no longer have children in the targeted age range cannot be excluded from the group of beneficiaries. After a while, the average leakage rate would be high, but leakage in new areas, where the system for identifying beneficiaries is again applied properly, could remain low.

All these arguments indicate the need to expand the analysis of the estimated marginal incidence properties of the programs being studied. Lanjouw and Ravallion (1998), Younger (2002), and others based their estimates on one cross-section, so they used heterogeneity across regions to infer marginal behavior. Here, I use heterogeneity over time to estimate the impact of a program expansion or contraction on the poor on the basis of individual data.[14] The idea is to estimate the following equation:

$$D_{iqt} = \alpha_q + \beta_q p_t + v_{qt} \qquad q = 1, \ldots, 5 \tag{14.1}$$

where i indexes the individual, t indexes the year of the survey, and q indexes the per capita expenditure quintiles. The dependent variable is the program participation dummy for each individual. The explanatory variables are quintile dummies and the interaction between these dummies and the program participation rate for a particular year; β_q can be interpreted as the marginal effect of an increase in program participation on the participation rate in a particular quintile; and $\beta_q > 1$ (< 1) would indicate that a general expansion (contraction) in coverage will cause a more than proportional increase (reduction) in participation for that quintile.

I estimate (14.1) imposing the following restrictions:

$$\sum_q \alpha_q = 0 \quad \text{and} \quad \sum_q \beta_q = 5$$

The estimated vector $\hat{\beta}_q$ is used to generate a concentration curve by plotting

$$\sum_j^q \hat{\beta}_j \Big/ 5$$

on q, so that we can check which program is marginally more pro-poor.[15]

The key issue is to analyze to what extent the marginal ranking differs from the average ranking. Programs A and B may have the same average level of leakage, but the marginal performance of program B may be substantially more pro-poor than that of program A. If that is so, cutting (expanding) program B will have a larger negative (positive) effect on the poor.[16]

Empirical Results

The LSMS questionnaire asks key respondents whether the household receives transfers from a large list of public programs and which household members benefit. It could be argued that individual identification is biased toward the age groups the programs target in the fear that surveyors could denounce the household to the program. We are in no position to check this, but we note that the LSMS survey is now run by a private firm, Instituto Cuánto, whose surveyors are trained to explain to respondents that none of the information revealed to them goes to any government agency. In that sense, such bias may not be important. Moreover, the survey results are very consistent with the characteristics of each program's delivery mechanisms.

Table 14.3 shows participation rates by quintile for each of the public programs studied here. The analysis is done at the individual and household levels. At the individual level, two estimates are presented, one that constructs quintiles on the whole population and a second that does it for those belonging to the target population.[17] At the individual level, the Vaso de Leche program achieves the largest coverage rate, 12.4 percent. The coverage of the school breakfast program is similar, at 10.4 percent. The ECHINP aggregate covers only 1.4 percent of the Peruvian population. Vaso de Leche was less pro-poor than the other two programs in 2000. Almost 4 percent of Peruvians in the least poor quintile, and not quite 19 percent in the poorest quintile, benefited from it. The ECHINP aggregate shows the lowest coverage but also the greatest pro-poor bias; the proportion of beneficiaries among the poorest is 17 times that of the least poor quintile.

Estimated coverage rates are naturally larger when analysis is restricted to the target population, and in that case the school breakfast program has the largest coverage, with 44.7 percent. In 2000 almost 31 percent of schoolchildren in the least poor quintile and more than 55 percent in the poorest quintile benefited from the program. The ECHINP aggregate again shows the lowest coverage but the greatest pro-poor bias; the proportion of beneficiaries among the poorest is 5.4 times greater than in the least poor quintile. At the household level, average global rates are similar to the latter individual rates for all programs, but differences by quintile are significant for Vaso

Table 14.3. *Coverage of Selected Social Programs by Per Capita Expenditure Quintile, Peru (percent)*

Level and program	Quintile					All quintiles
	1	2	3	4	5	
Individual level						
School breakfast	18.7	13.4	10.0	7.1	2.6	10.4
Vaso de Leche	18.8	15.3	13.0	10.7	3.9	12.4
Early childhood nutritional programs (ECHINP)[a]	3.4	1.6	1.2	0.5	0.2	1.4
Individual level, targeted population						
School breakfast[a]	55.1	55.5	42.9	39.4	30.7	44.7
Vaso de Leche[b]	31.4	26.7	30.8	23.5	15.0	25.5
Early childhood nutritional programs (ECHINP)[c,d]	19.4	16.9	13.9	4.8	3.6	11.7
Household level[e]						
School breakfast	67.1	58.5	48.3	41.1	29.4	48.9
Vaso de Leche	48.1	41.7	35.7	28.6	14.8	33.8
Early childhood nutritional programs (ECHINP)[c]	22.2	18.0	12.7	5.9	3.9	12.5

Source: LSMS 2000 (Instituto Cuánto 2000).

a. As a share of children age 4–13 who attend public school.

b. As a share of children under age 13 and women who are pregnant or breastfeeding.

c. Includes Nutritional Assistance Program for High-Risk Families, Infant Feeding Program, Wawa-Wasi, Programas no Escolarizados de Educación Inicial, and Cuna.

d. As a share of children under age three.

e. As a share of households with at least one member in the age and school restriction of each program.

de Leche, with the household data indicating a more pro-poor bias than do the individual data.[18]

Table 14.4 shows the individual-level leakage and undercoverage rates for the analyzed programs by type of location (urban or rural). The smallest leakage rate—that is, the lowest proportion of beneficiaries who are non-poor—is in the ECHINP aggregate (17.1 percent). The estimated leakage rates for the school breakfast and Vaso de Leche programs are closer to each other, between 28 and 32 percent.

Analyzed by type of location, most of the difference between the ECHINP aggregate and the other programs occurs in rural areas; the performance of the

Table 14.4. *Estimated Leakage and Undercoverage Rates, Selected Public Programs, Peru*
(percent)

Program	Leakage[a]			Undercoverage[b]		
	Global	Urban	Rural	Global	Urban	Rural
School breakfast	28.8	31.3	27.3	86.4	91.5	79.4
Vaso de Leche	31.4	33.0	30.1	84.3	88.0	79.3
Early childhood nutritional programs (ECHINP)[c]	17.1	22.5	15.9	97.9	99.4	95.9

Source: LSMS 2000 (Instituto Cuánto 2000).
a. Nonpoor beneficiaries as a share of total beneficiaries.
b. Poor beneficiaries as a share of total poor.
c. Includes Nutritional Assistance Program for High-Risk Families, Infant Feeding Program, Wawa-Wasi, Programas no Escolarizados de Educación Inicial, and Cunas.

programs is more similar in urban areas. All programs show lower leakage rates in rural areas. For the total beneficiary population, Vaso de Leche has the lowest undercoverage rate (84 percent), and the ECHINP aggregate has the highest. A special bias is observed toward rural areas, where the Vaso de Leche and school breakfast programs cover about 20 percent of the population.

In conclusion, there seems to be a systematic relation between the size of the program, in number of beneficiaries, and its performance as measured by the leakage rate. The ECHINP aggregate has the smallest programs and the programs with the smallest leakage rates. But before trying to interpret these results, we should analyze their robustness. The first issue to consider is that the estimated targeting errors in table 14.4 define as a leakage only a nonpoor beneficiary, not the cases in which the beneficiary does not fulfill the age and school restrictions. In the Vaso de Leche program, for example, benefits to poor children above age 13 are not considered leakage.

Because not all programs face the same additional restrictions, it is important to disentangle the effect of each factor on the estimated leakages. Table 14.5 compares the leakage estimates in table 14.4 with those that tighten the definition of a leakage. When the age and school restrictions are considered, Vaso de Leche still has the largest leakage rate, with 49.5 percent, but this estimated rate is now much larger than that of the school breakfast program, 38 percent, which in turn is not much different from that of the ECHINP aggregate, 41.5 percent.[19]

Table 14.5 also shows that for the school breakfast program, which delivers rations only in public schools, the age restriction is more important than the school restriction. When the age restriction is omitted, the leakage rate for the school breakfast program rises 4 percentage points, to 33 percent.

The largest age effects are found with the Vaso de Leche and ECHINP programs. In the Vaso de Leche program the leakage rate rises 18 percentage points, to 49.5 percent, indicating that two-fifths of the leaks reported in the last column of table 14.5 are to beneficiaries who are indeed poor but are over 13.[20] For the ECHINP aggregate, the age effect is even more important, since its omission implies a 25 percentage point increase in the estimated leakage rate, meaning that almost three out of every five ECHINP leaks are to poor beneficiaries who are over three years old.

In summary, the age and school restrictions are not that relevant for the school breakfast program, which is not surprising because delivery takes place in the school. The age restriction has a significantly larger effect on Vaso de Leche and the ECHINP aggregate. This latter result is important because it suggests that food programs which allow for consumption within the household permit reallocation of the rations for the benefit of members who are not within the age restrictions set by the program.[21] Actually, it can be argued that such deviations should not be called leakage, but we need to keep in mind that failure by policy planners to take into account these intra-household reallocations can reduce the effect of the transfer on the originally targeted population because the per capita ration shrinks when distributed among more individuals than planned.[22] Furthermore, it should make us think about the justification for a program that imposes its preferences on households, especially if we consider that health and nutritional vulnerability are indeed determined at the household level.

Targeting Errors and the Poverty Line

We presented a way of analyzing the robustness of the comparison between two programs to changes in the poverty line,[23] which focuses on the leakage rate and uses the concentration curve to compare two programs along the

Table 14.5. *Leakage Rates under Alternative Set of Restrictions, Selected Public Programs, Peru*
(percent)

Program	Poverty restriction only	No age restriction	No school restriction	All restrictions
School breakfast	28.8	33.0	37.1	38.0
Vaso de Leche	31.4	31.4	49.5	49.5
Early childhood nutritional programs (ECHINP)	17.1	17.1	41.5	41.5

Source: LSMS 2000 (Instituto Cuánto 2000).

whole expenditure distribution. Figure 14.2 plots the concentration curves for the three programs and shows that the ECHINP aggregate performs best, as its concentration curve dominates those of the other two. The school breakfast program seems to slightly outperform Vaso de Leche, but no clear difference is observed, especially around the first decile.

In conclusion, movement of the poverty line has a negligible effect on the comparison of the targeting performance of the three programs analyzed here. The ranking remains intact when we omit the age restriction, which results in the largest differences among programs (see table 14.5).

Several factors could explain the observed superiority of the ECHINP aggregate. It differs from the other two programs because its programs are the only ones that use individual targeting instruments and because the programs focus on younger children (up to age three), who tend to be more concentrated in poor families. One way to approximate the importance of differences in the age groups assisted by each program is to compare the concentration curve of each program's beneficiaries with the curve of the target age group. Figure 14.3 plots those two curves for each program. We can see that the pro-poorness of the ECHINP aggregate well exceeds the

Figure 14.2. *Concentration Curves, Selected Public Food Programs, Peru, 2000 (percent)*

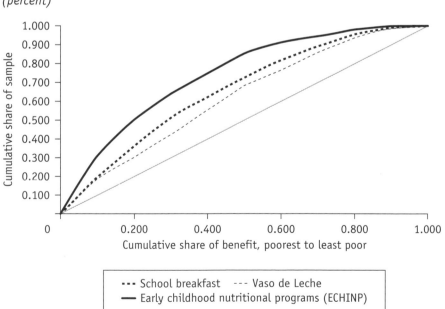

Source: LSMS 2000 (Instituto Cuánto 2000).

Figure 14.3. *Concentration Curves, Beneficiaries and Target Population, Selected Public Programs, Peru, 2000*
(percent)

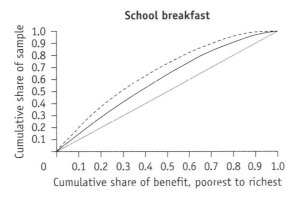

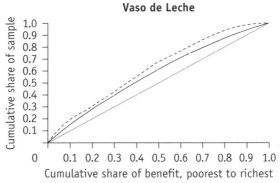

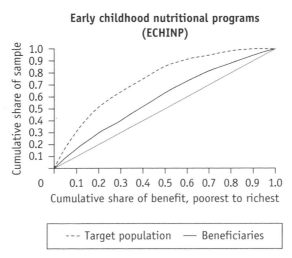

Source: LSMS 2000 (Instituto Cuánto 2000).

pro-poorness of the age group the programs work with, since the two curves for these programs are the farthest from each other. In the case of the other two programs, especially Vaso de Leche, the two curves are very close.[24]

The pattern observed in figure 14.3 suggests that something other than target group age has to be invoked to explain the superior performance of the ECHINP aggregate. One of these factors could be the ECHINP programs' use of specific individual targeting instruments, which could be of significant help, despite criticism about their subjectivity and sensitivity to political pressure. Nevertheless, our analysis cannot be considered proof positive. The observed feature may be less a property of the ECHINP programs than a result of the other two programs' targeting procedures. Accordingly, we focus next on those programs' targeting performance.

Marginal Incidence Analysis for the School Breakfast and Vaso de Leche Programs

As we have seen, average incidence analysis may not provide enough information to adjust the scale of an antipoverty program, as a number of factors could generate early or late capture by the nonpoor. With early capture, a program would have a large leakage rate, yet the effects of the reduction of that program could fall disproportionately on the poorest. We can estimate the marginal effect by using the variation of the coverage programs across quintiles and over time.

Here, we look at the results of the marginal analysis proposed above for two of the largest and oldest food programs in Peru: Vaso de Leche and the school breakfast program.[25] The exercise uses information from the 1997 and 2000 rounds of the LSMS. (See annex figure 14.1 for coverage rates by quintile and geographic area in both programs in both years.)

Figure 14.4 plots the concentration curves associated with the marginal effects estimated using expression (14.1) and compares them with the average effects.[26] The concentration curves for both programs, but especially the school breakfast program, show a stronger pro-poor bias at the margin than on average. This means that if the Vaso de Leche program were expanded, about 32 percent of the new beneficiaries would belong to the poorest quintile, so that marginal behavior is no different from average behavior. The estimates also suggest that 51 percent of the new beneficiaries would be in the second-poorest quintile, much larger than the proportion of current beneficiaries in that quintile (26 percent). In the case of the school breakfast program, 58 percent of the new beneficiaries would be concentrated in the

Figure 14.4. *Marginal and Average Effects, Vaso de Leche and School Breakfast Programs, Peru, 2000*

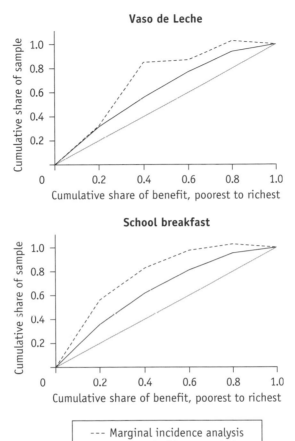

Vaso de Leche

School breakfast

--- Marginal incidence analysis
— Average incidence analysis

Source: LSMS 1997 and 2000 (Instituto Cuánto 1997, 2000).

poorest quintile and 23 percent in the second-poorest quintile. The averages are 38 and 22 percent, respectively.

The robustness of these results can be evaluated by looking at what happens when the analysis is repeated with regional averages instead of individual data. This approach was followed by Lanjouw and Ravallion (1998), using cross-sectional data. Annex table 14.2 includes those estimates. The school breakfast program estimates are similar. For the Vaso de Leche program the pro-poorness of the marginal effect is even larger for the three poorest quintiles. The pro-poorness of both programs at the margin is an interesting result, since it suggests that two programs with a fairly mediocre targeting performance on average have a significantly greater pro-poor behavior at the margin. The implication is that cutting (expanding) the programs would damage (benefit) the poorest much more than the average leakage rate would suggest.

How can we explain this dramatically different targeting performance at the margin? As observed above, many researchers have argued that the difference could result from mechanisms that facilitate or promote early capture by the nonpoor (Lanjouw and Ravallion 1998). One idea is that the less poor have more political power and can influence public officials to make them early beneficiaries. Later, as the program expands, the poor inevitably benefit more. We cannot test this hypothesis properly here, but we mention a possible alternative that has more to do with the dynamics of each program's beneficiary list.

As explained above, initial transfers are distributed according to the poverty level of the districts in which the schools or mothers' clubs are located. Once a public school is included in the registry, it is politically difficult to drop it when poverty is reduced in the surrounding neighborhood. In the Vaso de Leche program it is difficult to retire a mothers' club once the municipality has registered it as a beneficiary. It is also conceivable that after a family or household has been registered as a beneficiary, it is unlikely to be dropped from the registry if it moves out of poverty or has fewer children in the qualifying age range.[27] If that is true, a program will spring more and more leakage as time passes, no matter how good its system for the initial selection (identification) of beneficiaries is.

Disentangling these two mechanisms would be interesting, but the important thing is that either hypothesis would weaken the emphasis on the use of poverty maps and means-tested programs to identify the poorest. In the case of the second hypothesis, however, the focus shifts toward designing enforceable exit rules for pruning the beneficiary list, giving due consideration to the political economy of program delivery mechanisms managed on the ground by social organizations.

Summary of Results, Policy Implications, and Limitations

This study analyzes the targeting performance of selected public child nutrition programs in Peru: Vaso de Leche, the school breakfast program, and an aggregate of programs (ECHINP) focused on the nutrition of children in their first three years. These programs have large leakages—

between 40 and 50 percent of their beneficiaries fall outside the target group, either because they are not poor or because they are outside the age range. The leakages are larger for the Vaso de Leche program (50 percent) and in urban areas, where poverty rates are relatively lower. The numbers argue for urgent policy intervention to reduce these leaks. Nevertheless, a closer look suggests that improving poverty maps and means-tested programs may not be the right priority. Instead, priority should be given to defining delivery protocols that are consistent with program objectives and to addressing political distortions in their management so that appropriate exit rules for beneficiaries become feasible.

In analyzing the robustness of those results, I explore three key adjustments to the original estimates:

- restricting the definition of leakage to the poverty level of the individual or household, disregarding the age of the beneficiary
- exploring the effect of movements in the poverty line
- comparing the average with the marginal incidence estimates

With respect to the first adjustment, the effect of the age restriction is very important, especially for programs (Vaso de Leche and the ECHINP aggregate) that allow for consumption within the household. The results call into question the notion that in-kind transfers are preferable to cash transfers because they can be better directed to the target population. Indeed, when the age restriction is dropped, Vaso de Leche ceases to be the one with the worst targeting performance, and the ECHINP aggregate becomes by far the program with lowest leakage (17 percent). Furthermore, none of the analyzed programs have a leakage rate above 32 percent once the age restriction is disregarded.

The importance of the age-related leaks within households for Vaso de Leche and the ECHINP aggregate suggests that food programs which allow consumption of the food ration in the household cannot prevent distribution of the transfer among household members instead of to the targeted individuals. It is hard to argue that this is bad per se. On the contrary, the policy implication is that these intrahousehold reallocations need to be considered when defining the size of the transfer because otherwise they imply a reduction in the size of the transfer per capita and limit the possibility that the programs' transfers will improve nutrition within the target population.

Changes in the poverty line have little effect on ranking the targeting performance of the three programs analyzed here. In other words, the ECHINP aggregate has lower leakage than the others no matter where program officers draw the poverty line. The comparison of each ECHINP component's concentration curve with that of its target population also suggests that the superiority of the aggregate cannot be explained by differences in the distribution of the programs' target groups and supports the notion that the programs' targeting instruments perform better for some reason. What we do not know is how the small size of the programs considered within the ECHINP aggregate influences these results.

With respect to the marginal incidence analysis, the school breakfast and Vaso de Leche programs display very pro-poor behavior at the margin despite their mediocre targeting performance on average. This result suggests a need for caution about making decisions based on a program's average targeting performance. Even though a program shows large leakages on average, a cut (or expansion) could still damage (or benefit) the poor dispro-portionately.[28] For policy, this result implies that emphasis on improving the targeting instruments used by these two programs should be shifted to dealing with the political distortions that influence the selection of benefi-ciaries. Working with the political economy underlying the delivery mecha-nisms would seem to be a powerful way to get base organizations (mothers' clubs) to accept appropriate exit rules when beneficiaries escape poverty. Nevertheless, along the lines of Tullock's arguments, these leaks to the non-poor may be optimal, in the sense that they may be necessary to sustain the political support of the people who pay for the programs. If so, the political base for the programs will have to be changed before anything can be done about leakage.

Further research is definitely needed before any action is taken, and con-sidering the limitations of this study, its findings must be taken cautiously. One important limitation is our assumption that all beneficiaries receive the same kind of transfer, when they often do not, for several reasons. In the case of food programs involving daily rations, two individuals may identify themselves as beneficiaries of the program, but one receives more rations because she goes more regularly to the community center where meals are delivered. The content of the ration also varies significantly by region, and foods are often chosen for the convenience of local agricultural producers rather than for their nutritional value. We could try to homogenize transfers by assigning them a value, but assigning a unit value to a transfer is often complicated. A common solution is to use the unit production cost as the transfer value. Finally, when analyzing a program's benefits distribution, other sources of large leaks must be considered—for example, those associ-ated with large administrative costs or corruption, which may vary substan-tially among programs.

Annex Table 14.1. *Targeting Errors and the Poverty Line, Selected Public Programs, Peru*

Error and program	0.75	0.9	1.0 (poverty line)	1.1	1.25
Leakage					
School breakfast	56.6	43.2	38.0	32.9	28.1
Vaso de Leche	66.3	54.3	49.5	45.4	41.0
Early childhood nutritional programs (ECHINP)	57.1	47.8	41.5	39.1	37.4
Undercoverage					
School breakfast	50.0	51.2	52.1	52.6	53.5
Vaso de Leche	72.0	71.5	71.7	71.9	72.3
Early childhood nutritional programs (ECHINP)	83.9	82.2	85.3	85.8	86.5

Source: LSMS 2000 (Instituto Cuánto 2000).

Annex Table 14.2. *Marginal Effects by Quintile, Vaso de Leche and School Breakfast Programs, Peru, 1997–2000*

	With individual data		With regional averages	
Quintile/quarter	Vaso de Leche	School breakfast	Vaso de Leche	School breakfast
1 (poorest quintile)	1.601 $(2.83)^a$	2.804 $(12.37)^a$	2.113 $(1.64)^b$	2.219 $(3.44)^a$
2	2.605 $(4.61)^a$	1.337 $(5.90)^a$	3.176 $(3.82)^a$	1.289 $(4.10)^a$
3	0.141 (0.25)	0.736 $(3.25)^a$	1.533 $(1.81)^b$	0.635 $(1.69)^b$
4	0.753 (1.33)	0.263 (1.16)	−0.698 $(−0.53)$	0.737 $(1.62)^b$
5 (least poor quintile)	−0.101 $(−0.18)$	−0.139 $(−0.61)$	−1.124 $(−1.41)$	0.121 (0.27)

Source: LSMS 2000 (Instituto Cuánto 2000).
Note: Numbers in parentheses are absolute values of *t*-statistics.
a. Significant at 1 percent.
b. Significant at 10 percent.

Annex Figure 14.1. *Vaso de Leche and School Breakfast Program Coverage, by Quintile, Region, and Year, Peru*

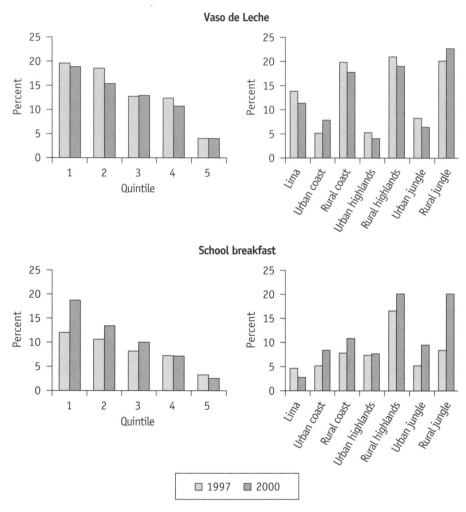

Sources: LSMS 1997 and 2000 (Instituto Cuánto 1997, 2000).

Notes

This chapter benefited from comments by two anonymous reviewers and by participants at the World Bank conference "Reaching the Poor with Effective Health, Nutrition, and Population Services: What Works, What Doesn't, and Why?" held in Washington, DC, in February 2004. In addition, I thank Gianmarco León for excellent research assistance, as well as Jorge Mesinas and Verónica Frisancho for their help in the initial stages of the project.

1. See *El Peruano* (2002: 223000). The norm does not include the Vaso de Leche program, which is administered by municipalities.

2. See Alcázar, Lópex-Cálix, and Wachtenheim (2003) and Stifel and Alderman (2003), which focus on the Vaso de Leche program. For a general evaluation of all public food programs, see STPAN (1999) and Instituto Cuánto (2001).

3. See STPAN (1999) or Instituto Cuánto (2001) for a detailed description of these programs and their evolution over time. In 2002 the regulation and supervision of most of these programs were unified under the National Institute of Health (NIH), which is part of the Ministry of Health. Later, the responsibility was transferred to PRONAA, a dependency of the Ministry for the Promotion of Women and Human Development (PROMUDEH).

4. Cueto and Montes (1999) find that most breakfasts are delivered between 9 AM and 11 AM because children are hungrier by that time than when they arrive at school.

5. Changes in the regulation have encouraged these adjustments, shifting purchases to local producers as part of program objectives.

6. Actually, the law indicates that older children (up to age 13), elders, and tuberculosis patients should be served after the needs of younger children and mothers are met.

7. See Alcázar, Lópex-Cálix, and Wachtenheim (2003). Local mothers' committees argue that they do not prepare the product because of lack of organization and resources but also because coming in daily for the ration is too burdensome for individuals who live in remote places. This way, recipients only have to come once a week (or once a month) to pick up the ration for the whole period.

8. The Programa de Complementación Alimentaria para Grupos en Mayor Riesgo (PACFO) is another nutritional program run by the Ministry of Health, but it is not included as a separate alternative in the LSMS questionnaire. Because it has the same objective and target population as PANFAR, some households that report benefiting from PANFAR may actually be PACFO beneficiaries.

9. An important difference is that the PANFAR basket does include some food for adults (for example, oil, rice) on the premise that the economic situation of the family is what puts the children at nutritional risk.

10. In some cases adjustments are made according to household composition, with the understanding that there are consumption economies of scale and differences in the needs of household members by age and gender (Deaton and Zaidi 1999). We disregard this practice, following Valdivia (2002), which reports a negligible effect for these adjustments when the value of relevant parameters remains within a reasonable range. Actually, the ranking of households does not change much, but poverty levels may still change substantially with these adjustments if the poverty line is kept fixed. We deal with that issue below when discussing the effect of movements in the poverty line over the estimated targeting performance of the analyzed programs.

11. One exception is the Vaso de Leche program, which also includes pregnant and breastfeeding mothers as part of the priority target population.

12. The curve can be above or below the 45° line of equality. Being above the line implies that the program has a pro-poor bias; being below the line implies a bias favoring the nonpoor.

13. This ordering is incomplete in the sense that not much can be said if concentration curves cross at some point.

14. See Younger (2002) for a discussion of the advantages of such a procedure.

15. Younger (2002) also suggests running a model with fixed effects at the department (or region) level, since departments of regions have different unobservable characteristics for department (region).

16. It should be kept in mind that budget adjustments cannot be based solely on these estimates because they do not take into account the marginal benefits and costs of the program.

17. For the target population, I restrict the analysis to individuals within the age and school restrictions set for each program. At the household level, the analysis is restricted to those having at least one member within the age and school restriction for each program. The comparison of these two levels of analysis is important for checking consistency with the findings of previous studies that focus on household-level data (Younger 2002; Stifel and Alderman 2003).

18. Household-level results are consistent with those reported in Stifel and Alderman (2003) but not with those in Younger (2002). I have not been able to identify the reasons for that discrepancy.

19. A disaggregated analysis by type of location is available on request. Observed patterns are similar in urban and rural areas.

20. This finding for the Vaso de Leche program is indeed consistent with the results of Alcázar, Lópex-Cálix, and Wachtenheim (2003). The authors use two Public Expenditure Tracking Surveys (PETS) to analyze the channeling of resources from the Vaso de Leche program and the educational programs in Peru. For Vaso de Leche, they find that the largest leakage occurs within the household because rations are actually distributed among all household members, not only among children under age six and pregnant and breastfeeding women. Only 41 percent of the ration assigned to the household actually reaches the target group.

21. Most programs in the ECHINP aggregate deliver *papillas,* which are supposed to be specifically for children in their first months. Nevertheless, according to anecdotal evidence, the *papillas* are dissolved in beverages and soups that are also consumed by household members outside the age range.

22. Stifel and Alderman (2003) do attempt to evaluate the nutritional impact of the Vaso de Leche program using a model with district fixed effects. They find no significant effect.

23. This analysis disregards the age restriction, defining a leak as occurring only when the individual is not poor.

24. The other feature we can observe from figure 14.3 is that the distribution of the target groups does not seem to differ much across programs.

25. Marginal analysis for the other ECHINP programs was not feasible because they were not singled out in the LSMS surveys before the one in 2000.

26. Annex table 14.2 shows the corresponding βs. The coefficients for the poorest three quintiles are significant.

27. Anecdotal evidence supporting this hypothesis is growing in Peru. The media report cases of beneficiaries of the Vaso de Leche program in neighborhoods that were once slums but are now residential neighborhoods, while new slums receive no transfers. If the program were expanded, the current slums, not the residential areas, would likely benefit the most. The problem is that neighborhoods and households work their way out of poverty, but the political economy of the program does not allow for appropriate revision of the list of beneficiaries.

28. In addition, targeting performance at the margin is not sufficient to determine program expansion or shrinkage. The answer to that question requires an analysis of the program's nutritional impact and cost.

References

Alcázar, Lorena, José López-Cálix, and Eric Wachtenheim. 2003. Las pérdidas en el camino: Fugas en las transferencias municipales, Vaso de Leche y educación. Instituto Apoyo, Lima.

Alderman, Harold, and Kathy Lindert. 1998. The potential and limitations of self-targeted food subsidies. *World Bank Research Observer* 13(2): 213–29.

Besley, Timothy, and Ravi Kanbur. 1993. The principles of targeting. In *Including the poor: Proceedings of a symposium organized by the World Bank and the International Food Policy Research Institute*, ed. Michael Lipton and Jacques van der Gaag. Washington, DC: World Bank.

Cueto, Santiago, and Iván Montes. 1999. Asistencia alimentaria a niños pre-escolares y de educación primaria en areas rurales. Grupo de Análisis para el Desarrollo, Lima.

Deaton, Angus, and Salman Zaidi. 1999. Guidelines for constructing consumption aggregates for welfare analysis. World Bank, Washington, DC.

Gilman, Josephine. 2003. "Managing for results. A nutrition program experience from Peru. Proyectos de Informática, Salud, Medicina, Agricultura, Lima.

Instituto Cuánto. 1997. Living Standards Measurement Survey 1997. Lima.

———. 2000. Living Standards Measurement Survey 2000. Lima.

———. 2001. Diseño de una estrategia de racionalización del gasto social público en alimentación nutricional. Final report. Lima.

Lanjouw, Peter, and Martin Ravallion. 1998. Benefit incidence and the timing of program capture. Policy Research Working Paper 1956, Development Research Group, Poverty and Human Resources, World Bank, Washington, DC.

Stifel, David, and Harold Alderman. 2003. The "Glass of Milk" subsidy program and malnutrition in Peru. Policy Research Working Paper 3089, Public Services, Development Research Group, World Bank, Washington, DC.

STPAN (Secretaría Técnica de Política Alimentaria Nutricional). 1999. Los programas de alimentación y nutrición: Consolidado y comparación de características. Lima.

Tullock, Gordon. 1982. Income testing and politics: A theoretical model. In *Income-tested transfer programs: The case for and against,* ed. Irwin Garfinkel. New York: Academic Press.

Valdivia, Martín. 2002. Acerca de la magnitud de la inequidad en salud en el Perú. Working Paper 37, Grupo de Análisis para el Desarrollo, Lima.

Younger, Stephen. 2002. Benefits on the margin: Observations on average vs. marginal benefit incidence. Cornell University, Food and Nutrition Policy Program, Ithaca, NY.

About the Authors

A. T. M. Iqbal Anwar, MPH, DPH, MBBS, has been a senior research investigator at the Centre for Health and Population Research, Bangladesh, since 2002. Among his previous positions were epidemiological information systems medical officer, Institute of Epidemiology, Disease Control and Research, Mohakhali Dhaka (1999–2000); operations research consultant, Thana Functional Improvement Pilot Project, Directorate General of Health Services, Dhaka (1997–9); medical officer, Epidemiology, Institute of Epidemiology Disease Control and Research, Dhaka (1995–7); divisional trainer, Extended Programme on Immunization (EPI), Office of the Director of Health, Khulna Division (1993–5); and medical officer at the Medical Officer, Office of the Civil Surgeon, Khulna (1992–3) and at the Thana Health Complex, Dacope, Khulna (1985–92). He has published and presented papers at international conferences on such topics as epidemiology, poverty, and health care–seeking behavior, particularly for obstetrical care.

Aluísio J. D. Barros is an associate professor at the Federal University of Pelotas, Brazil, and is director of the postgraduate program in epidemiology there. He trained as a physician at the State University of Campinas, where he was graduated in 1983. In 1990 he received a master's in statistics from the same university. That same year, he started his studies at the London School of Hygiene and Tropical Medicine, where he obtained an MS in medical statistics in 1991 and a PhD in epidemiology in 1996, at the Maternal and Child Epidemiology Unit. He then joined the Department of Social Medicine at the Federal University of Pelotas, where he has assumed the main responsibility for teaching statistical methods in postgraduate courses. During this period, he has coordinated several research projects, mostly related to child health, traffic accidents, and health inequalities. These projects were funded by Brazilian agencies (CNPq, Fapergs) and international agencies, including the U.K. Overseas Development Administration (now the Department for International Development), the Canadian International Development Research Centre, the Pan American Health Organization, the World Health Organization, and the World Bank.

Andréa D. Bertoldi is a doctoral student in the postgraduate program in epidemiology at the Federal University of Pelotas, Brazil, where she earned a master's in epidemiology in 2002. She was graduated in pharmacy and biochemistry from the Catholic University of Pelotas in 1984. Her main field of interest is pharmacoepidemiology, especially drug utilization at the population level and out-of-pocket expenditure on medicines by the poor.

Indu Bhushan is director of the Pacific Department of the Asian Development Bank (ADB). Earlier, he was principal economist in charge of ADB health sector operations in Cambodia and Vietnam. Before joining the ADB in 1997, he was a health economist in the Africa Region of the World Bank. He has also worked with the government of India in Rajasthan State, where he was involved in several community-based health projects. He holds a master's in health sciences and a PhD in public health economics from Johns Hopkins University.

Martha Campbell, a political scientist, has specialized in global population issues, health policy, and the economics of international health and family planning. Her degrees are from Wellesley College and the University of Colorado. In 1994 she joined the David and Lucile Packard Foundation, where she led the population program and developed its international component. In 2000 Ms. Campbell and colleagues founded the Center for Entrepreneurship in International Health and Development (CEIHD, pronounced "seed") in the School of Public Health, University of California at Berkeley. At the same time, she founded Venture Strategies for Health and Development, an independent nonprofit organization working in developing countries (www.venturestrategies.org). Ms. Campbell is completing four years of research on the broad range of barriers to fertility regulation methods around the world and is developing the new "ease" model of fertility decline as an alternative but closely related theory complementing current theoretical explanations for demographic transitions.

Juraci A. Cesar is an assistant professor at the University of Rio Grande, Brazil, and is working toward a PhD at the London School of Hygiene and Tropical Medicine. He has been doing research in the fields of maternal and child health (mainly relating to breastfeeding, antenatal care, malnutrition, and pneumonia) and health program evaluation regarding the activities of community health workers and the extension to households of integrated management of common illnesses in childhood.

John Chimumbwa, BS, MS, PhD holds a doctorate in malaria epidemiology from the University of Natal. Until 2004, he was manager of the Malaria

Program in Zambia's Ministry of Health. He then worked for NetMark AED, a pan-African project bringing together the public and private sectors to pioneer ways of ensuring sustainable delivery of good-quality, cost-effective insecticide-treated mosquito nets. In 2004 he moved to the Roll Back Malaria Partnership Secretariat, based at the United Nations Children's Fund (UNICEF), Eastern and Southern Africa Region, where he coordinates the Roll Back Malaria partnership in10 East African countries. He is currently a member of the Global Fund for HIV/AIDS, Tuberculosis and Malaria Technical Review Panel, on the malaria portfolio.

Mahbub-E-Elahi Khan Chowdhury, MS, PhD, has been senior research investigator in the Reproductive Health Unit, Public Health Sciences Division, Centre for Health and Population Research, Bangladesh, since December 2002. Before that, from 1994, he was a researcher at the Bangladesh Institute of Research for Promotion of Essential and Reproductive Health and Technologies. He has published in international journals, including *Tropical Medicine and International Health* and the *International Journal of Gynaecology and Obstetrics.*

Sushil Kanta Dasgupta, BS (honors), MS (statistics), diploma in information technology, has been a senior programmer analyst at the Centre for Health and Population Research, Bangladesh, since 2002. Previously he served as software development manager at Technohaven Co. Ltd., and as software developer for the Bangladesh Railway computerized seat reservation and ticketing system (1996–2002). He has developed software for Bangladesh Railway and for the Centre for Health and Population Research.

Nick Farrell is a public health adviser for the U.S. Centers for Disease Control and Prevention (CDC). He has extensive international experience in public health, most recently as a secondee to the International Federation of Red Cross and Red Crescent Societies in Geneva (IFRC). While serving as a health project officer, he established IFRC initiatives in polio eradication, measles control, HIV/AIDS, and malaria control. Currently, he serves in the CDC's Office of Global Health, where he manages a broad portfolio of international health activities.

Leonardo Gasparini, PhD in economics, Princeton University, is a professor at the Universidad Nacional de La Plata (UNLP) in Argentina and the director of the Center for Distributional, Labor and Social Studies. He teaches undergraduate and graduate courses in income distribution and labor economics at the UNLP and the Universidad de San Andrés. His articles on income distribution and labor issues have appeared in *Social Choice* *and Welfare, Applied Economics, Journal of Income Distribution, Latin American Journal of Economics, Desarrollo Económico,* and *Económica.* He has also contributed to several recent books on income distribution in Latin America, including the 2003 World Bank flagship report on inequality in the Latin America and Caribbean region. He has worked for the World Bank, the Inter-American Development Bank, the International Labour Organization, and the United Nations Development Programme. From 1999 to 2003 he was associate economist with the Fundación de Investigaciones Económicas Latinoamericana.

Mark Grabowsky, MD, MPH, is a technical adviser to the American Red Cross, Washington, DC., on loan from the U.S. Centers for Disease Control and Prevention. His professional interest has focused on childhood immunization and Africa and on developing effective public health delivery systems. In his current position he is responsible for the Measles Initiative, a partnership that has conducted vaccination campaigns to reduce measles mortality in half in Africa over three years at very low cost. Dr. Grabowsky is evaluating whether the operational approach used in measles campaigns may also be appropriate for delivering other commodities such as malaria bednets. He has served as chief medical officer for HIV Prevention Research and as chief of clinical development of HIV vaccines at the U.S. National Institutes of Health.

Davidson R. Gwatkin is a consultant on health and poverty to the World Bank, the Rockefeller Foundation, and other organizations. Previously, he was principal health and poverty specialist at the World Bank. For 15 years before that he directed the International Health Policy Program, a joint initiative of the Pew Charitable Trusts, the Carnegie Corporation of New York, the World Bank, and the World Health Organization, which provided long-term support to 15 policy development groups in 11 developing countries. In addition to the Reaching the Poor Program, his recent activities have included coordinating a project to produce basic data about socioeconomic disparities with respect to health, nutrition, and population in 56 developing countries and consulting with six global health initiatives to help them improve coverage of disadvantaged population groups.

Palak Joshi has worked since November 2002 as a research associate with SEWA Health, the health program of the Self-Employed Women's Association, where she is coordinating a project evaluating the functioning of village-based public health subcenters. Ms. Palak completed her undergraduate studies at the Centre for Environment Planning and Technology, Ahmedabad, and received her master's degree in environmental planning from the School of Planning and Architecture, New Delhi. Her previous research experience includes work on a World Health Organization–funded project that assessed hazardous waste management in Ahmedabad's Civil Hospital, one of the biggest hospitals in India.

Japhet Killewo, MBCHB, DPH, MSC, PhD, a physician and a public health professional, has been an associate professor of epidemiology at the University of Dar es Salaam since July 1996 and is affiliated with the Muhimbili University College of Health Sciences (MUCHS). He is trained in epidemiology and medical anthropology and has conducted teaching and research in many health fields since 1980. Dr. Killewo has held a number of administrative positions, including head of the MUCHS Epidemiology and Biostatistics Department (1986–97), program manager of the MUCHS Programme Management Unit (1997–9), and head of the Reproductive Health Programme at the Centre for Health and Population Research, Bangladesh (1999–2003). His research topics include infectious disease epidemiology, environmental health, reproductive health, and HIV/AIDS and other sexually transmitted diseases.

Anju Malhotra is group director, Social and Economic Development, International Center for Research on Women (ICRW). She leads the center's research and its work on social, economic, and demographic issues, particularly in the areas of women's empowerment, adolescence, reproductive health and rights, migration, and program evaluation. She holds a PhD and an MA, both of which are in sociology and demography, from the University of Michigan and has contributed to the field through numerous published articles, workshops, training courses, and participation in review committees. Before joining the ICRW, she was an assistant professor at the University of Maryland and a National Institutes of Health fellow at the University of North Carolina.

Sanyukta Mathur is a public health specialist on the Population and Social Transitions team at the International Center for Research on Women (ICRW). She has extensive expertise in adolescent reproductive health programs and the linkage of social, economic, and reproductive health issues. She has also worked on a number of projects focusing on HIV/AIDS, livelihoods, and social transitions in South Asia and East Africa. Prior to joining the ICRW, Ms. Mathur conducted a qualitative research study on women's status in rural Nepal. She holds a master of health science degree in international health, with a focus on disease control and prevention, from Johns Hopkins University.

Sandi Andrew Mbatsha is a researcher at the Health Economics Unit (HEU), University of Cape Town, South Africa. He joined the HEU as a research intern in 1998. His main areas of research interest include health and health system equity, health planning, health policy analysis, and health system development and financing.

Dominic Montagu is an assistant professor of epidemiology and biostatistics, Institute for Global Health, University of California at San Francisco. He is also the chief executive officer and cofounder of Healthspot Franchise International, an organization working to expand access to quality tuberculosis and HIV/AIDS care through private provider franchises in Africa. He holds an MBA and a DPH from the University of California at Berkeley. His primary areas of research concern private providers in developing countries, with a focus on interventions that improve the quality and availability of public health services. At Berkeley, he teaches courses on private sector delivery of health services and on international health. He is on the boards of a number of nonprofit organizations and foundations and has worked as a consultant on private sector–related projects throughout Asia and Africa.

Nelson A. Neumann trained as a physician and worked as a lay missionary in one of the poorest areas in Brazil for almost two years. He earned a master's in epidemiology at the Federal University of Pelotas in 1997 and a PhD in public health at the State University of São Paulo in 2000. Since 1989, he has been codirector of Pastoral da Criança (Pastorate of the Child), an internationally acclaimed nongovernmental organization.

Theresa Nobiya is the health program officer for the Ghana Red Cross. Her focus is on using community volunteers in social mobilization and service delivery in rural areas of Ghana. She has extensive experience in working with mothers' clubs and Red Cross volunteers in guinea worm eradication, vaccination campaigns, and community awareness.

Solomon Orero, MD, trained as a physician at the University of Nairobi and practiced obstetrics and gynaecology. He later studied international maternal health at the University of Uppsala. Dr. Orero has worked as a consultant on tropical reproductive health issues in program design and implementation, monitoring, and evaluation in low-resource settings in Eritrea, Kenya, Somalia, southern Sudan, and Tanzania. He has done training and has developed innovative approaches to solving maternal health problems, and he is a master trainer in the Sub-Saharan African region in emergency obstetric care services. Dr. Orero has worked with the Kisumu Medical and Educational Trust (KMET) on the design of microcredit financing for the private sector to improve reproductive health services, working with clinical providers and informal community-based health providers, and on the development of KMET Nutricare programs using local food ingredients to supplement the diets of people living with AIDS and on anti-retroviral therapy.

Natasha Palmer is a lecturer in the Health Economics and Financing Pro-gramme at the London School of Hygiene and Tropical Medicine (LSHTM). She holds a PhD in health economics from the London School of Hygiene and Tropical Medicine. She is involved in research on the role of nonstate providers of basic health services, contracting out of health services, and the motivations and incentives of different health care providers. Prior to join-ing the LSHTM in 1997, she worked for a number of years in Lesotho, Cam-bodia, and South Africa.

Mónica Panadeiros has a bachelor's degree in economics from the Univer-sidad de Buenos Aires and a master's in economics from the Instituto Torcu-ato Di Tella. She is a senior economist at the Fundación de Investigaciones Económicas Latinoamericana (FIEL). Her main fields of interests are in social policy, in particular health economics. She has been a professor of health care economics in various graduate programs (Universidad del Cema, Favoloro Foundation, Universidad de Buenos Aires) and a consul-tant for several international development bank and United Nations Devel-opment Programme projects and for the government of El Salvador. She has published articles on social and health issues in books and working papers edited by FIEL, Desarrollo Económico, and the Institute for Economic Research in Munich.

Rohini Pande is a social demographer with the Population and Social Tran-sitions team at the International Center for Research on Women (ICRW)., Her research expertise is in issues of gender and power, poverty and health, and monitoring and evaluation of adolescent reproductive health pro-grams. She has also worked on HIV-related stigma, child health, and girls' education in India and in East and West Africa. Before joining the ICRW, Ms. Pande served as a consultant to the World Bank and the Ford Foundation, was a Warren Weaver Fellow at the Rockefeller Foundation, and worked with CARE in Chad and with the URMUL Trust (a community-based non-profit organization) in India. Ms. Pande holds a doctor of science degree from the Department of Population Dynamics at the Johns Hopkins Bloomberg School of Public Health and a master's of public affairs from the Woodrow Wilson School of Public and International Affairs, Princeton Uni-versity.

David Peters, MD, MPH, DPH, is a public health physician and health systems specialist with extensive experience in international health policy, research, and management. His teaching and research focus on health sector performance in developing countries, including health and poverty linkages, the role of the private sector, quality of care, health personnel, technology assessment, and the diffusion of innovations. He has led many multidisciplinary research, policy, and operational teams in Africa and Asia. While working at the World Bank, he helped pioneer the first sectorwide approaches (SWAps) in health. He currently heads the academic program in health systems in the Department of International Health **at** Johns Hopkins Bloomberg School of Public Health.

Ndola Prata, MD, worked as a public health physician in Angola and was the head of the Social Statistics Department at the Angolan National Institute of Statistics. She holds an MS in medical demography from the London School of Hygiene and Tropical Medicine. Dr. Prata is currently a lecturer and specialist in the Health Policy and Management Division, School of Public Health, University of California at Berkeley (UCB). As the scientific coordinator for the Bixby Program in Population, Family Planning, and Maternal Health at Berkeley, she is involved in research projects in the areas of reproductive health, maternal mortality, and evaluation of public health programs. In addition, she is on special assignment with the Division of Reproductive Health, U.S. Centers for Disease Control and Prevention, providing technical support for survey research on reproductive health in developing countries. In the Berkeley graduate program, she coteaches courses on the international health core; family planning, population change, and health; and private sector health services in developing countries.

Jumana Qamruddin is a public health operations analyst with the Health, Nutrition, and Population Unit of the World Bank. Currently, she is working on global health policy, with a specific emphasis on the Millennium Development Goals for health and on acceleration of progress at the country level. Prior to joining the World Bank, Ms Qamruddin was based in Mali, developing and managing public health programs at the district and national levels.

G. N. V. Ramana, MD, is a public health physician with two decades of experience working in developing countries. His work in health policy has included assessing the burden of disease and the cost-effectiveness of health interventions and studying inequalities in the use of essential health services. He has led many research studies and operations in India and other developing countries. He is currently a senior public health specialist at the New Delhi office of the World Bank.

Kent Ranson is a lecturer in the Health Policy Unit, London School of Hygiene and Tropical Medicine, and a research coordinator at Self-Employed Women's Association Insurance (Vimo SEWA). Dr. Ranson has degrees in clinical medicine (MD, McMaster University), public health epidemiology and biostatistics (MPH, Harvard University), and health economics and financing (PhD, University of London). He currently heads a three-year research project that will assess the effect of several interventions aimed at optimizing the equity impact of Vimo SEWA. His other research interests include the cost-effectiveness of public health interventions (for example, against tobacco use, malaria, and trachoma blindness) and the identification and measurement of characteristics of health systems that prevent implementation of the theoretically most cost-effective interventions.

Krishna Rao is a health economist who has focused on the evaluation of health, nutrition, family planning, and development programs. He received his MS in economics from Cornell University and his PhD from the Johns Hopkins Bloomberg School of Public Health. He has worked at the World Bank, the Cornell International Institute for Food, Agriculture and Development, and Johns Hopkins University and is now based in New Delhi.

Eva Roca is a research assistant with the Population and Social Transitions team at the International Center for Research on Women (ICRW). She has worked on a number of projects in adolescent reproductive health, HIV/AIDS, social transitions, and program monitoring and evaluation. Prior to joining the ICRW, Ms Roca worked on the Horizons program at the Population Council. She holds a master's degree in health science from the Johns Hopkins Bloomberg School of Public Health, in international health with a focus on disease prevention and control.

J. Brad Schwartz is a lecturer in the Department of Economics at the University of North Carolina, Chapel Hill, and a consultant to the Asian Development Bank (ADB). He has more than 20 years' experience in the economics and financing of health care services, research, and technical assistance. He has served as a consultant to a number of multilateral and bilateral agencies, in addition to the ADB, in more than a dozen developing countries, mostly in Southeast Asia. He holds an MA in economics from the University of Iowa and a PhD in economics from the University of North Carolina.

Joel Selanikio, MD, is the president and cofounder of the DataDyne Group, a small consultancy devoted to bringing to bear the best applicable technologies to support public health in developing countries. A former medical officer at the U.S. Centers for Disease Control and Prevention, Dr. Selanikio is a pioneer in the use of handheld computers for field data collection. With the support of grants from the World Bank and the United Nations Foundation, he is currently developing public-domain software to support development organizations and health ministries with data collection, analysis, and distribution. Dr. Selanikio also maintains clinical medical competence as an assistant professor in the Department of Pediatrics, Georgetown University Hospital, Washington, DC.

Mittal Shah is the coordinator of the Self-Employed Women's Association (SEWA) Health Team. She is responsible for coordinating and supervising the work of 80 full-time health organizers, 100 part-time local women leaders (barefoot managers), 60 barefoot health workers, and 200 traditional midwives . SEWA Health's main activities are primary health care, delivered through 60 stationary health centers and mobile health camps; health education and training; capacity building among local SEWA leaders and dais; provision of high-quality, low-cost drugs through drug shops; and occupational health activities. Ms. Mittal is a member of the Executive Committee of SEWA Union, a trade union with nearly 500,000 members in Gujarat State. She has a diploma in pharmacy and 15 years of work experience with SEWA.

Yasmin Shaikh has worked with the Self-Employed Women's Association (SEWA) for the past eight years, since completing 12th grade. She is responsible for supervising the work of grassroots health care providers in Ahmedabad City and one rural district. These health care providers are involved in monitoring community health, providing preventive health care services and basic drugs, organizing health camps, and referring patients to the hospital. Besides working as a supervisor on the Reaching the Poor project, Ms. Shaikh has been involved in other research projects, including an assessment of the health and socioeconomic status of SEWA members, an annual evaluation of SEWA's health care services for presentation at the annual meeting, and a recent assessment of village-based public health subcenters.

Michael Thiede is deputy director of the Health Economics Unit, University of Cape Town. He holds a PhD in economics from the University of Kiel, Germany. As a senior researcher, he is involved in research projects in the areas of health system equity and pharmaceutical markets. Within the University of Cape Town's MPH (health economics) program, he teaches a course on microeconomics for the health sector. He serves on various committees of the South African Department of Health, including the Pharmaceutical Pricing Committee and the ARV Drug Negotiating Task Team. Before going to South Africa in 2002, Thiede worked in Germany as a health economics and policy consultant specializing in projects on hospital management, managed care, and reference pricing in social health insurance.

Martín Valdivia holds a PhD in applied economics from the University of Minnesota and has a senior research position at Grupo de Análisis para el Desarrollo (GRADE), Lima. His topics of interest include health, poverty, and social policies; microfinance; rural development; and governance and local development. He is a member of the advisory board of the International Society for Equity in Health (ISEQH) for 2004–6, an adviser to the technical committee on quantitative aspects of the Global Equity Gauge Alliance (GEGA), and general coordinator of the Alliance for Equity in Health in Peru (AES). In 2000 he served as academic director of the master's program in health economics at Centro de Investigación y Docencia Económicas (CIDE), México City. He has developed research projects and is a consultant to international agencies, including the Inter-American Development Bank, the World Bank, the World Health Organization, the Pan American Health Organization, the Food and Agriculture Organization, and the International Labour Organization.

Cesar G. Victora is professor of epidemiology at the Federal University of Pelotas, Brazil, which he joined in 1977 after earning his MD from the Federal University of Rio Grande do Sul in 1976. In 1983 he received a PhD in health care epidemiology from the London School of Hygiene and Tropical Medicine. He has conducted extensive research in the fields of maternal and child health and nutrition, equity issues, and the evaluation of health services. Dr. Victora has worked closely with the United Nations Children's Relief Fund and with the World Health Organization (WHO), where he is the senior technical adviser to the Multi-Country Evaluation of the Integrated Management of Childhood Illness Strategy and a member of the Advisory Committee on Health Research. In 1996 his unit was designated a WHO Collaborating Centre in Maternal Health and Nutrition. He is an honorary professor at the London School of Hygiene and Tropical Medicine.

Adam Wagstaff is a lead economist (health) in the World Bank's Development Research Group, Public Services Team, and the Human Development unit within the East Asia and Pacific Region. Prior to joining the Bank in 1998, Mr. Wagstaff was a full professor of economics at the University of Sussex. He holds a PhD in economics from the University of York, a pioneering institution in the field of health economics. He has been an associate editor of the *Journal of Health Economics* since 1989 and has published extensively on a variety of aspects of the field, including the valuation of health, the demand for and production of health, efficiency measurement, and illicit drugs and drug enforcement. Much of his recent work has involved conceptual and empirical studies of equity, poverty, and health. He has also published on efficiency measurement in the public sector, the measurement of trade union power, and the redistributive effect and sources of progressivity of the personal income tax. His current health research interests include health insurance and the targeting and impacts of public programs; his recent research outside the health field has included papers on income distribution and redistribution. Beyond his research, Mr. Wagstaff has been heavily involved in work on the Millennium Development Goals (he coauthored a recent Bank report on the subject) and on China's rural health sector.

Julia Walsh, MD, is an adjunct professor of maternal and child health and international health at the School of Public Health, University of California at Berkeley. She is a physician with an MS in tropical public health from the London School of Hygiene and Tropical Medicine. Her primary research interest concerns setting priorities for health policies and programs when resources are extremely limited. She also studies the private sector and ways to improve efficiency and effectiveness in health systems, especially with respect to vaccines and reproductive health. At Berkeley, she codirects the doctorate in public health program and teaches international health. She has acted as an expert adviser and consultant to several UN agencies and the U.S. Agency for International Development and has worked extensively in many poor countries, most recently on evaluation, health sector reform, and reproductive health.

Hugh Waters is a health economist and assistant professor at the Johns Hopkins Bloomberg School of Public Health. His areas of expertise are health insurance and health financing reforms, evaluation of the effects of health financing mechanisms on access to health care and equity, and costing of health care interventions. He has worked extensively as a consultant with the World Bank, the U.S. Agency for International Development, and the World Health Organization and teaches a course on comparative health financing systems.

Adam Wolkon is a public health adviser for the Malaria Branch of the U.S. Centers for Disease Control and Prevention. He joined the Malaria Branch in 2001 and has been involved as a technical adviser, program consultant, and evaluation specialist in malaria transmission reduction activities, focusing on insecticide-treated nets.

Abdo S. Yazbeck is lead health economist and leader of the Health Program at the World Bank Institute (WBI). His regional responsibilities cover South and East Asia, and his training responsibilities include health economics, equity analysis and policy, the private sector, and prioritization. He joined the WBI in 2001 after working in World Bank operations for Bangladesh, India, the Maldives, and Sri Lanka and serving as a coordinator of the Bank's Health and Poverty Thematic Group. Prior to joining the Bank, he taught economics at Texas A&M University and Rice University. Mr. Yazbeck has more than 15 years' experience in health economics and development economics and has worked on 22 countries in the former Soviet Union, the Middle East, North Africa, South Asia, and Sub-Saharan Africa. He has a PhD in economics from Rice University.

Index